Women in Sports and Exercise: From Health to Sports Performance

Women in Sports and Exercise: From Health to Sports Performance

Editors

Filipe Manuel Clemente
Ana Filipa Silva

MDPI • Basel • Beijing • Wuhan • Barcelona • Belgrade • Manchester • Tokyo • Cluj • Tianjin

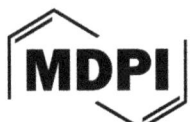

Editors
Filipe Manuel Clemente
Escola Superior de Desporto
e Lazer
Instituto Politécnico
de Viana do Castelo
Viana do Castelo
Portugal

Ana Filipa Silva
Escola Superior de Desporto
e Lazer
Instituto Politécnico
de Viana do Castelo
Viana do Castelo
Portugal

Editorial Office
MDPI
St. Alban-Anlage 66
4052 Basel, Switzerland

This is a reprint of articles from the Special Issue published online in the open access journal *International Journal of Environmental Research and Public Health* (ISSN 1660-4601) (available at: www.mdpi.com/journal/ijerph/special_issues/women_sports).

For citation purposes, cite each article independently as indicated on the article page online and as indicated below:

LastName, A.A.; LastName, B.B.; LastName, C.C. Article Title. *Journal Name* **Year**, *Volume Number*, Page Range.

ISBN 978-3-0365-3133-5 (Hbk)
ISBN 978-3-0365-3132-8 (PDF)

© 2022 by the authors. Articles in this book are Open Access and distributed under the Creative Commons Attribution (CC BY) license, which allows users to download, copy and build upon published articles, as long as the author and publisher are properly credited, which ensures maximum dissemination and a wider impact of our publications.

The book as a whole is distributed by MDPI under the terms and conditions of the Creative Commons license CC BY-NC-ND.

Contents

About the Editors vii

Preface to "Women in Sports and Exercise: From Health to Sports Performance" ix

Jose Manuel Jurado-Castro, Julián Campos-Pérez, M Ángeles Vilches-Redondo, Fernando Mata, Ainoa Navarrete-Pérez and Antonio Ranchal-Sanchez
Morning versus Evening Intake of Creatine in Elite Female Handball Players
Reprinted from: *Int. J. Environ. Res. Public Health* **2021**, *19*, 393, doi:10.3390/ijerph19010393 . . . 1

Reiko Momma, Yoshio Nakata, Akemi Sawai, Maho Takeda, Hiroaki Natsui and Naoki Mukai et al.
Comparisons of the Prevalence, Severity, and Risk Factors of Dysmenorrhea between Japanese Female Athletes and Non-Athletes in Universities
Reprinted from: *Int. J. Environ. Res. Public Health* **2021**, *19*, 52, doi:10.3390/ijerph19010052 13

Patricia Sánchez-Murillo, Antonio Antúnez, Daniel Rojas-Valverde and Sergio J. Ibáñez
On-Match Impact and Outcomes of Scoring First in Professional European Female Football
Reprinted from: *Int. J. Environ. Res. Public Health* **2021**, *18*, 12009, doi:10.3390/ijerph182212009 . 23

Laurent Chapelle, Chris Bishop, Peter Clarys and Eva D'Hondt
No Relationship between Lean Mass and Functional Asymmetry in High-Level Female Tennis Players
Reprinted from: *Int. J. Environ. Res. Public Health* **2021**, *18*, 11928, doi:10.3390/ijerph182211928 . 33

Yining Lu, Huw D. Wiltshire, Julien S. Baker and Qiaojun Wang
The Effects of Running Compared with Functional High-Intensity Interval Training on Body Composition and Aerobic Fitness in Female University Students
Reprinted from: *Int. J. Environ. Res. Public Health* **2021**, *18*, 11312, doi:10.3390/ijerph182111312 . 47

Lillian Gonçalves, Filipe Manuel Clemente, Joel Ignacio Barrera, Hugo Sarmento, Gibson Moreira Praça and André Gustavo Pereira de Andrade et al.
Associations between Physical Status and Training Load in Women Soccer Players
Reprinted from: *Int. J. Environ. Res. Public Health* **2021**, *18*, 10015, doi:10.3390/ijerph181910015 . 61

Abdel-Rahman Akl, Amr Hassan, Helal Elgizawy and Markus Tilp
Quantifying Coordination between Agonist and Antagonist Elbow Muscles during Backhand Crosscourt Shots in Adult Female Squash Players
Reprinted from: *Int. J. Environ. Res. Public Health* **2021**, *18*, 9825, doi:10.3390/ijerph18189825 . . . 71

Dawid Koźlenia and Jarosław Domaradzki
The Impact of Physical Performance on Functional Movement Screen Scores and Asymmetries in Female University Physical Education Students
Reprinted from: *Int. J. Environ. Res. Public Health* **2021**, *18*, 8872, doi:10.3390/ijerph18168872 . . . 81

Juan Gavala-González, Amanda Torres-Pérez and José Carlos Fernández-García
Impact of Rowing Training on Quality of Life and Physical Activity Levels in Female Breast Cancer Survivors
Reprinted from: *Int. J. Environ. Res. Public Health* **2021**, *18*, 7188, doi:10.3390/ijerph18137188 . . . 91

Kengo Ishihara, Naho Inamura, Asuka Tani, Daisuke Shima, Ai Kuramochi and Tsutomu Nonaka et al.
Contribution of Solid Food to Achieve Individual Nutritional Requirement during a Continuous 438 km Mountain Ultramarathon in Female Athlete
Reprinted from: *Int. J. Environ. Res. Public Health* **2021**, *18*, 5153, doi:10.3390/ijerph18105153 . . . **103**

Felipe García-Pinillos, Pascual Bujalance-Moreno, Carlos Lago-Fuentes, Santiago A. Ruiz-Alias, Irma Domínguez-Azpíroz and Marcos Mecías-Calvo et al.
Effects of the Menstrual Cycle on Jumping, Sprinting and Force-Velocity Profiling in Resistance-Trained Women: A Preliminary Study
Reprinted from: *Int. J. Environ. Res. Public Health* **2021**, *18*, 4830, doi:10.3390/ijerph18094830 . . . **119**

Lillian Gonçalves, Filipe Manuel Clemente, Joel Ignacio Barrera, Hugo Sarmento, Francisco Tomás González-Fernández and Markel Rico-González et al.
Exploring the Determinants of Repeated-Sprint Ability in Adult Women Soccer Players
Reprinted from: *Int. J. Environ. Res. Public Health* **2021**, *18*, 4595, doi:10.3390/ijerph18094595 . . . **129**

Felipe García-Pinillos, Pascual Bujalance-Moreno, Daniel Jérez-Mayorga, Álvaro Velarde-Sotres, Vanessa Anaya-Moix and Silvia Pueyo-Villa et al.
Training Habits of Eumenorrheic Active Women during the Different Phases of Their Menstrual Cycle: A Descriptive Study
Reprinted from: *Int. J. Environ. Res. Public Health* **2021**, *18*, 3662, doi:10.3390/ijerph18073662 . . . **141**

About the Editors

Filipe Manuel Clemente

Filipe Manuel Batista Clemente has been a university professor since the 2012/2013 academic year and is currently an assistant professor at Escola Superior de Desporto e Lazer de Melgaço (IPVC, Portugal). Filipe holds a Ph.D. in Sports Sciences –Sports Training from the University of Coimbra; his dissertation, entitled "Towards a new approach to match analysis: understanding football players' synchronization using tactical metrics", involved observation and match analysis in soccer.

As scientific merit, Filipe has had 264 articles published and/or accepted by journals indexed with an impact factor (JCR), as well as over 105 scientific articles that have been peer-reviewed indexed in other indexes. In addition to scientific publications in journals and congresses, he is also the author of six international books and seven national books in the areas of sports training and football. He has also edited various special editions subordinate to sports training in football in journals with an impact factor and/or indexed in SCImago. Additionally, he is a frequent reviewer for impact factor journals in quartiles 1 and 2 of the JCR.

Although he started producing research in 2011, he was included in the restricted list of the world's most-cited researchers in the world (where only eight other Portuguese researchers in sports sciences appear), which was published in the journal *Plos Biology* in 2020. In 2021, the list was updated, with Filipe Manuel Clemente being again included in the top 2% of the world researchers, in which was positioned in the second place in six Portugueses included in the area of sports sciences. Filipe M. Clemente's SCOPUS h-index is 24 (with a total of 2605 citations), and his Google h-index is 35 (5305 citations). In a list promoted by independent website Expert Escape, he was ranked 40th of 14,875 researchers of football (soccer) in 2020 and in 19th of 15949 in 2021.

Ana Filipa Silva

Ana Filipa Silva currently works as Assistant Professor in the Polytechnic Institute of Viana do Castelo (IPVC) in Melgaço, Portugal and as a researcher in Research Centre in Sports Sciences, Health Sciences and Human Development (CIDESD, Portugal). She has a European Ph.D. in Sport Sciences –Sports Training in Faculty of Sport, University of Porto, Porto, Portugal (2017, Portugal). Among others, her main publications are within the following topics: (i) motor control, (ii) youth sports performance, (iii) decision making in sports, and (iv) cognitive performance in sports. She is currently guest associate editor for Frontiers in Physiology, Frontiers in Sport and Active Living and Human Movement. She is guest editor of different Special Issues: (i) Training and Performance in Youth Sports at International Journal Environmental Research and Public Health; (ii) In Search of Individually Optimal Movement Solutions in Sport: Learning between Stability and Flexibility at Frontiers in Physiology and Frontiers in Sport and Active Living and Human Movement; (iii) Decision-Making in Youth Sport Flexibility at Frontiers in Physiology and Frontiers in Sport and Active Living and Human Movement; and (iv) Children's Exercise Physiology, Volume II at Frontiers in Physiology and Frontiers in Sport and Active Living and Human Movement.

Preface to "Women in Sports and Exercise: From Health to Sports Performance"

The creation of a consolidated body of knowledge about women's participation in sports and exercise should be prioritized, since the great majority of research in sports is still conducting in men. Despite a call for equity, consistent findings and research about women's physiology, performance, and response to exercise are still needed to increase the capacity to understand the specific opportunities to adjust the training process to women. The understanding of biological mechanisms and interactions with training load, recovery, and performance is determinant for increasing consolidated evidence. Therefore, this Special Issue provided more information about the impact of exercise and sports activities on women, allowing further advances in sports sciences and exercise.

Filipe Manuel Clemente, Ana Filipa Silva
Editors

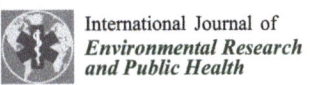

Article

Morning versus Evening Intake of Creatine in Elite Female Handball Players

Jose Manuel Jurado-Castro [1,2,*], Julián Campos-Pérez [3], M Ángeles Vilches-Redondo [4], Fernando Mata [5,6], Ainoa Navarrete-Pérez [7] and Antonio Ranchal-Sanchez [4,6,*]

1. Metabolism and Investigation Unit, Maimonides Biomedical Research Institute of Cordoba (IMIBIC), Reina Sofia University Hospital, University of Cordoba, 14004 Cordoba, Spain
2. Escuela Universitaria de Osuna (Centro Adscrito a la Universidad de Sevilla), 41640 Osuna, Spain
3. Department of Food Science and Technology, Rabanales University Campus, University of Cordoba, 14071 Cordoba, Spain; m02capej@uco.es
4. Department of Nursing, Pharmacology and Physiotherapy, Faculty of Medicine and Nursing, University of Cordoba, 14071 Cordoba, Spain; mariangelesvilches1@hotmail.com
5. Centro de Estudios Avanzados en Nutrición (CEAN), 14010 Cordoba, Spain; fmataor@gmail.com
6. Maimonides Biomedical Research Institute of Cordoba (IMIBIC), University of Cordoba, 14004 Cordoba, Spain
7. Neuroplasticity and Oxidative Stress, Maimonides Biomedical Research Institute of Córdoba (IMIBIC), University of Córdoba, 14004 Cordoba, Spain; ep2napea@uco.es
* Correspondence: juradox@gmail.com (J.M.J.-C.); en1rasaa@uco.es (A.R.-S.)

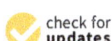

Abstract: A great deal of evidence has been gathered on the use of creatine as an ergogenic supplement. Recent studies show greater benefits when creatine ingestion is performed close in time to training, but few studies tackle the way that circadian rhythms could influence creatine consumption. The aim of this study was therefore to observe the influence circadian rhythms exert on sports performance after creatine supplementation. Our method involved randomly assigning fourteen women players of a handball team into two groups in a single-blind study: one that consumed the supplement in the morning and one that consumed it in the evening, with both groups following a specific training program. After twelve weeks, the participants exhibited a decreased fat percentage, increased body weight and body water, and improved performance, with these results being very similar in the two groups. It is therefore concluded that, although circadian rhythms may influence performance, these appear not to affect creatine supplementation, as creatine is stored intramuscularly and is available for those moments of high energy demand, regardless of the time of day.

Keywords: woman; female; sports training; sports performance; creatine; circadian rhythms; sports performance

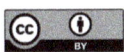

1. Introduction

Dietary supplements are a common strategy for achieving improved health status and benefiting athletic performance [1]. Extensive research has been conducted on the different types of ergogenic dietary supplements used in sport and their benefit for performance, with creatine (Cr), particularly Cr monohydrate, being one of the most widely studied and one with the most evidence [2].

Cr is a compound that is synthesised in the liver, kidneys, and pancreas from amino acids glycine, arginine, and methionine [3], but it can also be obtained through the diet by eating meat and fish, and it is also, in small amounts, found in some vegetables. Its absorption is favoured by the consumption of simple carbohydrates, and it accumulates mainly in skeletal muscle (95%), where 40% is in free form and 60% is in the form of phosphocreatine [4]. Under resting conditions, adenosine triphosphate (ATP) is formed in the mitochondria from adenosine diphosphate (ADP) through the process of oxidative phosphorylation. In muscles, ATP is used by the enzyme phosphorylcreatine kinase (CK) to convert Cr to Cr phosphate. This enzyme can reverse the reaction to obtain additional ATP, making Cr phosphate a temporary store of ATP under high energy demand conditions [5].

The importance of this compound lies in the fact that it provides energy when used in the resynthesis of ATP, giving it ergogenic potential (when consumed as a supplement), improving performance in athletes, specifically in high-intensity, short-duration exercise, increasing power and strength and improving body composition [4,5].

Although several studies have attempted to elucidate whether the best time to ingest Cr is before or after training [6], the results showed greater benefits when Cr was ingested close to the training sessions due to the increased blood flow, with significant improvements seen with post-training consumption [7] due to the fact that Cr can increase glycogen formation in the muscle and increase insulin sensitivity [8].

Another aspect to take into account when scheduling both training and sports supplementation is circadian rhythms. The time at which the physical activity is performed is another variable to consider, as a number of physiological changes occur that could affect sporting performance [9]. Therefore, based on the premise that an increase in body temperature seems to be strongly related to physical performance, the peak of body temperature coincides with the time of greatest activity and can cause variations in cardiorespiratory rate and muscle strength [10]. These variations are the result of the physiological, metabolic, and psychological rhythms synchronizing; the peak of these rhythms being in the early afternoon, when muscle hypertrophy increases due to increased hormone and growth factor binding protein levels (IGFBP-3). In addition to the increased muscle repair that results from elevated levels of creatine kinase and homocysteine, there are increased levels of antioxidant activity [9,11]. This may be influenced by the consumption of certain ergogenic substances used in sports supplements, which may enhance the ergogenic effect [12].

In view of the above, the aim of this study was to elucidate whether circadian rhythms could influence the ergogenic effect of Cr supplements by testing whether evening or morning intake improved athletic performance more in elite female athletes.

Therefore, it was hypothesized that Cr supplementation would improve the performance of female handball players regardless of a possible influence of the circadian rhythm.

2. Materials and Methods

2.1. Design

A randomized clinical trial was conducted on 14 female handball players competing in the highest national category. The study was designed according to the Consolidated Standards of Reporting Trials (CONSORT), with the appropriate adaptations (Table S1—CONSORT Checklist).

The effect Cr monohydrate supplements had on improving the performance of the players was evaluated by randomizing the sample into two groups, where half trained and took Cr in the morning (morning group) and the other half in the evening (evening group) for a period of twelve weeks, according to the protocol described below. All the variables were measured at baseline (week 0) and at the end of the intervention programme (week 12).

2.2. Participants

For this study, professional players were chosen from a women's handball team playing in the top Spanish league in the 2020/2021 season.

The inclusion criteria were the following: (1) age between 18 and 35 years; (2) possession of a federation membership in their club; (3) not suffering from any type of illness or injury that would prevent them from participating in the study. These inclusion criteria were verified through personal interviews.

Taking into account the possible influence an altered hormonal secretion could have on circadian rhythm, and that menstrual cycle could have influenced the sports performance of the players [9], information about the menstrual status of participants was collected.

They all presented physiologically normal periods without alterations. Furthermore, only one participant indicated taking oral contraceptives. The type of contraceptives was monophasic oral contraceptive with 3 mg of drospirenone and 0.02 mg ethinylestradiol.

2.2.1. Ethical Aspects

The participants recruited were briefed on the protocol and objective of the study, and they signed a mandatory written consent prior to the start of the research. The study was conducted in accordance with the Declaration of Helsinki [13], and the project protocol was approved by the Cordoba Provincial Research Ethics Committee on 26 April 2021, with code ARS2921.

2.2.2. Randomisation

The participants were randomly selected and assigned to two groups using the web page https://www.randomlists.com/team-generator (accessed on 30 April 2021): one group of which took the Cr supplement and trained in the morning and the other in the evening. The participation of a control group that did not consume the Cr supplement was not considered necessary given the high level of scientific evidence that exists on how Cr improves performance [2,14,15].

2.3. Intervention Procedure

The Cr monohydrate supplement was distributed to the participants by one of the researchers who explained how they should take it. They were instructed to dilute it in 250 mL of water and consume it after strength training according to their assigned group (morning or evening) or at the same time if they had a rest day.

The intake protocol consisted of a 5-day loading phase with a standard intake of 0.3 $g \cdot kg^{-1} \cdot day^{-1}$, followed by a maintenance phase with 0.03 $g \cdot kg^{-1} \cdot day^{-1}$ [8] after morning or evening training according to the assigned group, in order to achieve higher phosphocreatine reserves in skeletal muscle [15].

2.4. Training Protocol

In terms of training, all the participants generally carried out specific technical–tactical handball training sessions five days a week, each lasting an hour and a half. In addition, the participants underwent specific strength training and performed in the morning or in the evening, depending on the assigned group, supervised by a Physical Activity and Sports Science technician three times a week for at least one hour in which they worked on a "full-body" routine, performing 4 sets of 12 repetitions at 70% of one repetition maximum (1RM) of the following exercises: squats, bench press, dead weight, front pull-up, and military press. The 70% 1RM was estimated with a linear position transducer (encoder) (Speed4Lift v.4.1, Speed4Lift, Madrid, Spain) during the warm-up. In addition, at the weekend they played a competitive match lasting one hour (30 min each half). This frequency of training and matches was carried out throughout the season, regardless of the intervention.

2.5. Dietary Guidelines

As the diet of the players could affect energy metabolism during exercise, the participants were given nutritional guidelines to ensure that, during the study, they followed a dietary pattern with the following macronutrient distribution: 5.0 $g \cdot kg^{-1}$ fat-free mass·day^{-1} carbohydrate, 2.5 $g \cdot kg^{-1}$ fat-free mass·day^{-1} protein, and 1.0 $g \cdot kg^{-1}$ fat-free mass·day^{-1} fat [16]. Before starting the intervention, a nutritional session was carried out with the guidelines of the diet by exchanges. They were given tables of food groups and rations per exchange, calculated from their body weight. Thus, for 10 g of each macronutrient, there was 1 exchange of the food groups that contained this macronutrient in the majority, according to Russolillo et al. [17]. They were also explained the nutritional tool The Athlete's Plate, a guide to sports meals created by dietitians of the United States Olympic Committee. With this tool, the athletes could modify the size of portions and servings of each food group according to the duration and intensity of their training [18]. All participants followed an omnivore dietary pattern and a Mediterranean diet.

Moreover, all the participants were instructed to refrain from consuming other ergogenic substances while they were participating in the study. During training sessions and matches this could be verified by the researchers.

2.6. Study Variables

2.6.1. Body Composition and Anthropometric Measurements

The anthropometry and body composition of all the participants were measured at the beginning and end of the study, following the protocol established by the International Society for the Advancement of Kineanthropometry (ISAK) [19]. The participants' height was measured (Seca 214 portable stadiometer; Seca, Hamburg, Germany), as was their body composition, using bioelectrical bioimpedance analysis (Tanita MC-780MA; Tanita Corporation, Tokyo, Japan). The participants received specific indications for the standardization of the measurement [20].

Arm circumference was measured using a non-elastic flexible tape measure (Cescorf Scientific model, sensitivity 0.1 mm, Rio Grande do Sul, Brazil) and skinfold thickness with a plicometer (Holtain DIM-98.610ND, sensitivity 0.2 mm, Crymych, UK), measuring in defined areas, always avoiding muscle. The anthropometric measurements consisted of three skinfolds and the circumference of the triceps muscle of the dominant arm, with this at rest and parallel to the body [20]. All the anthropometric measurement data were collected by an ISAK certified technician (J.M.J-C.) with a technical measurement error of 0.57%. The technical error of measurement was within 5% agreement for skinfolds and within 1% for circumferences.

2.6.2. Lower Body

Back Squat Muscle Strength (One Repetition Max Test)

The 1RM test for the back squat was assessed on a Smith machine (Technogym, Barcelona, Spain), which ensured verticality. Each participant stopped after the eccentric phase (between 1 and 1.5 s), with the bar resting on a support that limited the countermovement, allowing greater control and reproducibility of the measurement in the concentric phase. The protocol used has been described previously [21].

The participants were instructed to refrain from any exercise other than their daily activities for at least 72 h before the measurement tests.

All the participants performed a general warm-up prior to the test, consisting of 7 to 10 min of light to moderate cardiovascular exercise until 75% of maximum heart rate was reached and maintained (Polar H10, Kempele, Finland). The players then performed an exercise-specific warm-up set for 12 to 15 repetitions at approximately 40% of the participants' perceived 1RM, with a load progression for each exercise of 3 to 6 load increments. Increments at each load were approximately 10% of 1RM until an average propulsive speed of 0.5 m·s^{-1} was reached, followed by increments of 5 to 10 kg until 1RM was achieved. The speed was controlled by means of a linear position transducer (encoder) (Speed4Lift v.4.1, Speed4Lift, Madrid, Spain), with a coefficient of variation (2.61%) with respect to the gold standard (V120: Trio; OptiTrack, NaturalPoint, Inc., Corvallis, OR, USA) [22].

The participants were urged to perform at their maximum speed in the concentric phase of each repetition to ensure the use of maximum muscle strength. A rest interval of three to five minutes was allowed between each successive attempt. For the test to be considered successful, each participant stood with their feet shoulder width apart and the bar at their shoulder blades with their hands gripping the bar, then flexed their knees to 90°, followed by extension to the original standing position [23]. The technique was observed by the researchers to verify that the exercise was being carried out correctly.

Power (Countermovement Jump)

After a three-minute rest, a specific warm-up consisting of three countermovement jumps (CMJ) at a moderate intensity (60–70% of perceived maximum performance) was performed. Subsequently, with two minutes rest in between, three CMJs were performed, with a recovery period of 45 s between jumps, observed by an evaluator who stood at a distance of 1.5 m in the frontal plane to monitor correct execution of the jump and to record the maximum height (cm) reached in the three attempts [24]. The participants were instructed to start each jump in a squatting position, with their knees bent at a 90° angle, while keeping their hands on their hips with their trunk upright, taking care not to interrupt the movement from the start of the jump to the end. The height reached was recorded using an infrared measurement sensor (ADR jumping, Ciudad Real, Spain) provided by the Department of Nursing, Pharmacology, and Physiotherapy at the Faculty of Medicine and Nursing (University of Cordoba).

2.6.3. Upper Body

Muscle Strength (Medicine Ball Throws)

To assess the strength of the extensor muscles in the upper limbs, a standing medicine ball throw test was used (weight of ball: 5 kg). Prior to the start of the test, a two-minute warm-up was performed involving joint mobility exercises (flexo-extension and shoulder circumduction) as well as three ball throws at submaximal intensities (40, 60, 80% intensity, respectively). For this technique, the participants had to stand behind a line with their feet shoulder-width apart and throw the ball with both hands behind their heads. To perform this throw correctly, they had to bend their legs and extend their trunk to give themselves momentum, as well as extending their heels without taking their feet off the ground. This test was repeated three times, with a 30 s break in between, with the distance achieved (cm) for each throw being noted [25].

Grip Strength (Dynamometry)

Using a calibrated handgrip dynamometer (Takei TKK 5001, Takei Scientific Instruments Co. Ltd., Niigata, Japan), three maximal voluntary isometric contractions were measured to determine grip strength with the right and left hands, respectively [26]. To measure this correctly, the participants had to stand with their arm parallel to the body with their hand in a neutral position.

2.7. Sample Size

As the 1RM back squat was one of the main outcomes for this study, the sample size was determined by calculating the statistical power based on a previous study [27], with a power of 0.80 and a two-tailed α level set to 0.05; the minimum number of participants required to detect a 10% difference in 1RM back squat performance was estimated as 14.

2.8. Statistical Analysis

We ran a Shapiro–Wilk test for normality of variables and Levene's test for equality of variances with a normal distribution of two groups as result. We then compared the mean results between the baseline measurements for the two groups (morning and evening) using a Student's t-test. To compare baseline and final measurements, a repeated-measures test with the group as a fixed factor was carried out. The effect size (ES) of the repeated measures test was calculated using partial eta squared (η_p^2), with small considered to be under 0.25, medium as 0.26–0.63, and large above 0.63 [28]. A difference-in-difference (DD) analysis was performed to compare the changes in the intervention between the morning and evening groups. For the results to have practical significance of DD analysis, the relative ES was calculated as Hedge's g [29] with its corresponding confidence interval (CI). The ES was considered to be large (ES > 0.8), moderate (ES = 0.8 to 0.5), small (ES = 0.5 to 0.2), or trivial (ES < 0.2). The results are expressed as the mean ± the standard deviation or the mean relative differences (Δ). The level of statistical significance was set as $p < 0.05$. All

3. Results

Fourteen female players completed the study and were included in the analyses, seven in the morning group (25.71 ± 3.90 years; 173.86 ± 6.47 cm) and seven in the evening group (22.71 ± 3.90 years; 169.43 ± 7.55 cm). Two participants (one in the morning group and one in the evening group) decided not to proceed with the intervention (Figure 1).

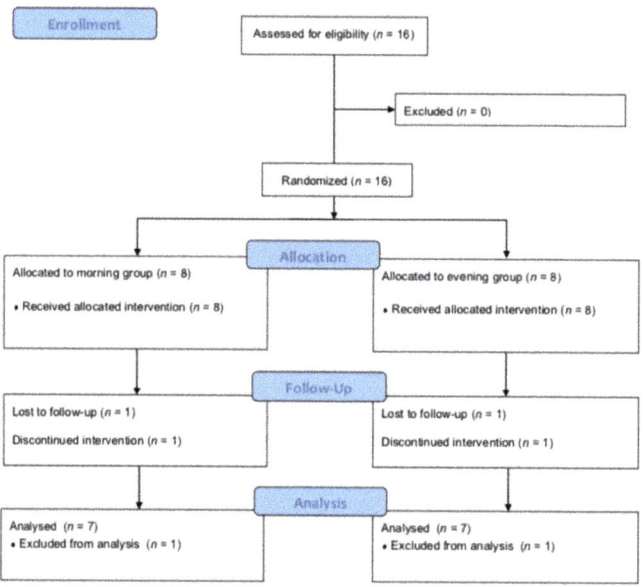

Figure 1. Flow Diagram CONSORT.

No significant differences ($p > 0.05$) were observed in body composition or in any study variable between the two groups (morning vs. evening) at the baseline (Table 1).

Table 1. Changes in body composition and sports performance variables in the morning and evening groups of female handball players after 12 weeks of intervention.

Variables	Group	Measurements		Δ	η_p^2
		Baseline (Week 0)	Final (Week 12)		
Weight (kg)	Morning	65.33 ± 5.99	65.66 ± 4.96	0.33 ± 1.69	0.045
	Evening	63.27 ± 9.10	63.40 ± 9.72	0.12 ± 1.45	0.009
BMI	Morning	21.91 ± 1.62	22.08 ± 1.12	0.16 ± 0.54	0.104
	Evening	22.02 ± 2.65	22.11 ± 2.56	0.09 ± 0.52	0.033
% Fat	Morning	27.43 ± 2.40	22.55 ± 4.21	−0.88 ± 3.36 *	0.717
	Evening	27.22 ± 5.79	24.50 ± 4.61	−2.38 ± 6.34	0.202
Lean Body Mass (kg)	Morning	47.38 ± 4.25	48.36 ± 4.35	0.97 ± 2.67	0.138
	Evening	46.12 ± 8.47	45.62 ± 6.25	−0.49 ± 2.41	0.048

Table 1. Cont.

Variables	Group	Measurements		Δ	η_p^2
		Baseline (Week 0)	Final (Week 12)		
% Body Water	Morning	51.46 ± 3.27	57.60 ± 3.24	6.13 ± 2.37 *	0.889
	Evening	50.31 ± 2.89	55.54 ± 3.36	5.22 ± 3.11 *	0.767
Arm Circumference (cm)	Morning	27.30 ± 1.61	26.70 ± 0.82	−0.59 ± 0.92	0.332
	Evening	27.52 ± 2.53	26.69 ± 2.98	−0.83 ± 1.21	0.353
Tricipital Skinfold (mm)	Morning	17.86 ± 5.81	10.10 ± 1.74	−7.75 ± 5.60 *	0.697
	Evening	14.17 ± 4.60	11.64 ± 3.07	−2.53 ± 3.97	0.321
1RM Saddle Squats (kg)	Morning	98.80 ± 22.86	112.79 ± 23.35	13.98 ± 12.86 *	0.579
	Evening	89.95 ± 12.32	104.01 ± 23.30	14.05 ± 14.36 *	0.527
CMJ (cm)	Morning	36.11 ± 6.07	38.32 ± 5.54	2.21 ± 1.81 *	0.635
	Evening	35.22 ± 6.86	37.81 ± 8.16	2.58 ± 2.13 *	0.631
Ball Throw (m)	Morning	4.98 ± 0.34	5.35 ± 0.50	0.37 ± 0.25 *	0.709
	Evening	4.66 ± 0.34	5.03 ± 0.44	0.37 ± 0.28 *	0.683
Dynamometer (kg)	Morning	36.57 ± 5.14	37.42 ± 5.28	0.85 ± 1.64	0.241
	Evening	33.66 ± 5.67	34.08 ± 5.06	0.41 ± 0.99	0.174

BMI, body mass index; 1RM, repetition maximum; CMJ, countermovement jump; η_p^2, partial eta squared; Δ, change between baseline and final measurement; * Indicated statistical significance between baseline and final measurement ($p < 0.05$).

After the 12-week intervention period, a reduction in body fat percentage was observed in the morning group, as well as a reduction in the tricipital skinfold in the same group. Improved performance between the initial assessment and the end of the study was also observed in the two groups, with improvements in strength (1RM squat) and lower body power (CMJ), as well as medicine ball throwing. However, no improvement was observed in the upper body results associated with the dynamometer test (Table 1).

No differences were observed in the DD analysis between the morning and evening group for any of the variables studied (Table 2).

Table 2. Comparison of body composition and sports performance variables in the morning vs. evening group after a 12-week intervention in female handball players.

Variables	Mean (Δ1–Δ2)	Difference in Differences (DD) *	ES
Weight (kg)	0.33 to 0.13	0.20	0.645
BMI	0.17 to 0.09	0.08	0.909
% Fat	−4.88 to −2.72	−2.16	0.387
Lean Body Mass (kg)	0.98 to −0.50	1.48	0.235
% Body Water	6.14 to 5.23	0.91	0.632
Arm Circumference (cm)	−0.60 to −0.83	0.23	0.461
Tricipital Skinfold (mm)	−7.76 to −2.53	−5.23	0.116
1RM Saddle Squats (kg)	13.99 to 14.06	−0.07	1.000
CMJ (cm)	2.21 to 2.59	−0.38	0.549
Ball Throw (m)	0.37 to 0.37	0.00	0.970
Dynamometer (kg)	0.85 to 0.42	0.43	0.617

BMI, body mass index; 1RM, one repetition maximum; CMJ, countermovement jump; Δ1, change between baseline and final measurement of the morning group; Δ2, change between baseline and final measurement of the evening group; DD, difference-in-differences. * No differences were observed in the DD analysis between the morning and evening group for any of the variables studied.

4. Discussion

The aim of this study was to investigate whether circadian rhythms influence Cr monohydrate supplementation in order to observe whether morning or evening intake of

Cr monohydrate has a greater effect on the performance of elite female handball players with respect to the variables studied.

The results of this study indicate, in terms of the physical tests, that Cr monohydrate supplements improved performance in the 1RM squat, CMJ, and medicine ball tests in both groups (morning and evening), which was to be expected due to the already demonstrated effects of Cr on sports performance [1]. Although no differences in absolute values were found between the morning and evening groups, the evening group achieved a superior performance with respect to the morning group (1RM squat: 14.36 vs. 12.86; CMJ: 2.13 vs. 1.81; ball throwing: 0.28 vs. 0.25). Although performance increased in the above tests, no statistically significant differences were observed in the dynamometer test. These latter results are not in line with the published literature, given that various studies report an improvement in hand grip strength after Cr intake [30], which could be due to the type of sport, the time of the study, or the training program followed by our participants. Other studies, in turn, argue that grip strength is closely related to hand length [31], and given that this is not affected by Cr intake, this could explain why there is a discrepancy between our results and the existing literature. It would be worthwhile further investigating the importance of Cr intake in the improvement in handball dynamometry test results, particularly given the importance of the ball catching manoeuvre in this sport.

Studies such as those by Bonilla et al. [5] and Mills et al. [32] used similar variables to those in this study to determine what effect Cr supplements had on athletic performance. The results obtained in the present study are in line with those published in these two articles, with improvements being found in the 1RM squat, CMJ, and medicine ball throwing tests. With respect to the study by Chirosa-Ríos et al. [33], no significant differences were observed in the CMJ, which could be due to factors such as the type of training or the fact that there was no pre-loading phase. Given that our research involved female athletes, the results are within what would be expected according to the information found in various studies on performance improvement for both sexes [3,32,34] as well as in others carried out specifically on women [35–37], work showing increased muscle strength and higher load volumes in women after ingesting Cr.

In terms of body composition, the results of the study show a reduction in the percentage of body fat in both the morning (-4.88 ± 3.36) and evening groups (-2.38 ± 6.34), with a greater reduction in the percentage of adipose tissue in the morning group. This reduction in body fat percentage was accompanied by a reduced arm circumference (morning: -0.59 ± 0.92; evening: -0.83 ± 1.21), as well as the tricipital skinfold (morning: -7.75 ± 5.60; evening: -2.53 ± 3.97), in both groups, with the tricipital skinfold improvement once again being greater in the morning group. This may indicate that creatine supplements, in conjunction with a strength training programme, can improve body composition by reducing fat tissue without negatively affecting muscle mass. However, taking into account the difference in body composition results between the two groups, as well as the previous scientific evidence, which does not suggest that creatine alone can help weight loss, these reductions in fat percentage, tricipital fold, and arm circumference may be due to factors other than creatine, such as the training program followed, in addition to the possible influence of the time of training and of the dietary recommendations that were given to the players, which would explain the differences between the two groups.

Indeed, with respect to the influence of circadian rhythms, it is known that there is an individual biological preference for activity and rest influenced by chronotype (morning, intermediate, and evening), which is of particular importance when trying to improve performance in athletes [9]. Changes in performance related to factors that depend on circadian rhythms, such as temperature, blood pressure, energy metabolism, and hormone secretion, among other physiological variables, have been reported in the literature [10]. In relation to these changes, the increase in body and muscle temperature that occurs in the afternoon has been observed to improve ATP-PC and glycolytic ATP turnover, leading to greater muscle activation and strength [11].

Numerous studies argue that athletes perform better when training in the afternoon and that this is the result of the synchronization (chronotype) between physiological, psychological, and metabolic rhythms, which reach their peak in the early afternoon, in coordination with cardiovascular processes, which also show a circadian pattern [9]. This fact makes it reasonable to think that taking Cr supplements in the afternoon could be beneficial.

However, the results obtained show that no significant differences were found between the consumption of Cr supplements in the morning or in the evening. This lack of difference could be explained by the fact that Cr supplementation aids the intramuscular storage of Cr, keeping it available in case it is needed when there is a greater energy demand [38], whether this is in the morning or the evening. In addition, other studies have reported limited changes in performance with respect to the time of day the supplement is taken [39], and likewise, no differences have been demonstrated in terms of recovery from anaerobic exercise in the morning vs. the evening [11]. These results suggest the need for further studies on diurnal fluctuations and exercise performance, especially in well-trained athletes.

This study included some limitations, some of them being that there was no control group to compare the effect of Cr, so the results should be interpreted with caution. However, Cr has been successfully and extensively shown to be effective in enhancing athletic performance [2,15]. Moreover, this study did not have a daily dietary monitoring on the nutrition of the athletes, therefore being another limitation of the study. In future studies that compare the influence of the circadian rhythm and timing in supplementation and elite athletes, it would be interesting to carry out a nutritional monitoring that guarantees the dietary pattern. The consumption of protein, especially consumption of animal protein, is a covariate of special importance for future studies that delve into moments of Cr ingestion as a supplement for elite athletes.

Another limitation of our study was the relatively small size of the sample. Although clinical trials with a larger sample size are needed to confirm these findings, we can state that the results of the present study are in line with recent research on the optimal timing of Cr intake, which suggests that greater performance is achieved when Cr supplementation is performed after strength training [6,8,38]. Factors that could have influenced the different results obtained are the level of training of the participants and the initial amount of Cr present in their muscles. Given that the initial level of Cr in the muscles was not measured in this study, an attempt was made to correct any bias by carrying out a prior loading phase to try to homogenize the sample and ensure that all the participants started with similar levels of Cr reserves.

On the other hand, future research could focus on how the menstrual cycle affects Cr metabolism in female athletes and the repercussions this has on their performance [40], with a view to analysing whether Cr supplementation could achieve greater benefits and make up for the energy deficit that is allocated to other physiological processes in order to use it to improve performance.

5. Conclusions

In conclusion, the results confirm the ergogenic effect of Cr supplements in improving sporting performance in elite female handball players according to the specific physical tests of lower limb and upper limb strength carried out. Handball is a sport that has short duration and high intensity actions, such as direction changes, jumps, and throws, where the phosphocreatine system plays an important physiological role in the generation of ATP. The specific improvement in the strength and power of the lower limbs is important in many of these actions where this musculature is required for jumping or repeated high intensity sprints.

However, no significant differences in performance were observed between morning vs. evening intake of Cr following the supplementation protocol in the sample of players analysed.

Supplementary Materials: The following are available online at https://www.mdpi.com/article/10.3390/ijerph19010393/s1, Table S1: CONSORT 2010 checklist of information to include when reporting a randomised trial.

Author Contributions: Conceptualization, J.M.J.-C. and A.R.-S.; methodology J.M.J.-C. and A.R.-S.; software, J.M.J.-C., J.C.-P. and A.R.-S.; validation, J.M.J.-C. and A.R.-S.; formal analysis, J.M.J.-C.; investigation, J.M.J.-C., J.C.-P. and A.R.-S.; resources, J.M.J.-C. and A.R.-S.; data curation, J.M.J.-C.; writing—original draft preparation, J.M.J.-C., J.C.-P., M.Á.V.-R. and A.R.-S.; writing—review and editing, J.M.J.-C., J.C.-P., M.Á.V.-R., F.M., A.N.-P. and A.R.-S.; visualization, J.M.J.-C., J.C.-P., M.Á.V.-R., F.M., A.N.-P. and A.R.-S.; supervision, J.M.J.-C. and A.R.-S.; project administration, J.M.J.-C. and A.R.-S.; funding acquisition, A.R.-S. All authors have read and agreed to the published version of the manuscript.

Funding: This research was supported by Departamento de Enfermería, Farmacología y Fisioterapia (Facultad de Medicina y Enfermería, Universidad de Córdoba).

Institutional Review Board Statement: The study was conducted according to the guidelines of the Declaration of Helsinki, and the study was approved by the Cordoba Provincial Research Ethics Committee on 26 April 2021 (protocol code ARS2921).

Informed Consent Statement: Informed consent was obtained from all subjects involved in the study.

Acknowledgments: We acknowledge "Clínica CIMDE +" for the support given in the creatine donation, and to "Nursing, Pharmacology and Physiotherapy Department" from Cordoba University for the ADR jumping technical support.

Conflicts of Interest: The authors declare no conflict of interest.

References

1. Baltazar-Martins, G.; Brito de Souza, D.; Aguilar-Navarro, M.; Muñoz-Guerra, J.; Plata, M.D.M.; Del Coso, J. Prevalence and patterns of dietary supplement use in elite Spanish athletes. *J. Int. Soc. Sports Nutr.* **2019**, *16*, 30. [CrossRef] [PubMed]
2. Australian Institute of Sport: Sports Supplement Framework. 2019. Available online: https://www.sportaus.gov.au/ais/nutrition/supplements (accessed on 27 February 2021).
3. Kalhan, S.C.; Gruca, L.; Marczewski, S.; Bennett, C. Whole body creatine and protein kinetics in healthy men and women: Effects of creatine and amino acid supplementation. *Amino acids* **2016**, *48*, 677–687. [CrossRef] [PubMed]
4. Greenhaff, P.L. The nutritional biochemistry of creatine. *J. Nutr. Biochem.* **1997**, *8*, 610–618. [CrossRef]
5. Bonilla, D.A.; Kreider, R.B.; Petro, J.L.; Romance, R.; García-Sillero, M.; Benítez-Porres, J.; Vargas-Molina, S. Creatine Enhances the Effects of Cluster-Set Resistance Training on Lower-Limb Body Composition and Strength in Resistance-Trained Men: A Pilot Study. *Nutrients* **2021**, *13*, 2303. [CrossRef]
6. Ribeiro, F.; Longobardi, I.; Perim, P.; Duarte, B.; Ferreira, P.; Gualano, B.; Roschel, H.; Saunders, B. Timing of Creatine Supplementation around Exercise: A Real Concern? *Nutrients* **2021**, *13*, 2844. [CrossRef] [PubMed]
7. Ciccone, J.A.; Ciccone, V. The effects of pre versus post workout supplementation of creatine monohydrate on body composition and strength. *J. Int. Soc. Sports Nutr.* **2013**, *10*, 36. [CrossRef]
8. Jurado-Castro, J.M.; Navarrete-Pérez, A.; Ranchal-Sánchez, A.; Ordóñez, F.M. Timing óptimo en la suplementación con creatina para la mejora del rendimiento deportivo. *Arch. Med. Deporte.* **2020**, *38*, 48–53. [CrossRef]
9. Ayala, V.; Martínez-Bebia, M.; Latorre, J.A.; Gimenez-Blasi, N.; Jimenez-Casquet, M.J.; Conde-Pipo, J.; Bach-Faig, A.; Mariscal-Arcas, M. Influence of circadian rhythms on sports performance. *Chronobiol. Int.* **2021**, *38*, 1522–1536. [CrossRef]
10. Chtourou, H.; Souissi, N. The effect of training at a specific time of day: A review. *J. Strength Cond. Res.* **2012**, *26*, 1984–2005. [CrossRef]
11. Dumar, A.M.; Huntington, A.F.; Rogers, R.R.; Kopec, T.J.; Williams, T.D.; Ballmann, C.G. Acute Beetroot Juice Supplementation Attenuates Morning-Associated Decrements in Supramaximal Exercise Performance in Trained Sprinters. *Int. J. Environ. Res. Public Health* **2021**, *18*, 412. [CrossRef]
12. Cribb, P.J.; Hayes, A. Effects of supplement-timing and resistance exercise on skeletal muscle hypertrophy. *Med. Sci. Sports Exerc.* **2006**, *38*, 1918–1925. [CrossRef]
13. World Medical Association Declaration of Helsinki. Ethical principles for medical research involving human subjects. *Bull. World Health Organ.* **2001**, *79*, 373–374.
14. Kreider, R.B.; Kalman, D.S.; Antonio, J.; Ziegenfuss, T.N.; Wildman, R.; Collins, R.; Candow, D.G.; Kleiner, S.M.; Almanda, A.L.; Lopez, H.L. International Society of Sports Nutrition position stand: Safety and efficacy of creatine supplementation in exercise, sport, and medicine. *J. Int. Soc. Sports Nutr.* **2017**, *14*, 1–18. [CrossRef] [PubMed]

15. Antonio, J.; Candow, D.G.; Forbes, S.C.; Gualano, B.; Jagim, A.R.; Kreider, R.B.; Rawson, E.S.; Smith-Ryan, A.E.; VanDusseldorp, T.A.; Willoughby, D.S.; et al. Common questions and misconceptions about creatine supplementation: What does the scientific evidence really show? *J. Int. Soc. Sports Nutr.* **2021**, *18*, 13. [CrossRef] [PubMed]
16. Campbell, B.; Kreider, R.; Ziegenfuss, T.; Bounty, P.; Roberts, M.; Burke, D.; Landis, J.; Lopez, H.; Antonio, J. International society of sports nutrition position stand: Protein and exercise. *J. Int. Soc. Sports Nutr.* **2007**, *4*, 8. [CrossRef] [PubMed]
17. Russolillo Femenías, G.; Marques Lopes, I. Listas de intercambio de alimentos españoles para la confección de dietas y planificación de menús. *Act. Dietética* **2009**, *13*, 137–139. [CrossRef]
18. Reguant-Closa, A.; Harris, M.M.; Lohman, T.G.; Meyer, N.L. Validation of the Athlete's Plate Nutrition Educational Tool: Phase I. *Int. J. Sport Nutr. Exerc. Metab.* **2019**, *29*, 628–635. [CrossRef]
19. Marfell-Jones, M.J.; Stewart, A.D.; de Ridder, J.H. *International Standards for Anthropometric Assessment*, 1st ed.; International Society for the Advancement of Kinanthropometry: Wellington, New Zealand, 2012.
20. Alvero-Cruz, J.R.; Gómez, L.C.; Ronconi, M.; Vázquez, R.F.; i Manzañido, J.P. La bioimpedancia eléctrica como método de estimación de la composición corporal: Normas prácticas de utilización. *Rev. Andal. Med. Deporte.* **2011**, *4*, 167–174.
21. Ranchal-Sanchez, A.; Diaz-Bernier, V.M.; De La Florida-Villagran, C.A.; Llorente-Cantarero, F.J.; Campos-Perez, J.; Jurado-Castro, J.M. Acute Effects of Beetroot Juice Supplements on Resistance Training: A Randomized Double-Blind Crossover. *Nutrients* **2020**, *12*, 1912. [CrossRef]
22. Pérez-Castilla, A.; Piepoli, A.; Delgado-García, G.; Garrido-Blanca, G.; García-Ramos, A. Reliability and concurrent validity of seven commercially available devices for the assessment of movement velocity at different intensities during the bench press. *J. Strength Cond. Res.* **2019**, *33*, 1258–1265. [CrossRef]
23. Caulfield, S.; Berninger, D. Exercise technique for free weight and machine training. In *Essentials of Strength Training and Conditioning*, 4th ed.; Haff, G., Triplett, T., Eds.; Human Kinetics: Champaign, IL, USA, 2016; Volume 4, pp. 735–736.
24. Markovic, G.; Dizdar, D.; Jukic, I.; Cardinale, M. Reliability and factorial validity of squat and countermovement jump tests. *J. Strength Cond. Res.* **2004**, *18*, 551–555. [CrossRef]
25. Cervera, V.O. *Entrenamiento de Fuerza y Explosividad Para la Actividad Física y el Deporte de Competición*; Editorial Inde: Barcelona, Spain, 1999.
26. Härkönen, R.; Piirtomaa, M.; Alaranta, H. Grip Strength and hand positions of the dynamometer in 204 Finnish. *J. Hand Surg.* **1993**, *18*, 129–132. [CrossRef]
27. Izquierdo, M.; Ibañez, J.; González-Badillo, J.J.; Gorostiaga, E.M. Effects of creatine supplementation on muscle power, endurance, and sprint performance. *Med. Sci. Sports Exerc.* **2002**, *34*, 332–343. [CrossRef]
28. Ferguson, C.J. An Effect Size Primer: A Guide for Clinicians and Researchers. *Prof. Psychol. Res. Pract.* **2009**, *40*, 532–538. [CrossRef]
29. Hedges, L.V. Distribution theory for Glass's estimator of effect size and related estimators. *J. Educ. Stat.* **1981**, *6*, 107–128. [CrossRef]
30. Soyal, M.; Çelik, N. Comparing the hand grip power and creatine kinase levels of U-17 judo national team athletes before and after a 6-week strength training. *Pedagog. Phys. Cult.* **2020**, *24*, 163–168. [CrossRef]
31. Helena, M.; Suárez, V.; Pedro, E. Características cineantropométricas y la fuerza en jugadores juveniles de balonmano por puestos específicos. *Arch. de Medicina del Deporte* **2008**, *25*, 167–177.
32. Mills, S.; Candow, D.G.; Forbes, S.C.; Neary, J.P.; Ormsbee, M.J.; Antonio, J. Effects of Creatine Supplementation during Resistance Training Sessions in Physically Active Young Adults. *Nutrients* **2020**, *12*, 1880. [CrossRef] [PubMed]
33. Chirosa-Rios, L.J.; Chirosa-Rios, I.; Padial, P.; Pozo, A. Efecto del suplemento oral de creatina a jugadores de Balonmano para la mejora del salto. *Eur. J. Hum. Mov.* **1999**, *5*, 25–34.
34. Tarnopolsky, M.A.; MacLennan, D.P. Creatine monohydrate supplementation enhances high-intensity exercise performance in males and females. *Int J. Sport Nutr. Exerc. Metab.* **2000**, *10*, 452–463. [CrossRef] [PubMed]
35. Aguiar, A.F.; Januário, R.S.B.; Junior, R.P.; Gerage, A.M.; Pina, F.L.C.; Do Nascimento, M.A.; Padovani, C.R.; Cyrino, E.S. Long-term creatine supplementation improves muscular performance during resistance training in older women. *Eur. J. Appl. Physiol.* **2013**, *113*, 987–996. [CrossRef] [PubMed]
36. Ayoama, R.; Hiruma, E.; Sasaki, H. Effects of creatine loading on muscular strength and endurance of female softball players. *J. Sports Med. Phys. Fit.* **2003**, *43*, 481. [CrossRef]
37. Ramírez-Campillo, R.; González-Jurado, J.A.; Martínez, C.; Nakamura, F.Y.; Peñailillo, L.; Meylan, C.M.; Caniuqueo, A.; Cañas-Jamet, R.; Alonso-Martínez, A.M.; Izquierdo, M. Effects of plyometric training and creatine supplementation on maximal-intensity exercise and endurance in female soccer players. *J. Sci. Med. Sport* **2016**, *19*, 682–687. [CrossRef]
38. Forbes, S.C.; Candow, D.G. Timing of creatine supplementation and resistance training: A brief review. *J. Exerc. Nutr.* **2018**, *1*. Available online: https://journalofexerciseandnutrition.com/index.php/JEN/article/download/33/26 (accessed on 28 December 2021).
39. Deschenes, M.R.; Sharma, J.V.; Brittingham, K.T.; Casa, D.J.; Armstrong, L.E.; Maresh, C.M. Chronobiological effects on exercise performance and selected physiological responses. *Eur J. Appl. Physiol. Occup. Physiol.* **1998**, *77*, 249–256. [CrossRef] [PubMed]
40. Muccini, A.M.; Tran, N.T.; de Guingand, D.L.; Philip, M.; Della Gatta, P.A.; Galinsky, R.; Sherman, L.S.; Kelleher, M.A.; Palmer, K.R.; Berry, M.J.; et al. Creatine Metabolism in Female Reproduction, Pregnancy and Newborn Health. *Nutrients* **2021**, *13*, 490. [CrossRef] [PubMed]

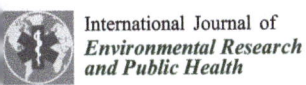

Article

Comparisons of the Prevalence, Severity, and Risk Factors of Dysmenorrhea between Japanese Female Athletes and Non-Athletes in Universities

Reiko Momma [1], Yoshio Nakata [2], Akemi Sawai [3], Maho Takeda [1], Hiroaki Natsui [4], Naoki Mukai [2] and Koichi Watanabe [2,*]

1. Graduate School of Comprehensive Human Sciences, University of Tsukuba, 1-1-1 Tennodai, Tsukuba, Ibaraki 3058574, Japan; monrei015@gmail.com (R.M.); m.clepa13@gmail.com (M.T.)
2. Faculty of Health and Sport Sciences, University of Tsukuba, 1-1-1 Tennodai, Tsukuba, Ibaraki 3058574, Japan; nakata.yoshio.gn@u.tsukuba.ac.jp (Y.N.); mukai.naoki.fu@u.tsukuba.ac.jp (N.M.)
3. Research Institute of Physical Fitness, Japan Women's College of Physical Education, 8-19-1 Kitakarasuyama, Setagaya, Tokyo 1578565, Japan; sawai.akemi@jwcpe.ac.jp
4. Faculty of Sports and Health Sciences, Japan Women's College of Physical Education, 8-19-1 Kitakarasuyama, Setagaya, Tokyo 1578565, Japan; natsui.hiroaki@jwcpe.ac.jp
* Correspondence: watanabe.koichi.ga@u.tsukuba.ac.jp; Tel.: +81-29-853-5902

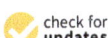

Abstract: This study aimed to investigate the difference in the prevalence, severity, and risk factors of dysmenorrhea between Japanese female athletes and non-athletes in universities. The participants were 18 to 30 years old with no history of a previous pregnancy and/or childbirth. After application of the exclusion criteria, the cohort comprised 605 athletes and 295 non-athletes. An anonymous questionnaire, which included self-reported information on age, height, weight, age at menarche, menstrual cycle days, menstrual duration, dysmenorrhea severity, sleeping hours, dietary habits, exercise habits, training hours, and competition level was administered. Compared with athletes, non-athletes had a higher prevalence of dysmenorrhea (85.6% in athletes, 90.5% in non-athletes, $p < 0.05$); non-athletes also demonstrated increased severity (none/mild 27.8%, moderate 19.3%, and severe 52.9% in athletes; none/mild 21.2%, moderate 17.2%, and severe 61.6% in non-athletes; $p < 0.05$). Factors related to severe dysmenorrhea in athletes included long training hours, early menarche, and prolonged menstrual periods. In non-athletes, short menstrual cycle days and extended menstrual periods were related to severe dysmenorrhea. The prevalence and severity of dysmenorrhea were higher among non-athletes than among athletes; different factors were related to severe dysmenorrhea in these two groups. Thus, different strategies are necessary to manage dysmenorrhea for athletes and non-athletes in universities.

Keywords: menstruation disturbances; menstrual cycle; athletes; women's health; exercise

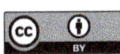

1. Introduction

Dysmenorrhea is an important women's health problem. It is experienced during menstruation and is associated with pain and discomfort such as headaches, abdominal pain, and back pain [1]. There are two types of dysmenorrhea: primary dysmenorrhea, which is caused by excessive prostaglandin secretion without an organic uterine disease, and secondary dysmenorrhea, which is caused by an organic disease of the uterus [2]. Previous studies have demonstrated that the prevalence of dysmenorrhea is approximately 80% among young women; 77.6% among working women (aged 25–55 years) [3]; 83.6% among college students [4]; and 89% among adolescent girls [5]. Moreover, dysmenorrhea is a severe problem in young women because it negatively impacts their lives; for example, it is a cause of absenteeism from school and work and decreased health-related quality of life [6,7].

Bad lifestyle habits may potentially be important risk factors of dysmenorrhea. Short sleeping hours and not having breakfast regularly were associated with moderate-to-severe dysmenorrhea in a previous study [8]. In addition, caffeine consumption [9], alcohol consumption, and smoking [10] were also associated with dysmenorrhea. Moreover, mental stress [11–13] and a lack of exercise [14] were related to the severity of dysmenorrhea. Therefore, lifestyle changes may be a potential strategy to manage dysmenorrhea.

Armor et al. reported that dysmenorrhea lowered athletic performance during training and competitions [15]. Another study showed that the dysmenorrhea pain score was higher in athletes than in sedentary students [16]. Additionally, an interview-based study reported that menstruation-related symptoms reduce athletic performance in athletes [17]. In a previous study, athletes had a lower prevalence of dysmenorrhea than non-athletes (39.44% in athletes and 43.88% in non-athletes), although the difference was not significant [18]. An additional study showed that exercise can reduce dysmenorrhea [14]; however, the participants in this study were women with no exercise habits. Research on dysmenorrhea in athletes and non-athletes has therefore not yielded consistent results.

To address this issue, the present study aimed to investigate the difference in the prevalence, severity, and risk factors of dysmenorrhea between Japanese female athletes and non-athletes in universities. The present study hypothesized that athletes show an increased prevalence of severe dysmenorrhea relative to non-athletes and that different factors are associated with severe dysmenorrhea between these two groups of women.

2. Materials and Methods

2.1. Study Design

We conducted a cross-sectional, anonymous questionnaire survey administered from October 2019 to March 2020. The participants were recruited using a snowball sampling method, and all individuals consented to participating in this study. The Ethics Review Board of the Faculty of Health and Sport Sciences at the University of Tsukuba approved the study protocol (approval number: 19–85) on 19 September 2019.

2.2. Participants

Our cohort of participants included 961 athletes and 423 non-athletes who were recruited with the help of faculty members from six Japanese universities located in Tokyo (three universities), Ibaraki (two universities), Chiba (one university), and Okayama (one university). The athlete group consisted of university students who majored in physical education or sports science and/or who belonged to athletic clubs. The non-athlete group consisted of university students who majored in subjects other than sports science, such as nutrition and nursing, and/or those who did not participate in athletic competitions, such as managers of athletic clubs. This study included women who were aged 18 to 30 years, those who had never been pregnant and/or given birth, those who did not take oral contraceptives, and those who did not have irregular menstruation or secondary amenorrhea. University athletes were defined as those who belonged to an athletic club (not a recreational club), participated in competitions on a regular basis, and trained at least 3 days per week. As shown in Figure 1, 356 women in the athlete group and 126 women in the non-athlete group were excluded owing to the following exclusion criteria: those taking oral contraceptives (n = 22 and n = 15 in the athlete and non-athlete groups, respectively), those with irregular menstruation or secondary amenorrhea (n = 49 and n = 20, respectively), those who trained less than 3 days a week (n = 62 in the athlete group), and those with incomplete data (n = 223 and n = 93, respectively). The final analysis dataset comprised data from 605 athletes and 295 non-athletes. The athletes played basketball (n = 98), track and field (n = 88), lacrosse (n = 62), handball (n = 62), volleyball (n = 44), soccer (n = 33), rhythmic gymnastics (n = 32), dance (n = 32), softball (n = 27), kendo (n = 23), judo (n = 23), swimming (n = 19), badminton (n = 14), baseball (n = 13), tennis (n = 12), cheerleading (n = 9), gymnastics (n = 6), wheel gymnastics (n = 5), and wrestling (n = 3).

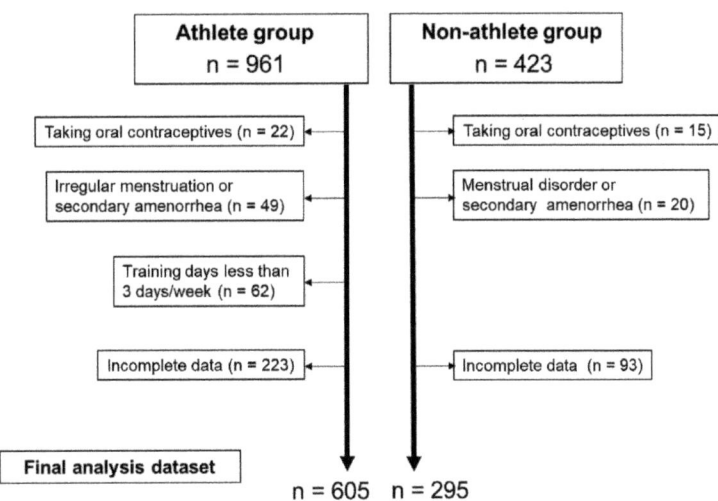

Figure 1. Participant flow diagram.

2.3. Questionnaire

A questionnaire that included questions related to age, height, weight, age at menarche, menstrual cycle days, menstrual duration, dysmenorrhea severity (none: 0 to heavy pain: 10), sleeping hours, dietary habits (skipping meals), exercise habits (in non-athletes), training hours (per week), and competition level (1: international, 2: national, 3: regional, 4: prefectural, 5: other, in athletes) was prepared. Body mass index (BMI) was calculated using the following formula: weight (kg) divided by the square of height (m^2). The following question was asked about the prevalence and severity of dysmenorrhea. "What is the degree of pain you experience during menstruation? Please circle the number between 0 and 10 that is reflective of the pain you experience." Those with a severity score of ≥ 1 were defined as having dysmenorrhea. With reference to a previous study [19], the severity of dysmenorrhea was classified into three categories, namely, none/mild (0 to 3), moderate (4 to 6), and severe (7 to 10). Additionally, gynecological age was calculated by subtracting the age at menarche from the calendar age [20]. The severity of dysmenorrhea was compared between competition levels or sport types in university athletes.

2.4. Statistical Analysis

Data were analyzed using SPSS version 26 (SPSS Inc., Chicago, IL, USA). The Kolmogorov–Smirnov normality test was used to examine normality. Because all variables were not normally distributed, the Mann–Whitney test was conducted to compare the characteristics of the participants, and the chi-square test was conducted to compare the prevalence and severity of dysmenorrhea between athletes and non-athletes, between sport types, and between competition levels. The Kruskal–Wallis test was used to compare the characteristics of the participants according to the severity of dysmenorrhea in athletes and non-athletes, followed by a Bonferroni post hoc test. The effect sizes were calculated and expressed as ES [21]. A logistic regression model was used to identify risk factors for severe dysmenorrhea (severe or not); the severity of dysmenorrhea was the dependent variable in the athlete and non-athlete groups. Independent variables were age, BMI, sleeping hours, skipping meals, age at menarche, menstrual cycle, menstrual period, training hours (in athletes), competition level (in athletes), and exercise hours (in non-athletes). The odds ratio and 95% confidence interval (95% CI) were calculated for each variable. Data are expressed as median (interquartile range) or frequency (%).

3. Results

3.1. Participant Characteristics

As shown in Table 1, some characteristics differed significantly between athletes and non-athletes. Athletes were taller, heavier, and higher in BMI and had shorter menstrual periods, a younger gynecological age, and longer sleeping hours than non-athletes. The prevalence of dysmenorrhea was significantly higher in non-athletes than in athletes ($p = 0.04$, ES = 0.07).

Table 1. The characteristics of the study participants.

	Athletes (n = 605)		Non-Athletes (n = 295)		p	ES
Age (years)	20.0	[19.0–21.0]	20.0	[19.0–21.0]	0.82	0.01
Height (cm)	161.0	[157.0–165.0]	158.0	[155.0–162.0]	<0.01	0.23
Weight (kg)	55.5	[52.0–60.0]	50.0	[47.0–54.0]	<0.01	0.40
BMI (kg/m^2)	21.5	[20.3–22.8]	19.8	[18.8–21.3]	<0.01	0.34
Sleeping hours (hours)	7.0	[6.0–7.8]	6.0	[5.5–7.0]	<0.01	0.19
Skipping meals (yes, %)	124	(20.5%)	76	(25.8%)	0.07	0.06
Age at menarche (years)	13.0	[12.0–14.0]	12.0	[11.0–14.0]	<0.01	0.20
Menstrual cycle (days)	30.0	[28.0–30.0]	30.0	[28.0–31.0]	0.03	0.07
Menstrual period (days)	5.0	[5.0–7.0]	6.0	[5.0–7.0]	<0.01	0.10
Gynecological age (years)	7.0	[6.0–8.5]	8.0	[6.0–10.0]	<0.01	0.16
Prevalence of dysmenorrhea (yes, %)	518	(85.6%)	267	(90.5%)	0.04	0.07
Training/exercise hours (hours/week)	18.0	[12.5–24.0]	0.0	[0.0–0.0]	<0.01	0.37
Competition level (n, %)						
International	49	(8.1%)				
National	323	(53.4%)				
Regional	142	(23.5%)				
Prefectural	75	(12.4%)				
Other	16	(2.6%)				

Data are expressed as median [interquartile range] or frequency (%). BMI, body mass index; ES, effect size.

3.2. Dysmenorrhea Severity

As shown in Figure 2, the severity of dysmenorrhea differed significantly between athletes and non-athletes ($p = 0.04$, ES = 0.09). Dysmenorrhea was shown to be more severe in non-athletes (none/mild 21.2%, moderate 17.2%, and severe 61.6%) than in athletes (none/mild 27.8%, moderate 19.3%, and severe 52.9%).

Tables 2 and 3 present characteristics by the severity of dysmenorrhea in athletes and non-athletes, respectively. In athletes, there were significant differences in age, age at menarche, menstrual period, and gynecological age between the dysmenorrhea severity groups. However, there were no differences in these variables between competition levels or between sport types. In non-athletes, there were no significant differences in these variables between the dysmenorrhea severity groups.

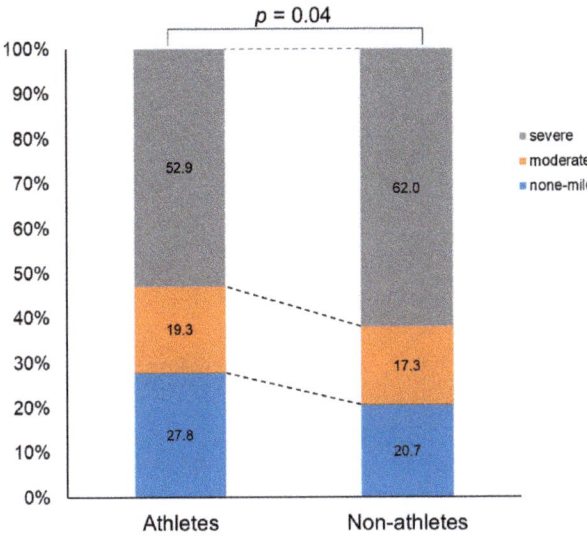

Figure 2. Severity of dysmenorrhea in athletes and non-athletes.

Table 2. Characteristics by severity of dysmenorrhea in athletes.

	No/Mild (n = 168)		Medium (n = 117)		Severe (n = 320)		ES	
Age (years)	20.0	[19.0–21.0]	20.0	[19.0–21.0]	20.0	[20.0–21.0]	0.02	#
Height (cm)	161.0	[157.5–166.0]	160.2	[155.9–164.2]	161.0	[157.0–165.0]	<0.01	
Weight (kg)	55.1	[51.0–60.0]	55.0	[52.0–60.0]	56.0	[52.0–61.0]	<0.01	
BMI (kg/m^2)	21.4	[20.1–22.6]	21.3	[20.2–22.8]	21.6	[20.4–22.9]	<0.01	
Sleeping hours (hours)	6.8	[6.0–7.5]	7.0	[6.1–7.9]	7.0	[6.0–7.8]	<0.01	
Skipping meals (yes, %)	30	(17.9%)	18	(15.4%)	76	(23.8%)	0.09	
Age at menarche (years)	14.0	[12.0–15.0]	13.0	[12.0–14.0]	13.0	[12.0–14.0]	0.03	#
Menstrual cycle (days)	30.0	[28.0–30.0]	30.0	[28.0–30.0]	30.0	[28.0–30.0]	<0.01	
Menstrual period (days)	5.0	[4.0–6.0]	5.0	[4.0–6.0]	6.0	[5.0–7.0]	0.03	#$
Gynecological age (years)	7.0	[5.0–8.0]	7.0	[6.0–9.0]	7.0	[6.0–9.0]	0.05	*#
Training hours(hours/week)	18.0	[12.0–24.0]	18.0	[12.3–21.0]	18.0	[12.5–24.0]	<0.01	
Competition level (n, %)							0.10	
International	12	(7.1%)	12	(10.3%)	25	(7.8%)		
National	90	(53.6%)	64	(54.7%)	169	(52.8%)		
Regional	46	(27.4%)	23	(19.7%)	73	(22.8%)		
Prefectural	15	(8.9%)	14	(12.0%)	46	(14.4%)		
Other	5	(3.0%)	4	(3.4%)	7	(2.2%)		

Data are expressed as median [interquartile range] or frequency (%). *: no/mild vs. medium ($p < 0.01$), #: no/mild vs. severe ($p < 0.01$), $: medium vs. severe ($p < 0.05$). BMI, body mass index; ES, effect size.

Table 3. Characteristics by severity of dysmenorrhea in non-athletes.

	No/Mild (n = 61)		Medium (n = 51)		Severe (n = 183)		ES
Age (years)	20.0	[19.0–21.0]	20.0	[19.0–22.0]	20.0	[19.0–21.0]	0.01
Height (cm)	158.0	[153.6–161.1]	158.7	[155.4–161.0]	158.0	[155.0–162.0]	<0.01
Weight (kg)	50.0	[48.0–54.0]	51.0	[47.8–54.0]	50.0	[47.0–54.2]	<0.01
BMI (kg/m^2)	20.4	[19.1–21.4]	20.0	[19.0–21.0]	19.6	[18.7–21.3]	0.01
Sleeping hours (hours)	6.0	[5.1–7.0]	6.5	[5.8–7.5]	6.0	[5.5–7.0]	<0.01
Skipping meals (yes, %)	14	(23.0%)	14	(27.5%)	48	(26.2%)	0.03
Age at menarche (years)	13.0	[11.0–14.0]	12.0	[12.0–14.0]	12.0	[11.0–13.0]	0.01
Menstrual cycle (days)	30.0	[28.0–31.0]	30.0	[28.0–35.0]	30.0	[28.0–30.0]	0.01
Menstrual period (days)	5.0	[4.8–7.0]	5.0	[5.0–6.0]	6.0	[5.0–7.0]	0.03
Gynecological age (years)	8.0	[6.0–9.0]	8.0	[6.0–10.0]	8.0	[7.0–10.0]	0.01
Exercise hours (hours/week)	0.0	[0.0–0.3]	0.0	[0.0–0.0]	0.0	[0.0–0.0]	0.01

Data are expressed as median [interquartile range] or frequency (%). BMI, body mass index; ES, effect size.

3.3. Factors Related to Severe Dysmenorrhea

Tables 4 and 5 illustrate the coefficients at 95% CIs generated from the logistic regression model using dysmenorrhea severity (severe or not) as the dependent variable in athletes and non-athletes, respectively. In athletes, long training hours, early menarche, and a long menstrual period were significantly related to severe dysmenorrhea (Table 4). In non-athletes, a short menstrual cycle and a long menstrual period were significantly related to severe dysmenorrhea (Table 5).

Table 4. Factors related to the severity of dysmenorrhea in athletes.

	B	Exp(B)	95% CI		p
Age (years)	0.123	1.130	0.977	1.308	0.10
BMI (kg/m^2)	0.051	1.052	0.968	1.144	0.23
Sleeping hours (hours)	−0.047	0.954	0.832	1.094	0.50
Skipping meals (yes)	0.386	1.471	0.957	2.262	0.07
Age at menarche (years)	−0.160	0.852	0.765	0.950	<0.01
Menstrual cycle (days)	−0.018	0.982	0.956	1.009	0.19
Menstrual period (days)	0.269	1.309	1.154	1.484	<0.01
Training hours (hours/week)	0.026	1.026	1.004	1.048	0.02
Competition level (low)	0.117	1.124	0.923	1.368	0.25

BMI, body mass index; CI, confidence interval; Exp(B), odds ratio.

Table 5. Factors related to the severity of dysmenorrhea in non-athletes.

	B	Exp(B)	95% CI		p
Age (years)	0.115	1.122	0.908	1.386	0.29
BMI (kg/m^2)	−0.066	0.936	0.834	1.052	0.27
Sleeping hours (hours)	−0.067	0.935	0.743	1.177	0.57
Skipping meals (yes)	0.170	1.185	0.665	2.114	0.57
Age at menarche (years)	−0.119	0.888	0.758	1.040	0.14
Menstrual cycle (days)	−0.044	0.957	0.918	0.997	0.04
Menstrual period (days)	0.355	1.426	1.161	1.752	<0.01
Exercise hours (hours/week)	−0.067	0.935	0.843	1.038	0.20

BMI, body mass index; CI, confidence interval; Exp(B), odds ratio.

4. Discussion

The present study investigated the difference in the prevalence, severity, and risk factors of dysmenorrhea between Japanese female athletes and non-athletes in universities. The prevalence of dysmenorrhea was higher in non-athletes (90.5%) than in athletes (85.6%) ($p = 0.04$, ES = 0.07). Furthermore, the severity of dysmenorrhea was higher in non-athletes than in athletes ($p = 0.04$, ES = 0.09). Although the effect sizes were small, significances were observed. The factors associated with severe dysmenorrhea were different between athletes and non-athletes. As mentioned earlier, long training hours, early menarche, and long menstrual periods were significant risk factors among athletes, while short menstrual cycles and long menstrual periods were shown to be significant risk factors among non-athletes. Therefore, different strategies may be necessary to address severe dysmenorrhea in athletes and non-athletes in universities.

Most previous studies have reported the prevalence of dysmenorrhea among the general population. Polat et al. reported that the prevalence of dysmenorrhea among adult university students in Turkey was 87.8% [22]. In contrast, Ortiz et al. reported a prevalence of 48.4% among Mexican high school students [23]. This inconsistency is partly due to the different definitions of dysmenorrhea. The former study defined dysmenorrhea as having pain during menstruation; the latter defined dysmenorrhea as having painful menstruation for the past 3 months. It is necessary to focus on this point when interpreting the prevalence of dysmenorrhea. The definition from the former study was used in the present study, and the prevalence of dysmenorrhea was similar in both [22].

Few previous studies have reported the prevalence of dysmenorrhea among athletes. Homai et al. compared the prevalence of dysmenorrhea between athletes and non-athletes (39.44% in athletes and 43.88% in non-athletes) [16]. However, they used a different definition of dysmenorrhea. The present study showed that the prevalence of dysmenorrhea was higher in non-athletes (90.5%) than in athletes (85.6%). While the prevalence of dysmenorrhea was much higher in the present study than in the previous study, the rank relationship noted in the present study was comparable to that reported in the previous study [16].

Many previous studies have reported the severity of dysmenorrhea among the general population of women; however, few previous studies compared differences in severity between athletes and non-athletes. Some observational studies reported that women without exercise habits had a high prevalence and severity of dysmenorrhea [8,14,24]. Some intervention studies demonstrated that an exercise intervention improved the severity of dysmenorrhea in sedentary women [25–28]. Therefore, exercise might be a potential strategy to manage dysmenorrhea in the general population of women.

However, very frequent training may be a risk factor for severe dysmenorrhea in athletes. Czajkowska et al. reported that premenstrual syndrome (PMS) might worsen in athletes due to high-intensity training and an extended competition history [29]. A previous study showed a correlation between the severity of PMS and the severity of dysmenorrhea [30]. Therefore, the present study hypothesized that the prevalence of severe dysmenorrhea is higher in athletes owing to consistent, high-intensity training. However, in the present study, the prevalence of severe dysmenorrhea was shown to be higher in non-athletes (61.6%) than in athletes (52.9%), which is not in line with the initial hypothesis. In addition, there was no difference in the severity of dysmenorrhea between competition levels or sport types in the present study. Further studies are necessary to be conducted in different populations.

The present study also examined the factors related to severe dysmenorrhea in athletes and non-athletes. In athletes, long training duration was a risk factor for severe dysmenorrhea, and this finding is similar to that of a previous study that reported that long training hours are associated with PMS [29]. Although the prevalence of severe dysmenorrhea was lower in athletes than in non-athletes, frequent training may be a risk factor for severe dysmenorrhea. Low-intensity exercises, such as yoga and Pilates, are thought to be beneficial for improving dysmenorrhea because it lowers the levels of cortisol, which in turn inhibits prostaglandin synthesis [31,32]. However, prolonged high-intensity exercise, which is performed by athletes, may increase the levels of inflammatory cytokines, which in turn may increase prostaglandin synthesis and increase the severity of dysmenorrhea [33]. Therefore, the management of training hours might be a crucial factor in controlling dysmenorrhea in athletes.

Long menstrual periods were a common risk factor for dysmenorrhea in university athletes and non-athletes. This result was consistent with those of previous studies conducted on the general population [23,34,35]. In non-athletes, short menstrual cycles were shown to be an important risk factor for dysmenorrhea, while, in contrast to previous studies, exercise habits were not [8,14,24]. Although the risk factors in athletes and non-athletes were examined separately, the previous studies may have included both athletes and non-athletes in the study population. Therefore, the difference in study designs and study populations might have resulted in different findings in these studies.

There were some limitations in this study. First, the study participants were not a representative sample. Athlete and non-athlete participants were recruited separately. Therefore, the overall sample included in this study could not be analyzed. Second, the participants were recruited from a limited number of universities, and the participants were pursuing studies in physical education, nursing, or nutrition. In addition, we enrolled athletes from many sports in this study. Third, self-reported data were collected using a questionnaire, which contained questions that required participants to recollect events that had happened in the past; this might have led to recall bias. Fourth, primary dysmenorrhea was not differentiated from secondary dysmenorrhea. The causes are different: primary dysmenorrhea is caused by prostaglandins and secondary dysmenorrhea is caused by an organic disease. As the causative mechanisms of primary and secondary dysmenorrhea are different, future studies involving the collection of the history of gynecological consultations and previous medical history are needed. In addition, the diseases that may cause dysmenorrhea were not investigated. Fifth, the validity and reliability of the questionnaires were not tested. Sixth, a detailed survey on the nutritional status of the participants was not conducted. Thus, caution is necessary when generalizing the results of this study.

5. Conclusions

The present study compared the prevalence and severity of dysmenorrhea between female university athletes and non-athletes in Japanese universities and investigated the risk factors. The prevalence and severity of dysmenorrhea were higher in non-athletes than in athletes. The risk factors for severe dysmenorrhea were long training hours, early menarche, and long menstrual periods in athletes. In contrast, short menstrual cycles and long menstrual periods were shown to be significant risk factors in non-athletes. Therefore, different strategies may be necessary to address dysmenorrhea in athletes and non-athletes in universities.

Author Contributions: Study concept and design: R.M., A.S., H.N., M.T., N.M. and K.W. Acquisition of data: R.M., A.S., M.T. and H.N. Analysis and interpretation: R.M., Y.N. and K.W. Writing the first draft: R.M. and Y.N. All authors have critically reviewed the article and agreed on the journal to which the article will be submitted. All authors have reviewed and agreed on all versions of the article before submission, during revision, the final version accepted for publication, and any significant changes introduced at the proofing stage. All authors have agreed to take responsibility and be accountable for the contents of the article. All authors have read and agreed to the published version of the manuscript.

Funding: The Total Conditioning Research Project of Japan Sport Council financially supported this research.

Institutional Review Board Statement: The Ethics Review Board of the Faculty of Health and Sport Sciences at the University of Tsukuba approved the study protocol (approval number: 19–85) on 19 September 2019.

Informed Consent Statement: Informed consent was obtained from all participants involved in the study.

Data Availability Statement: The data presented in this study are not publicly available in compliance with the investigation confidentiality and are available from the corresponding author on reasonable request.

Acknowledgments: We want to thank the participants for their cooperation and the collaborative faculty members for recruiting the participants.

Conflicts of Interest: The authors report no conflict of interest in this work.

References

1. Sultan, C.; Gaspari, L.; Paris, F. Adolescent dysmenorrhea. *Endocr. Dev.* **2012**, *22*, 171–180. [PubMed]
2. Zaiei, S.; Faghihzadeh, S.; Sohrabvand, F.; Lamyian, M.; Emamgholy, T. A randomised placebo-controlled trial to determine the effect of vitamin E in treatment of primary dysmenorrhoea. *BJOG* **2001**, *108*, 1181–1183.
3. Nohara, M.; Momoeda, M.; Kubota, T.; Nakabayashi, M. Menstrual cycle and menstrual pain problem and related risk factors among Japanese workers. *Ind. Health* **2011**, *49*, 228–234. [CrossRef] [PubMed]
4. Ameade, K.P.E.; Amalba, A.; Mohammed, S.B. Prevalence of dysmenorrhea among university students in Northern Ghana, its impact and management strategies. *BMC Women's Health* **2018**, *18*, 39. [CrossRef]
5. Soderman, L.; Edlund, M.; Marions, L. Prevalence and impact of dysmenorrhea in Swedish adolescent. *Acta Obstet. Gynecil. Scan.* **2019**, *98*, 215–221. [CrossRef]
6. Lacovides, S.; Avidon, I.; Bentley, A.; Baker, F. Reduced quality of life when experiencing menstrual pain in women with primary dysmenorrhea. *Acta Obstet. Gynecil. Scan.* **2014**, *93*, 213–217. [CrossRef]
7. Quick, F.; Mohammad-Alizadeh-Charandab, S.; Mirghafourvand, M. Primary dysmenorrhea with and without premenstrual syndrome: Variation in quality of life over menstrual phases. *Qual. Life Res.* **2019**, *28*, 99–107. [CrossRef]
8. Kazama, M.; Maruyama, K.; Nakamura, K. Prevalence of dysmenorrhea and Its correlating lifestyle factors in Japanese female junior high school students. *Tohoku J. Exp. Med.* **2015**, *236*, 107–113. [CrossRef]
9. Hashim, T.R.; Alkhalifah, S.S.; Alsalman, A.A.; Alfaris, D.M.; Alhussaini, A.M.; Qasim, R.S.; Shaik, S.A. Prevalence of primary dysmenorrhea and its effect on the quality of life amongst female medical students at King Saud University, Riyadh, Saudi Arabia. *Saudi Med. J.* **2020**, *41*, 283–289. [CrossRef]
10. Qin, L.-L.; Hu, Z.; Kaminga, A.C.; Luo, B.-A.; Xu, H.-L.; Feng, X.-L.; Liu, J.-H. Association between cigarette smoking and the risk of dysmenorrhea: A meta-analysis of observational studies. *PLoS ONE* **2020**, *15*, e0231201. [CrossRef]
11. Ju, H.; Jones, M.; Mishra, G. The prevalence and risk factors of dysmenorrhea. *Epidemiol. Rev.* **2014**, *36*, 104–113. [CrossRef]
12. Wang, L.; Wang, X.; Wang, W.; Chen, C.; Ronnennberg, A.G.; Guang, W.; Huang, A.; Fang, Z.; Zang, T.; Wang, L.; et al. Stress and dysmenorrhoea: A population based prospective study. *Occup. Environ. Med.* **2004**, *61*, 1021–1026. [CrossRef]
13. Rafique, N.; Al-Sheikh, H.M. Prevalence of menstrual problems and their association with psychological stress in young female students studying health sciences. *Saudi Med. J.* **2018**, *39*, 67–73. [CrossRef] [PubMed]
14. Khotimah, K.; Jauzak, R.R.R.A.; Nurunniyah, S.; Maharani, O.; Wahyuningsih, W. Association of BMI and Sport activity habits with dysmenorrhea. *J. Ners Dan Kebidanan Indones.* **2020**, *7*, 96–104. [CrossRef]
15. Armour, M.; Parry, K.A.; Steel, K.; Smith, C.A. Australian female athlete perceptions of the challenges associated with training and competing when menstrual symptoms are present. *J. Sports Sci. Coach.* **2020**, *15*, 316–323. [CrossRef]
16. Kartal, B.; Kissal, A.; Kaya, M. Comparison of Athletes and Sedentary Students in Terms of Premenstrual Syndrome and Dysmenorrhea. *Ordu Univ. J. Nurs. Stud.* **2020**, *3*, 125–135.
17. Findlay, J.R.; Marcrae, H.E.; Whyte, Y.I.; Easton, C.; Forrest, J.L. How the menstrual cycle and menstruation affect sporting performance: Experiences and perceptions of elite female rugby players. *Br. J. Sports Med.* **2020**, *54*, 1108–1113. [CrossRef]
18. Homai, H.M.; Shafai, F.S.; Zoodfekr, L. Comparing menarche age, menstrual regularity, dysmenorrhea and analgesic consumption among athletic and non-athletic female students at universities of Tabriz-Iran. *Int. J. Women's Health Reprod. Sci.* **2014**, *2*, 307–310. [CrossRef]
19. Bourdel, N.; Alves, J.; Pickering, G.; Ramilo, I.; Roman, H.; Canis, M. Systematic review of endometriosis pain assessment: How to choose a scale? *Hum. Reprod.* **2015**, *21*, 136–152. [CrossRef]
20. Arafa, A.E.; Senosy, S.A.; Helmy, H.K.; Mohamed, A.A. Prevalence and patterns of dysmenorrhea and premenstrual syndrome among Egyptian girls (12–25 years). *Middle East. Fertil. Soc. J.* **2018**, *23*, 486–490. [CrossRef]
21. Tomczak, M.; Tomczac, E. The need to report effect size estimates revisited. An overview of some recommended measures of effect size. *TRENDS Sport Sci.* **2014**, *1*, 19–25.
22. Polat, A.; Celik, H.; Gurates, B.; Kaya, D.; Nalbant, M.; Ebru, K.; Hanay, F. Prevalence of primary dysmenorrhea in young adult female university students. *Arch. Gynecol. Obset.* **2009**, *279*, 527–532. [CrossRef]
23. Ortiz, I.M.; Rangel-Flores, E.; Carrillo-Alarcón, C.L.; Veras-Godoy, A.H. Prevalence and impact of primary dysmenorrhea among Mexican high school students. *Int. J. Gynaecol. Obstet.* **2009**, *107*, 240–270. [CrossRef]
24. Bavil, A.D.; Dolatian, M.; Mahmoodi, Z.; Baghban, A.A. A comparison of physical activity and nutrition in young women with and without primary dysmenorrhea [version 1, peer review: 2 approved, 1 approved with reservations]. *F1000Research* **2019**, *7*, 59. [CrossRef]
25. Tsai, S.-Y. Effect of yoga exercise on premenstrual symptoms among female employees in Taiwan. *Int. J. Environ. Res. Public Health* **2016**, *13*, 721. [CrossRef]

26. Motahari-Tabari, N.; Shirvani, A.M.; Alipour, A. Comparison of the effect of stretching exercises and mefenamic acid on the reduction of pain and menstruation characteristics in primary dysmenorrhea: A randomized clinical trial. *Oman Med. J.* **2017**, *32*, 47–53. [CrossRef]
27. Zeinab, K.A.; Mohamadreza, T.M.; Alireza, J.K. The effects of pilates exercise and careway supplementation on the levels of prostaglamdin E2 and perception dysmenorrhea in adolescent girls non-athlete. *Asian Exerc. Sport Sci. J.* **2017**, *1*, 1–6.
28. Dehnavi, M.Z.; Jafarnejad, F.; Kamali, Z. The Effect of aerobic exercise on primary dysmenorrhea: A clinical trial study. *J. Educ. Health Promot.* **2018**, *7*, 3. [CrossRef]
29. Czajkowska, M.; Drosdzol-Cop, A.; Galazka, I.; Naworska, B.; Skrzypulec-Plinta, V. Menstrual cycle and the prevalence of premenstrual syndrome/premenstrual dysphoric disorder in adolescent athletes. *Pediatr. Adolesc. Gynecol.* **2015**, *28*, 492–498. [CrossRef]
30. Kitamura, M.; Takeda, T.; Koga, S.; Nagase, S.; Yaegashi, N. Relationship between premenstrual symptoms and dysmenorrhea in Japanese high school students. *Arch. Womens Ment. Health.* **2012**, *15*, 131–133. [CrossRef]
31. Pascoe, M.C.; Thompson, D.R.; Ski, C.F. Yoga, mindfulness-based stress reduction and stress-related physiological measures: A meta-analysis. *Psychoneuroendocrinology* **2017**, *86*, 152–168. [CrossRef]
32. Casey, M.L.; MacDonald, P.C.; Mitchell, M.D. Despite a massive increase in cortisol secretion in women during parturition, there is an equally massive increase in prostaglandin synthesis. A paradox? *J. Clin. Investig.* **1985**, *75*, 1852–1857. [CrossRef]
33. Febbraio, M.A. Exercise and inflammation. *J. Appl. Physiol.* **2007**, *103*, 376–377. [CrossRef] [PubMed]
34. Fernandez-Martinez, E.; Onieva-Zafra, M.D.; Parra-Fernandez, M.L. Lifestyle and prevalence of dysmenorrhea among Spanish female university students. *PLoS ONE* **2018**, *13*, e0201894. [CrossRef]
35. Kural, M.R.; Noor, N.N.; Pandit, D.; Joshi, T.; Patil, A. Menstrual characteristics and prevalence of dysmenorrhea in college going girls. *J. Family Med. Prim. Care* **2015**, *4*, 426–431.

International Journal of
Environmental Research and Public Health

Article

On-Match Impact and Outcomes of Scoring First in Professional European Female Football

Patricia Sánchez-Murillo [1], Antonio Antúnez [1], Daniel Rojas-Valverde [2,3,*] and Sergio J. Ibáñez [1,*]

1. Research Group in Optimization of Training and Performance Sports, Faculty of Sport Sciences, University of Extremadura, 10005 Cáceres, Spain; psanchezmy@alumnos.unex.es (P.S.-M.); antunez@unex.es (A.A.)
2. Centro de Investigación y Diagnóstico en Salud y Deporte (CIDISAD), Escuela Ciencias del Movimiento Humano y Calidad de Vida (CIEMHCAVI), Universidad Nacional, 86-3000 Heredia, Costa Rica
3. Clínica de Lesiones Deportivas (Rehab&Readapt), Escuela Ciencias del Movimiento Humano y Calidad de Vida (CIEMHCAVI), Universidad Nacional, 86-3000 Heredia, Costa Rica
* Correspondence: drojasv@una.cr (D.R.-V.); sibanez@unex.es (S.J.I.)

Abstract: Background: Scoring first seems to be a determinant in professional football playing; several factors could influence the development of the match and the outcome. This study aimed to identify which factors could influence scoring first and impact match outcomes in professional European female football. Methods: There were 504 official matches held on 74 match days during the 2018–2019 professional female European football seasons (*Primera Iberdrola, D1 Féminine*, and *Frauen-Bundesliga*), analysed using a notational and inferential assessment. Results: There was a direct positive relationship ($p < 0.05$) between scoring first and winning the match; 75.9% of the winning teams scored first. Moreover, those teams that usually scored first had a better final league classification ($p < 0.05$). These relationships were not influenced by home or away conditions. Conclusions: Scoring first is a determinant in the outcomes of professional European female football matches. Physical and tactical training and programming should focus on those variables, leading female teams to score first.

Keywords: women; football; final score; winning; match result; situational variables

Citation: Sánchez-Murillo, P.; Antúnez, A.; Rojas-Valverde, D.; Ibáñez, S.J. On-Match Impact and Outcomes of Scoring First in Professional European Female Football. *Int. J. Environ. Res. Public Health* **2021**, *18*, 12009. https://doi.org/10.3390/ijerph182212009

Academic Editors: Paul B. Tchounwou, Filipe Manuel Clemente and Ana Filipa Silva

Received: 12 October 2021
Accepted: 12 November 2021
Published: 16 November 2021

Publisher's Note: MDPI stays neutral with regard to jurisdictional claims in published maps and institutional affiliations.

Copyright: © 2021 by the authors. Licensee MDPI, Basel, Switzerland. This article is an open access article distributed under the terms and conditions of the Creative Commons Attribution (CC BY) license (https://creativecommons.org/licenses/by/4.0/).

1. Introduction

Football is well-known as one of the most played and popular sports worldwide. This sport attracts millions of fans, and the economic and social interest in related events, tournaments, and matches continues to grow. Curiously, despite its attractiveness, football match outcomes are often determined by relatively few critical actions, leading to small final scores. Usually, football matches have an average of 2.7 goals per game [1]. This reduced number of goals, which determines the final match result is the primary rationale of a study on the influence of scoring first in professional football [2].

Several studies analyse the impact of scoring first in male football [3–5]; but little studies focused on female teams [3]. All of the scientific evidence suggested that scoring first in female and male football is critical; this advantage increases the probability of winning the matches. In male football, 65–75% of the matches are won by the first-scoring teams, whereas female football lacks the evidence to summarise the real impact and benefits of scoring first.

Some factors may be determinant to scoring first, such as the home advantage, team league classification, and if the goal was scored in the first or second half of the match. The home advantage is understood as the relative advantage of being the match host. Previous studies in male football suggested that, when playing at home, the home team has winning odds of 74% [4]. Contrarily, if the visiting team scores first, the winning odds are 50% [5] to 63% [4]. These odds also seem to apply to women's football [6]; in an analysis of the top Spanish league, those female teams that scored first in the match won in more than 80 to 90% of cases, depending on the team's classification (top three vs. top ten) [7]. Additionally, in top European male football leagues, if the home team scores first, the winning odds are 62% [5].

The scoring-first effect on match outcome was studied in other sports, such as baseball and hockey. Scoring first (66.3%) and being the home team (61.7%) are determinants of the final score in baseball [8]. In hockey, the psychological momentum of scoring first causes a marked increase in the likelihood of winning the matches [9].

The abovementioned studies highlighted the second determinant of scoring first, proposing that the best-classified teams usually scored first during female matches [7]. This was also the cases in male football, where the best-ranked teams usually scored first and, as expected, won their matches [10]. Some evidence in male football suggested that higher-budget teams are more likely to win (14%) [11]. Additionally, the competitive balance, understood as the balance in the sport capabilities of teams, could influence the match outcome [12]. Additionally, other team characteristics, such as overall quality and overall ranking, are determinants in team sports [13,14].

Additionally, analyses of the top European championships (UEFA Champions League and European League) show that the first goal scored between 16 and 45 min of match time is more determinant in the outcome than those scored during the first 15 min of the match [15]. This evidence was confirmed by recent studies, suggesting that the team that scored its first goal during the final minutes of a game is usually the winner [1].

All of these situational factors could define the outcome of a match, and they are usually explained by a series of tactical and psychological reasons. Tactical passivity, decreased motivation and confidence, and reduced crew tactical structure and cohesion are common issues for losing teams after conceding a goal [16]. Additionally, with regard to the basic physiological differences [17], female football, as opposed to male football, has particular characteristics that could influence the match outcome and first goal, as budget disparities (competitive balance), quality, and technical and tactical skills differ between teams. To better understand female professional players' psychological, tactical, and physical behaviour and acknowledge the lack of studies on women's football, this study aimed to identify which factors could influence scoring first and how they could impact match outcomes in professional European female football.

2. Materials and Methods

2.1. Sample

This study was defined as observational since the authors did not influence the natural behaviour of the matches, using an ex post facto analysis [18]. All official matches were recorded and explored using a systematic notational analysis.

A total of 504 official matches held on 74 match days during the 2018–2019 top female European football seasons (*Primera Iberdrola*, *D1 Féminine*, and *Frauen-Bundesliga*) were assessed. The distribution of the matches by league was as follows: Primera Iberdrola = 240, D1 Féminine = 132 and Frauen-Bundesliga = 132. The French and German leagues included 12 teams and a total of 22 match days, while the Spanish league included 16 teams and a total of 30 match days. Consequently, a total of 1008 cases were analysed. The format of all leagues defined the champion as the team with the most points (best-ranked) following both home and away matches.

All of the data analysed were extracted from a digital database, accessible to the public from the leagues' official websites (e.g., www.laliga.es). This task was performed by two experts and was contrasted. If there were inconsistencies, both experts agreed after a consensus and final review of the databases.

2.2. Variables

Based on the previous literature, the selected variables were chosen as independent: first-scorer team (first scorer vs. the second scorer,) and the following as dependent variables: match time when the first goal was scored (e.g., 0–15 min, 16–30 min, 30–45 min, 45–60 min, 60–75 min, 75–90 min, 90+ min), league (*Primera Iberdrola* vs. *D1 Féminine* vs. *Frauen-Bundesliga*), local conditions (home vs. away). Other quantitative variables were used, including final ranking (top 1–4 vs. positions 5–12 and 13–16 for Primera Iberdrola; 5–8 and 9–12 for Frauen-Bundesliga and D1 Féminine), number of goals scored (0–11 per team), and number of yellow (0–6 per team) and red cards (0–1 per team).

2.3. Statistical Analysis

The observational data collection was performed using a data sheet (Excel, Microsoft Office 365, Mountain View, CA, United States). Analyses were made using the Statistical Package for Social Sciences (SPSS v.21.0, Chicago, IL, USA).

The normality of the data was explored by Kolmogorov–Smirnov test. Categorical variables were treated as non-parametrical data. The data were presented using descriptive analysis and frequency distribution for qualitative variables; for quantitative variables, the data were presented as mean, minimum, maximum and typic deviations [19]. Inferential analyses were used to explore the potential influence of independent variables on the dependent variable. Association between variables was explored using chi-squared (X^2) and Cramer's V (V). The relationship between variables using X^2 was understood as $p < 0.05$. Cramer's V was interpreted using previous criteria [20], as follows: trivial (<0.10), small (0.10–0.29), moderate (0.30–0.49) and large (>0.50).

The relationship level between variables was established using the *adjusted standardised residuals (ASR)* and different contingency tables (Field, 2009). Those residuals greater than 1.96 confirmed the association between variables, the interpretation made based on previous criteria [21].

Differences in goals, yellow cards, and red cards between first and non-first scorers were explored using a one-way analysis of variance (F value) (1 × 3).

3. Results

The descriptive results of match outcome, local conditions and the match time when the first goal was scored are presented by league (see Table 1). In the Primera Iberdrola League, the winning teams scored first in 77.3% of cases ($X^2 = 393.5$, $p < 0.01$; $V = 0.6$ *(large)*, $p = 0 < 0.01$, $ASR = 15.2$), D1 Féminine teams in 94.0% of cases ($X^2 = 192.8$, $p < 0.01$; $V = 0.6$ *(large)*, $p < 0.01$, $ASR = 10.9$) and Frauen-Bundesliga in 95.0% of the matches ($X^2 = 174.0$, $p < 0.01$; $V = 0.6$ *(large)*, $p < 0.01$, $ASR = 11.1$).

Moreover, must of those teams that scored first did so in the first 15 min (36.9% for Primera Iberdrola, 36% for D1 Féminine and 43.8% for Frauen-Bundesliga). Additionally, the home teams and first scorers won in 52.9%, 55.2% and 53.9% of cases, respectively. There was no statistical evidence suggesting a clear probability of winning when scoring at a specific match time for any league (Primera Iberdrola: $X^2 = 1.5$, $p = 0.4$; $V = 0.1$ *(small)*, $p = 0.5$, $ASR = 1.2$; D1 Féminine: $X^2 = 12.7$, $p = 0.3$; $V = 0.1$ *(small)*, $p = 0.3$, $ASR = 1.6$; Frauen-Bundesliga: $X^2 = 1.6$, $p = 0.5$; $V = 0.1$ *(small)*, $p = 0.5$, $ASR = 1.2$).

Table 1. Descriptive analysis of the result, time point when the first goal was scored, and local status by the league and first scorer.

League	First Scorer	Result Won n (%)	Result Loss n (%)	Result Draw n (%)	No Goal (%)	First Goal Time Point 0–15 min n (%)	16–30 min n (%)	31–45 min n (%)	45–60 min n (%)	61–75 min n (%)	75–90 min n (%)	Local Status Home n (%)	Visit n (%)
Primera Iberdrola	Yes	174.0 (77.3)	23.0 (10.2)	28.0 (12.4)	0.0 (0.0)	83.0 (36.9)	44.0 (19.6)	46.0 (20.4)	21.0 (9.3)	20.0 (8.9)	11.0 (4.9)	119.0 (52.9)	106.0 (47.1)
	No	23.0 (10.2)	174.0 (77.3)	28.0 (12.4)	225.0 (100.0)	0.0 (0.0)	0.0 (0.0)	0.0 (0.0)	0.0 (0.0)	0.0 (0.0)	0.0 (0.0)	106.0 (47.1)	119.0 (52.9)
	Draw	0.0 (0.0)	0.0 (0.0)	30.0 (100)	30.0 (100.0)	0.0 (0.0)	0.0 (0.0)	0.0 (0.0)	0.0 (0.0)	0.0 (0.0)	0.0 (0.0)	15.0 (50.0)	15.0 (50.0)
D1 Féminine	Yes	94.0 (75.4)	13 (10.4)	18.0 (14.4)	0.0 (0.0)	45.0 (36.0)	31.0 (24.8)	25.0 (20.0)	9.0 (7.2)	10.0 (8.0)	5.0 (4.0)	69.0 (55.2)	56.0 (44.8)
	No	13.0 (10.4)	94.0 (75.2)	18.0 (14.4)	125.0 (100.0)	0.0 (0.0)	0.0 (0.0)	0.0 (0.0)	0.0 (0.0)	0.0 (0.0)	0.0 (0.0)	56.0 (44.8)	69.0 (55.2)
	Draw	0.0 (0.0)	0.0 (0.0)	14.0 (100.0)	14.0 (100.0)	0.0 (0.0)	0.0 (0.0)	0.0 (0.0)	0.0 (0.0)	0.0 (0.0)	0.0 (0.0)	7.0 (50)	7.0 (50)
Frauen-Bundesliga	Yes	95.0 (74.2)	10.0 (7.8)	23.0 (18.0)	0.0 (0.0)	56.0 (43.8)	31.0 (24.2)	20.0 (15.6)	14.0 (10.9)	4.0 (3.1)	3.0 (2.3)	69.0 (53.9)	59.0 (46.1)
	No	10.0 (7.8)	95.0 (74.2)	23.0 (18.0)	128.0 (100.0)	0.0 (0.0)	0.0 (0.0)	0.0 (0.0)	0.0 (0.0)	0.0 (0.0)	0.0 (0.0)	59.0 (46.1)	69.0 (53.9)
	Draw	0.0 (0.0)	0.0 (0.0)	8.0 (100.0)	8.0 (100.0)	0.0 (0.0)	0.0 (0.0)	0.0 (0.0)	0.0 (0.0)	0.0 (0.0)	0.0 (0.0)	4.0 (50)	4.0 (50)

In Table 2, the descriptive data are shown relative to the number of goals and yellow/red cards, considering if the team scored first or not. First scorers scored a mean of 2.7 goals per match, significantly higher than non-first scorers. There were statistical differences in goals where first scorers scored more goals ($F = 239.6$, $p < 0.01$). No differences were found in number of yellow ($F = 1.4$, $p = 0.2$) or red ($F = 0.1$, $p = 0.9$) cards.

Table 2. Descriptive data of final number of goals and red/yellow cards by the first scorer.

First Scorer	Variable	n Cases	Minimum	Maximum	Mean	Typical Deviation
Yes	Goals (n)	478	1.0	11.0	2.7	1.8
	Yellow cards (n)	478	0.0	6.0	1.1	1.1
	Red cards (n)	478	0.0	1.0	0.1	0.2
No	Goals (n)	478	0.0	10.0	0.8	1.1
	Yellow cards (n)	478	0.0	5.0	1.3	1.0
	Red cards (n)	478	0.0	1.0	0.1	0.20
No goal	Goals (n)	52	0.0	0.0	0.0	0.0
	Yellow cards (n)	52	0.0	4.0	1.2	1.0
	Red cards (n)	52	0.0	1.0	0.1	0.2

Finally, the better-ranked teams usually scored first in all leagues. The association between variables for the best-ranked teams was as follows: (Primera Iberdrola: $X^2 = 43.5$, $p < 0.01$; $V = 0.2$ (small), $p = 0 < 0.01$, $ASR = 5.9$; D1 Féminine: $X^2 = 30.3$, $p < 0.01$; $V = 0.2$ (small), $p < 0.01$, $ASR = 5.1$; Frauen-Bundesliga: $X^2 = 43.9$, $p < 0.01$; $V = 0.3$ (moderate), $p < 0.01$, $ASR = 5.3$).

4. Discussion

This study aimed to identify which factors could influence scoring first and match outcomes in professional European female football. The results of the analyses suggested that scoring first in female professional football was critical to winning. Female football teams in top European leagues who scored first won in 77–95% of the matches and were better ranked, significantly different results from non-first scorers. More than a third of the first scorers' teams scored in the first 15 min (36–43% of cases) but with no statistical differences compared to other match time points. First scorers scored more goals, but no differences were found in the number of yellow or red cards. Local status also did not influence the final match outcome.

The results of the study confirmed the critical role of scoring first in female professional football. Scoring the first goal may create an advantage, psychologically, tactically, and physically. The evidence suggests that when male football teams are winning, the team usually creates a positive psychological momentum and mindset that makes winning more probable [9]. When scoring first, the conceding team tend to have a higher ball possession than when drawing or wining [22,23]. Additionally, losing teams tend to make more mistakes (e.g., ball interceptions by a rival, fewer clearances) [24] and show more high-intensity actions [14,25], positioning the losing team in a technically and tactically disadvantageous position. Moreover, female losing teams make more tackles, lose the ball more often and accumulate more yellow and red cards than the winning teams [26].

Compared to other sports (50–65%) [8], in female football (77–95%) the odds of winning after scoring first are higher. Compared to male football (65–75%) [3–5], the probability of scoring first in female football is slightly higher. Additionally, these odds depend on the league and could be explained by the greater difference in the teams' quality and the competitive imbalance of female football compared to male football. This could be explained by the higher heterogeneity in the quality of female football compared to male football, with professional and semi-professional female players competing in the same league.

Furthermore, the match time point in which the first goal is scored is also a variable that was studied [4]. Critical moments of the match were identified as essential and are in accordance with the results of this study. The first 15 min of both halves and the last

15 min of the match are critical periods regarding scoring first [27]. These critical moments in the female matches usually see an increase in match workload; depending on the game situation, this increase can be between 20 and 25% [28]. This increase in some periods of the match should be considered when addressing periodisation and strategies to achieve the first goal.

Finally, the evidence suggests that home advantage depends more on the quality of the home team and its rival than on a home effect per se [29]. Indeed, the results of this study indicate that being the first scorer is a determinant regardless of whether the scoring team is the home or the away team. It is also known that teams playing at home tend to show a higher ball possession than teams playing away [22]. Nonetheless, when playing against a stronger opponent, the opposing team must perform better [30], which may cause physical exhaustion and alterations to tactics. In this sense, the best quality team have a more stable pattern of play [13], improving their ability to perform consistent high-intensity actions (e.g., sprints, high-speed running, accelerations, changes of direction), which are essential for physical improvements in female football [31,32].

In female football, the home advantage effect was not as high as in male football. It seems that, in the European leagues, the home advantage in female football is reflected in winning odds of 51–59%; in male football the odds are almost 60% [6]. Some factors could explain these differences, such as the crowd effect (size, intensity and density) on players and referees (referee bias) and gender perceptions of territorial protection and competitive balance [33], usually greater in male football [6]. The aggressivity of the sport and intensity of the match also influence the home advantage. These plausible reasons are supported by other sports studies of the differences in home advantage by gender (e.g., water polo, handball) [34,35]. In Western European football, the evidence suggests a decrease in the home advantage, compared to that of recent decades, due to changes in rules, sport structure and diffusion since the 1980s, leading to a competitive balance [33,36].

Finally, recent studies proposed some tactical, technical and physical factors that may increase the likelihood of winning in female football and could influence scoring first. For example, one-quarter of goals are scored from crosses [37], and so free kicks should be made by a direct free kick or a direct shot on goal [38], pass accuracy should be increased, and a better performance in offensive and defensive duels should be demonstrated [39]. These are technical and tactically significant contributors to victory. Therefore, these actions and situations should be incorporated into training and improved upon to increase the odds of scoring the first goal and winning the match. Additionally, regarding tactics, the winning teams often intercept and recover the ball in more advanced regions of the field than the losing teams [40]; this could suggest the need for some deep pressure strategies during the match, resulting in a higher number of goal attempts. Additionally, some key indicators, such as the high-intensity actions of sprinting, running distances, high ball possession and optimal attacking organisation could influence the match outcome [41]. A home disadvantage is supported by a hypothesis underlying the pressure of winning in front of a supportive audience (expectation of winning). There is a diffusion of responsibility among team members in football compared to other sports, such as basketball or baseball [42]. In other sports, such as hockey and rugby, there is a hypothesis regarding the inhibition of anxiety, which reduces pressure on the home team due to high physical contact [42].

Due to the common playing dynamics and considering that football is a low-scoring sport, with an average of three or fewer goals [1], being the first scoring team seems determinant in female professional football leagues [27]. Scoring first has a strong positive effect that influences the match outcome. These findings can be fundamental for football coaches when developing strategic and tactical planning to enhance the performance of their players, with regard to the different situational variables that their teams may face during the matches.

Limitations

The main limitation of this study is due to the insufficient number of published scientific articles, which analyse the situational and contextual variables that influence female professional football, specifically those focusing on official match analyses and those factors that impact the final match outcomes. Several studies explored the situational and conditional factors that could influence performance in male football. Based on the basic physiological, genetic, social and cultural differences between women and men [17], such information must be collected and analysed concerning performance and the factors that influence performance in the female sphere. This gender gap reveals the need to better explore female performance in professional football in future studies.

Additional limitations are based on the limited data availability of the different official web pages, with regard to the specification of players' characteristics, weather conditions, and other situational information that could affect the interpretation of the data. While this study analysed the 2018–2019 tournaments of the Spanish, German and French female professional football leagues, recent data are not available or conclusive due to the season cancellations cause by the COVID-19 pandemic.

5. Conclusions

Scoring first determines the outcomes of official matches from top female European leagues and impacts the final number of goals in a match and the final ranking of the league team. Additionally, it is well known that scoring first provides an advantage during matches and could condition game dynamics, tactics, and programming during a tournament. The top-ranked teams usually have better preparation processes and resources available to develop physical, psychological and tactical skills; these advantages allow them to score the first goal in most cases.

Practical Applications

Considering the impact of being the first scorer in a female football match, coaches may plan training sessions, bearing in mind that there are physical and psychological aspects to focus on that may boost team performance during the opening minutes of a match, and design tasks that may help achieve the first goal. Different offensive strategies may also help when taking into account physical conditioning, the quality of the opposing team, the available players and their abilities.

Additionally, some training strategies may be devised to overcome a situation where the team is not the first scorer, thus avoiding negativity and encouraging confidence in solving this issue. Moreover, those teams at the bottom of the table may focus their training towards achieving the first goal as a condition that may change the outcome of the matches.

The teams from minor divisions should be aware of these results and consider the critical opening minutes of a match as a determinant for winning the match, and thus the fundamental role of scoring first. Finally, coaches may analyse these tactical and physical situations where the team scores the first goal to understand how it was achieved to boost future performance, considering the variables that may help accomplish the first goal.

The internal and external variables mediating the scoring of the first goal or the offensive tactics that may lead to it should be monitored and considered when planning physical and conditioning training (e.g., high-intensity actions, accelerations, changes of direction).

Future studies could focus on the teams who score first, considering psychological, tactical and physical conditions. Additionally, studies could explore how female footballers, whose teams are losing during a match, can overturn the match outcome.

Author Contributions: Conceptualisation, P.S.-M., A.A. and S.J.I.; methodology, P.S.-M. and S.J.I.; software, P.S.-M. and D.R.-V.; validation, A.A., D.R.-V. and S.J.I.; formal analysis, P.S.-M. and D.R.-V.; investigation, P.S.-M.; resources, P.S.-M., A.A. and S.J.I.; data curation, P.S.-M., A.A. and D.R.-V.; writing—original draft preparation, P.S.-M. and D.R.-V.; writing—review and editing, P.S.-M., D.R.-V.

and S.J.I.; visualisation, P.S.-M., A.A. and D.R.-V.; supervision, S.J.I.; project administration, S.J.I.; funding acquisition, S.J.I. All authors have read and agreed to the published version of the manuscript.

Funding: This study was partially subsidised by the Aid for Research Groups (GR18170) from the Regional Government of Extremadura (Department of Employment, Companies and Innovation), with a contribution from the European Funds for Regional Development of the European Union.

Institutional Review Board Statement: Not applicable.

Informed Consent Statement: Not applicable.

Data Availability Statement: Not applicable.

Conflicts of Interest: The authors declare no conflict of interest.

References

1. Anderson, C.; Sally, D. *The Numbers Game: Why Everything You Know about Football Is Wrong*; Penguin: London, UK, 2013. ISBN 978-0-241-96363-0.
2. Paulis, J.C. Conocer el pasado del futbol para cambiar su futuro. *Acciónmotriz* **2009**, *2*, 39–53.
3. Ibáñez, S.J.; Pérez-Goye, J.A.; Courel-Ibáñez, J.; García-Rubio, J. The Impact of Scoring First on Match Outcome in Women's Professional Football. *Int. J. Perform. Anal. Sport* **2018**, *18*, 318–326. [CrossRef]
4. Lago-Peñas, C.; Gómez-Ruano, M.; Megías-Navarro, D.; Pollard, R. Home Advantage in Football: Examining the Effect of Scoring First on Match Outcome in the Five Major European Leagues. *Int. J. Perform. Anal. Sport* **2016**, *16*, 411–421. [CrossRef]
5. Martínez, F.D.M.; García, H.G. Efecto de marcar primero y la localización del partido en las principales ligas del fútbol europeo (Effect of scoring first and match location in the main European football leagues). *Retos* **2019**, *35*, 242–245. [CrossRef]
6. Pollard, R.; Gómez, M.A. Comparison of Home Advantage in Men's and Women's Football Leagues in Europe. *Eur. J. Sport Sci.* **2014**, *14* (Suppl. S1), S77–S83. [CrossRef]
7. Ibañez, S.J.; García-Rubio, J.; Gómez, M.-Á.; Gonzalez-Espinosa, S. The Impact of Rule Modifications on Elite Basketball Teams' Performance. *J. Hum. Kinet.* **2018**, *64*, 181–193. [CrossRef]
8. Courneya, K.S. Importance of Game Location and Scoring First in College Baseball. *Percept. Mot Skills* **1990**, *71*, 624–626. [CrossRef]
9. Jones, B. Scoring First and Home Advantage in the NHL. *Int. J. Perform. Anal. Sport* **2009**, *9*, 320–331. [CrossRef]
10. Hewitt, A.; Norton, K.; Lyons, K. Movement Profiles of Elite Women Soccer Players during International Matches and the Effect of Opposition's Team Ranking. *J. Sports Sci.* **2014**, *32*, 1874–1880. [CrossRef]
11. Liu, T.; García-de-Alcaraz, A.; Wang, H.; Hu, P.; Chen, Q. Impact of Scoring First on Match Outcome in the Chinese Football Super League. *Front. Psychol.* **2021**, *12*, 1617. [CrossRef] [PubMed]
12. Szymanski, S. Income Inequality, Competitive Balance and the Attractiveness of Team Sports: Some Evidence and a Natural Experiment from English Soccer. *Econ. J.* **2001**, *111*, F69–F84. [CrossRef]
13. Lago-Peñas, C.; Dellal, A. Ball Possession Strategies in Elite Soccer According to the Evolution of the Match-Score: The Influence of Situational Variables. *J. Hum. Kinet.* **2010**, *25*, 93–100. [CrossRef]
14. Lago-Peñas, C.; Lago-Ballesteros, J. Game Location and Team Quality Effects on Performance Profiles in Professional Soccer. *J. Sports Sci. Med.* **2011**, *10*, 465–471. [PubMed]
15. Martínez, F.D.M.; García, H.G. Efecto de marcar primero en la final de la UEFA Champions League y la UEFA Europa League. *Retos* **2020**, *37*, 134–138.
16. Bar-Eli, M.; Tenenbaum, G.; Geister, S. Consequences of Players' Dismissal in Professional Soccer: A Crisis-Related Analysis of Group-Size Effects. *J. Sports Sci.* **2006**, *24*, 1083–1094. [CrossRef]
17. Carroll, C. The Performance Gap in Sport Can Help Determine Which Movements Were Most Essential to Human Evolution. *Front. Physiol.* **2019**, *10*, 1412. [CrossRef] [PubMed]
18. Montero, I.; León, O.G. A guide for naming research studies in Psychology. *Int. J. Clin. Health Psychol.* **2007**, *7*, 847–862.
19. Delgado, S.C.; Marín, B.M.; Sánchez, J.L.R. *Métodos de Investigación y Análisis de Datos en Ciencias Sociales y de la Salud*; Pirámide: Madrid, Spain, 2011; ISBN 978-84-368-2462-9.
20. Crewson, P. *Applied Statistics*, 1st ed.; AcaStat Software: Winter Garden, FL, USA, 2014.
21. Merino, A.P.; Díaz, M.Á.R. *SPSS 11: Guía Para el Análisis de Datos*; Mc Graw Hill: Aravaca, Spain, 2002; ISBN 978-84-481-3750-2.
22. Lago, C.; Martín, R. Determinants of Possession of the Ball in Soccer. *J. Sports Sci.* **2007**, *25*, 969–974. [CrossRef] [PubMed]
23. Lago, C. The Influence of Match Location, Quality of Opposition, and Match Status on Possession Strategies in Professional Association Football. *J. Sports Sci.* **2009**, *27*, 1463–1469. [CrossRef] [PubMed]
24. Taylor, J.B.; Mellalieu, S.D.; James, N.; Shearer, D.A. The Influence of Match Location, Quality of Opposition, and Match Status on Technical Performance in Professional Association Football. *J. Sports Sci.* **2008**, *26*, 885–895. [CrossRef]
25. Lago-Peñas, C.; Lago-Ballesteros, J.; Dellal, A.; Gómez, M. Game-Related Statistics That Discriminated Winning, Drawing and Losing Teams from the Spanish Soccer League. *J. Sports Sci. Med.* **2010**, *9*, 288–293.

26. Kubayi, A.; Larkin, P. Technical Performance of Soccer Teams According to Match Outcome at the 2019 FIFA Women's World Cup. *Int. J. Perform. Anal. Sport* **2020**, *20*, 908–916. [CrossRef]
27. Jong, L.M.S.; de Gastin, P.B.; Angelova, M.; Bruce, L.; Dwyer, D.B. Technical Determinants of Success in Professional Women's Soccer: A Wider Range of Variables Reveals New Insights. *PLoS ONE* **2020**, *15*, e0240992. [CrossRef]
28. Williams, J.H.; Hoffman, S.; Jaskowak, D.J.; Tegarden, D. Physical Demands and Physiological Responses of Extra Time Matches in Collegiate Women's Soccer. *Sci. Med. Footb.* **2019**, *3*, 307–312. [CrossRef]
29. Lago-Peñas, C. The Role of Situational Variables in Analysing Physical Performance in Soccer. *J. Hum. Kinet.* **2012**, *35*, 89–95. [CrossRef]
30. Sarmento, H.; Marcelino, R.; Anguera, M.T.; CampaniÇo, J.; Matos, N.; LeitÃo, J.C. Match Analysis in Football: A Systematic Review. *J. Sports Sci.* **2014**, *32*, 1831–1843. [CrossRef]
31. Datson, N.; Drust, B.; Weston, M.; Gregson, W. Repeated High-Speed Running in Elite Female Soccer Players during International Competition. *Sci. Med. Footb.* **2019**, *3*, 150–156. [CrossRef]
32. Vescovi, J.D. Sprint Profile of Professional Female Soccer Players during Competitive Matches: Female Athletes in Motion (FAiM) Study. *J. Sports Sci.* **2012**, *30*, 1259–1265. [CrossRef] [PubMed]
33. Gómez, M.A.; Pollard, R.; Luis-Pascual, J.-C. Comparison of the Home Advantage in Nine Different Professional Team Sports in Spain. *Percept. Mot. Ski.* **2011**, *113*, 150–156. [CrossRef] [PubMed]
34. Prieto, J.; Gómez, M.-Á.; Pollard, R. Home Advantage in Men's and Women's Spanish First and Second Division Water Polo Leagues. *J. Hum. Kinet.* **2013**, *37*, 137–143. [CrossRef] [PubMed]
35. Gutiérrez Aguilar, O.; Saavedra García, M.; Fernández Romero, J.J. Measuring Home Advantage in Spanish Handball. *Percept. Mot. Ski.* **2012**, *114*, 329–338. [CrossRef] [PubMed]
36. Pollard, R.; Gómez, M.A. Home Advantage in Football in South-West Europe: Long-Term Trends, Regional Variation, and Team Differences. *Eur. J. Sport Sci.* **2009**, *9*, 341–352. [CrossRef]
37. Mara, J.K.; Wheeler, K.W.; Lyons, K. Attacking Strategies That Lead to Goal Scoring Opportunities in High Level Women's Football. *Int. J. Sports Sci. Coach.* **2012**, *7*, 565–577. [CrossRef]
38. Alcock, A. Analysis of Direct Free Kicks in the Women's Football World Cup 2007. *Eur. J. Sport Sci.* **2010**, *10*, 279–284. [CrossRef]
39. Soroka, A.; Bergier, J. Actions with the Ball That Determine the Effectiveness of Play in Women's Football. *J. Hum. Kinet.* **2010**, *26*, 97–104. [CrossRef]
40. Barreira, D.; Garganta, J.; Machado, J.; Anguera, M.T. Effects of Ball Recovery on Top-Level Soccer Attacking Patterns of Play. *Rev. Bras. Cineantropometria Desempenho Hum.* **2014**, *16*, 36–46. [CrossRef]
41. Liu, T.; Yang, L.; Chen, H.; García-de-Alcaraz, A. Impact of Possession and Player Position on Physical and Technical-Tactical Performance Indicators in the Chinese Football Super League. *Front. Psychol.* **2021**, *12*, 4246. [CrossRef]
42. Loignon, A.; Gayton, W.F.; Brown, M.; Steinroeder, W.; Johnson, C. Home Disadvantage in Professional ICE Hockey. *Percept. Mot. Ski.* **2007**, *104*, 1262–1264. [CrossRef]

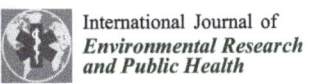

Article

No Relationship between Lean Mass and Functional Asymmetry in High-Level Female Tennis Players

Laurent Chapelle [1],*, Chris Bishop [2], Peter Clarys [1] and Eva D'Hondt [1,3]

1. Department of Movement and Sport Sciences, Faculty of Physical Education and Physiotherapy, Vrije Universiteit Brussel, 1050 Brussels, Belgium; peter.clarys@vub.be (P.C.); eva.dhondt@vub.be (E.D.)
2. London Sport Institute, Middlesex University, London NW4 4BT, UK; c.bishop@mdx.ac.uk
3. Department of Movement and Sports Sciences, Faculty of Medicine and Health Sciences, Ghent University, 9000 Ghent, Belgium
* Correspondence: laurent.chapelle@vub.be

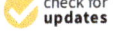

Citation: Chapelle, L.; Bishop, C.; Clarys, P.; D'Hondt, E. No Relationship between Lean Mass and Functional Asymmetry in High-Level Female Tennis Players. *Int. J. Environ. Res. Public Health* **2021**, *18*, 11928. https://doi.org/10.3390/ijerph182211928

Academic Editors: Filipe Manuel Clemente and Ana Filipa Silva

Received: 23 September 2021
Accepted: 11 November 2021
Published: 13 November 2021

Publisher's Note: MDPI stays neutral with regard to jurisdictional claims in published maps and institutional affiliations.

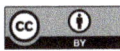

Copyright: © 2021 by the authors. Licensee MDPI, Basel, Switzerland. This article is an open access article distributed under the terms and conditions of the Creative Commons Attribution (CC BY) license (https://creativecommons.org/licenses/by/4.0/).

Abstract: The relationship between lean mass and functional asymmetry in terms of their magnitude and direction was examined in 22 high-level female tennis players (20.9 ± 3.6 years). Lean mass of both upper and lower extremities was examined using Dual X-ray Absorptiometry. Functional asymmetry was assessed using a battery of field tests (handgrip strength, seated shot-put throw, plate tapping, single leg countermovement jump, single leg forward hop test, 6 m single leg hop test, and 505 change of direction (time and deficit)). Paired sample *t*-tests compared the dominant (overall highest/best (performance) value) against the non-dominant value (highest/best (performance) value of the opposing extremity). Linear regressions were used to explore the relationship between lean mass and functional asymmetry magnitudes. Kappa coefficients were used to examine the consistency in direction between the extremity displaying the highest lean mass value and the extremity performing dominantly across tests. Significant asymmetry magnitudes ($p < 0.05$) were found for all upper and lower extremity lean mass and functional values. No relationship was apparent between lean mass and functional asymmetry magnitudes (*p*-value range = 0.131–0.889). Despite finding perfect consistency in asymmetry direction (k-value = 1.00) for the upper extremity, poor to fair consistency (k-value range = −0.00–0.21) was found for the lower extremity. In conclusion, lean mass and functional asymmetries should be examined independently.

Keywords: women; performance; unilateral; racket sport

1. Introduction

As one of the most popular sports globally, tennis is characterised by short high-intensity efforts which are alternated by bouts of recovery [1,2]. During these high-intensity efforts, tennis strokes are performed during which the preferred upper extremity of the player (i.e., the upper extremity holding the racket) is exposed to greater mechanical loading compared to the opposing upper extremity (i.e., the non-preferred upper extremity) [3]. Consequently, this predominantly unilateral sport is ideally suited to examine the occurrence of lean mass asymmetries (i.e., side-to-side differences in lean mass, expressed as a percentage) [4,5]. For instance, using Dual X-ray Absorptiometry (DXA), significant asymmetries between the preferred and non-preferred upper extremity in terms of lean mass (i.e., which includes muscle mass and body water) have previously been reported in both male (i.e., 9.7%) and female (i.e., 6.8%) tennis players [6,7].

In addition to the upper limbs, the lower extremities of tennis players are also subjected to asymmetrical loading due to their specific role in the kinetic chain when performing the various tennis strokes [8,9]. Several previous studies have examined lower extremity lean mass asymmetries by means of DXA in male youth [10], professional male adult [11] and high-level female adult tennis players [6], but reported varying results. For instance, the two beforementioned studies examining (youth) male tennis players indicated no significant lower extremity lean mass asymmetries (i.e., 0.6–0.8%), whilst the study examining female tennis players demonstrated significant lower extremity lean mass asymmetries (i.e., 4.8%). An important consideration, however, is that the latter study did not relate these significant side-to-side differences in lower extremity lean mass to players' tennis-specific physical performance (which may increase our knowledge regarding the impact of lean mass asymmetries). Hence, and in addition to the reported contradictory results, more research into (lower extremity) lean mass asymmetries in female tennis players is warranted.

Along with the occurrence of lean mass asymmetry, the presence of functional asymmetry (i.e., side-to-side differences in physical performance (e.g., strength or power), again expressed as a percentage) has also been established. Consequently, significant magnitudes of upper (i.e., 8.9–15.2%) and lower extremity (i.e., 1.8–9.4%) functional asymmetries have previously been reported in high-level female tennis players [12]. When examining functional asymmetries, it is essential to use a composite test battery (as opposed to isolated testing) given the direction specificity of asymmetries (i.e., which extremity displays higher values and/or is dominant in performance) between different sporting tasks [13]. For instance, the beforementioned study in high-level female tennis players reported that the preferred upper extremity consistently demonstrates superior performances compared to the opposing upper extremity. In contrast, the lower extremity was found to display poor levels of agreement as to which leg performed better across tests (i.e., the kappa coefficients ranged from -0.07 to 0.17), illustrating the direction specificity of lower extremity functional asymmetries [12].

It is important to note that both lean mass and functional asymmetries have, albeit separately, been associated with a decreased sport-specific performance, in addition to an increased injury risk [13–15]. However, no study has simultaneously examined both types of asymmetry. As a result, research regarding the relationship between lean mass asymmetry and functional asymmetry, both at the upper and lower extremity level, is currently lacking. More specifically, it is unknown whether a high(er) magnitude of lean mass asymmetry implies a high(er) magnitude of functional asymmetry (i.e., which could be the case since muscle mass (which entails lean mass) is reported to be a key determinant of functional strength and power) [16]. Similarly, regarding the agreement in direction between lean mass and functional asymmetry, it is unknown whether the extremity that displays the highest lean mass value also displays the best performance across body sides. As a result, the mutual relationship and the agreement in direction between both lean mass asymmetry and functional asymmetry remains to be investigated. Due to the lack of previous research in this respect (especially in female tennis players), this study aimed to examine the relationship between lean mass and functional asymmetry in terms of their magnitude and direction in high-level female tennis players.

2. Materials and Methods

2.1. Participants

Twenty-two high-level Belgian female tennis players aged between 17 and 27 years participated in this observational cross-sectional study. To be eligible for participation, these female tennis players had to be injury-free at the time of measurement and either have an international tennis ranking (i.e., Women's Tennis Association or International Tennis Federation) or a high national tennis ranking (i.e., being in the top 200 of the Belgian circuit ranking). Our study protocol was approved by the local university's medical ethics committee prior to data collection (B.U.N. 143201836107). The female tennis players, together with their legal guardians if they were still minor, were informed about the purposes of this study and signed an informed consent upon participation.

2.2. Procedures and Experimental Design

Data collection took place in the local university's biometry and biomechanics laboratory facilities between March 2019 and September 2020. Firstly, the female tennis players were asked to fill in a questionnaire to provide basic demographic and sport-specific information (i.e., date of birth, dominant upper extremity, starting age of tennis play and average weekly training volume over the last year). Next, after voiding their bladder and whilst being barefoot in light sports clothing, participants' body height and weight were measured to the nearest 0.1 cm and 0.002 kg using a stadiometer (SECA 217, Hamburg, Germany) and precision scale (RADWAG WLT 60/120/X/L3, All scales Europe, Veen, The Netherlands), respectively. Table 1 presents the demographic, sport-specific and anthropometric information of the 22 female tennis players included in our study sample.

Table 1. Demographic, sport-specific and anthropometric information of the high-level female tennis players (N = 22).

	High-Level Female Tennis Players
Age (years)	20.9 ± 3.6
Height (cm)	169.5 ± 4.8
Weight (kg)	62.5 ± 8.3
Starting age of tennis play (years)	6.1 ± 1.4
Training volume (hours/week)	10.2 ± 6.2
Handedness (n, right/left)	21/1

Note: Data are presented as n or mean ± standard deviation.

2.3. Lean Mass

DXA research scans (Norland Elite, Swissray, Fort Atkinson, WI, USA) of both the preferred and non-preferred upper extremity as well as the right and left lower extremity were conducted by the same researcher, who was intensively trained by the DXA scan manufacturer upon data collection, in order to determine participants' regional lean mass to the nearest 0.1 g. The DXA scanner was calibrated in accordance with the manufacturer's guidelines before each test session. Participants were instructed to lie as straight and still as possible in a supine position on the DXA scan table after the removal of all metal objects (e.g., earrings). The scan width was set to 6 × 6 mm, whilst a scan speed of 130 mm/s was applied. The upper extremity region included the upper arm, lower arm and hand, and was separated from the trunk by an inclined line passing through the scapula-humeral joint. The lower extremity region included the upper leg, lower leg and foot, and was separated from the trunk by an inclined line passing just below the pelvis [11]. The DXA research scans were analysed with the Norland Illuminatus software (Swissray, Fort Atkinson, WI, USA).

2.4. Functional Test Battery

A physical performance field-based test battery was used to examine the magnitude of functional asymmetry. Participants were instructed to wear their normal tennis outfit and sports shoes whilst performing the test battery, consisting of 8 different unilateral tests. A standardised 10-min warm-up, involving light running exercises and dynamic stretches, was implemented before completing the test battery. The different tests were always completed in the same order, ensuring alternation in testing the upper and lower extremities. The participants were guided through the test battery by the same well-trained researcher. Each participant was given three attempts per body side for every test. The first attempt of a test was always performed with the right body side, whereas the second attempt was always performed with the left body side, ensuring alteration between both sides of the body during testing. Participants were given 60 s of rest between attempts and 3 min of rest between tests to ensure adequate recovery.

Handgrip strength: Participants were instructed to squeeze as hard as possible (for three seconds) in a digital handheld dynamometer with an accuracy of 0.1 kg (Jamar

Plus, Patterson Medical, Nottinghamshire, UK), while being seated in a chair without armrests. The elbow of the participants had to remain 90 degrees flexed throughout every attempt [17].

Seated shot-put throw: Participants were seated on the ground with their back against a wall and their hips, knees and ankles parallel to the ground. The non-throwing arm was placed on the opposite (i.e., throwing) shoulder. From this position, participants had to throw a 3-kg medicine ball as far as possible in a forward direction. The distance where the medicine ball landed on to the ground was measured to the nearest 1 cm using a tape measure [18].

Plate tapping: Two discs (with a diameter of 20 cm) were placed with their centres 60 cm apart on a table together with a 10 × 20 cm rectangle (which was placed in between the two discs). Participants started the test with one hand placed on one of the two discs, whilst the other hand was placed on the rectangle in the middle. The aim of the plate tapping test was to move one hand back and forth between both discs over the other hand (which was on the rectangle) as fast as possible. This action was repeated for 25 full cycles (i.e., 50 taps on the discs) and the time needed to complete this test was recorded to the nearest 0.01 s using a hand-held stopwatch [19].

Single leg countermovement jump: Participants were instructed to jump up as high as possible on one leg. Throughout the jump, they were instructed to hold their hands on their hips. Swinging of the non-jumping leg was not allowed and the jumping leg had to remain completely extended throughout the flight phase. Participants needed to keep their balance on one leg after landing, otherwise an extra attempt was provided. Jumping height was determined to the nearest 0.1 cm using the Optojump Next system (Microgate Bolzano, Italy) [20].

Single leg forward hop test: Participants stood on one leg behind a tape line whilst holding their hands on the hips. They had to jump as far as possible in a forward direction landing on the same foot without losing their balance (e.g., moving their foot on which they land or planting the other foot on to the ground). If participants were not able to maintain their balance on one leg after landing, an extra attempt was provided. The covered distance from the starting line to the heel of the participants' landing foot was measured to the nearest 1 cm using a tape measure [21].

6 m single leg hop test: Participants were instructed to cover 6 m as fast as possible whilst hopping on one leg. The time needed to cover these 6 m was measured to the nearest 0.001 s using electronic timing gates (Witty Wireless Training Timer, Microgate, Bolzano, Italy). These timing gates were placed at hip height and participants had to start behind a tape line which was located 30 cm from the first timing gate.

505 change of direction time (505 COD time) and deficit (505 COD deficit): First, participants' 10 m sprint time was measured to the nearest 0.001 s using electronic timing gates (Witty Wireless Training Timer, Microgate, Bolzano, Italy). Next, their 505 COD time was determined to the nearest 0.001 s based on performing the 505 COD test, which consisted of a 5 m sprint, followed by a 180° turn to either the left or the right side, and a 5 m sprint back to the starting line. Participants' 505 COD deficit was then calculated by deducting their 10 m sprint time from their 505 COD time [22].

2.5. Asymmetry Calculations

The dominant value was defined as the highest lean mass value or the best (i.e., highest or fastest) value for a test of the functional test battery. The non-dominant value was defined as the highest or best result of the same outcome measure for the opposing upper or lower extremity [23]. The magnitude of lean mass and functional asymmetry was calculated for every outcome measure and expressed as a percentage by using the percentage difference method (PDM): (dominant value − non-dominant value)/dominant value) × 100 [24].

2.6. Statistical Analyses

Data analysis was conducted using SPSS version 27.0 (IBM, Chicago, IL, USA). Normality of distribution was examined for every outcome measure using the Shapiro–Wilk test. Variability and reliability of every outcome measure was verified by calculating the coefficient of variation (CV) and a two-way random intraclass correlation coefficient (ICC) with 95% confidence intervals. CV values of less than 10% were considered acceptable and ICC values were classified as poor (<0.50), moderate (0.50–0.74), good (0.75–0.89) and excellent (>0.90) [25,26]. Paired sample t-tests were used for within-subject comparisons of the dominant against the non-dominant values for every outcome measure. Effect size analyses using Hedges' g were conducted of the side-to-side difference between the dominant and non-dominant values and classified as trivial (<0.20), small (0.20–0.49), medium (0.50–0.79) or large (>0.80) [27]. A linear regression analysis, adjusting for the participants' age, was used to examine the relationship between the magnitude of lean mass asymmetry and the magnitude of functional asymmetry [28]. Lastly, the consistency in direction as to which extremity displayed the dominant lean mass value and which extremity performed dominantly across the different field tests of the functional test battery was examined using Kappa coefficients. These Kappa coefficients were classified as poor (≤0), slight (0.01–0.20), fair (0.21–0.40), moderate (0.41–0.60), substantial (0.61–0.80), almost perfect (0.81–0.99) and perfect (1.00) [29]. All data are presented as means ± standard deviations and p-values <0.05 were considered statistically significant.

3. Results

Every outcome measure showed acceptable reliability (i.e., all CVs were below 10%) and excellent reliability (i.e., all ICCs were above 0.90) as presented in Table 2. The lean mass and functional asymmetry values for our study sample of high-level female tennis players are displayed in Table 3. Significant magnitudes of lean mass and functional asymmetry for all outcome measures were found (t-value range = 4.027–8.638; $p < 0.001$). Effect sizes between the side-to-side differences of the dominant and non-dominant values ranged from small to large.

Table 2. Variability and reliability of the DXA research scans and the unilateral tests of the functional test battery.

	CV	ICC (95% CI)
DXA research scan		
Upper extremity lean mass	2.3	0.99 (0.99, 1.00)
Lower extremity lean mass	2.3	0.98 (0.98, 1.00)
Functional test battery		
Upper extremity field tests		
Handgrip strength	2.9	0.96 (0.95, 0.98)
Seated shot-put throw	4.8	0.95 (0.91, 0.98)
Plate tapping	3.8	0.94 (0.89, 0.97)
Lower extremity field tests		
Single leg countermovement jump	5.9	0.97 (0.95, 1.00)
Single leg forward hop test	3.5	0.98 (0.96, 1.00)
6 m single leg hop test	2.4	0.98 (0.95, 1.00)
505 changes of direction		
Time	1.5	0.98 (0.96, 1.00)
Direction	3.9	0.97 (0.92, 1.00)

Note: DXA = Dual X-ray Absorptiometry; CV = coefficient of variation; ICC = intraclass correlation coefficient; 95% CI = 95% confidence interval.

Table 3. Upper and lower extremity lean mass and functional asymmetry values of the high-level female tennis players (N = 22).

	Dominant Value	Non-Dominant Value	ES (95% CI)	PDM (%)
Lean mass				
Upper extremity (g)	2069.9 ± 356.8	1935.1 ± 299.1	0.41 (−0.10, 0.90)	7.1 ± 4.8 *
Lower extremity (g)	8453.8 ± 1226.0	8060.7 ± 1225.8	0.31 (−0.18, 0.81)	4.8 ± 2.9 *
Functional test battery				
Upper extremity				
Handgrip strength (kg)	38.9 ± 6.7	33.8 ± 5.8	0.80 (0.28, 1.31)	13.2 ± 8.3 *
Seated shot-put throw (cm)	328.2 ± 45.9	296.8 ± 44.0	0.70 (0.18, 1.20)	9.5 ± 5.0 *
Plate tapping (sec)	10.24 ± 1.50	11.47 ± 1.75	0.74 (0.23, 1.25)	11.1 ± 6.0 *
Lower extremity				
Single leg countermovement jump (cm)	15.0 ± 3.5	13.7 ± 3.0	0.40 (−0.11, 0.89)	8.4 ± 6.3 *
Single leg forward hop test (cm)	142.7 ± 16.7	136.1 ± 18.5	0.37 (−0.13, 0.87)	4.8 ± 4.2 *
6 m single leg hop test (sec)	1.938 ± 0.168	2.010 ± 0.172	0.42 (−0.09, 0.84)	3.6 ± 3.2 *
505 change of direction				
Time (sec)	3.249 ± 0.174	3.311 ± 0.181	0.34 (−0.16, 0.84)	1.9 ± 1.7 *
Deficit (sec)	1.144 ± 0.109	1.207 ± 0.120	0.54 (−0.03, 1.04)	5.0 ± 4.3 *

Note: Data are presented as mean ± standard deviation; ES = effect size; 95% CI = confidence interval; PDM = percentage difference method; * Significant ($p < 0.05$) magnitude of asymmetry between body sides.

For every field-based test, the corresponding individual lean mass asymmetry magnitudes alongside functional asymmetry magnitudes are displayed in Figure 1 for the upper extremity and in Figure 2 for the lower extremity. No significant relationship between the magnitude of lean mass asymmetry and the magnitude of functional asymmetry (F-value range = 0.021–3.461; r-value range = −0.232–0.254; p-value range = 0.131–0.889) was found as lean mass asymmetry magnitude could only explain 0.1 to 15.9% of the functional asymmetry magnitude.

The consistency in direction between the upper extremity displaying the dominant lean mass value and the upper extremity performing dominantly on the tests of the functional test battery was classified as perfect. For the lower extremity, the consistency between the lower extremity displaying the dominant lean mass value and the lower extremity performing dominantly across tests were classified from poor to fair (Table 4).

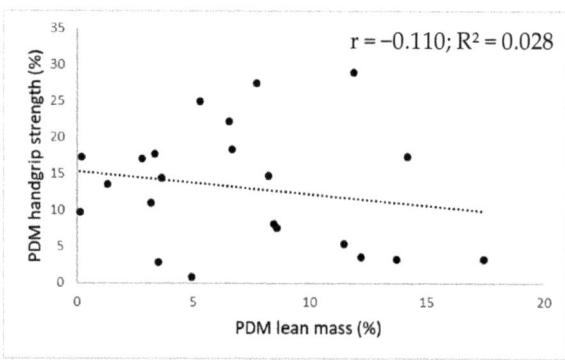

Figure 1. Cont.

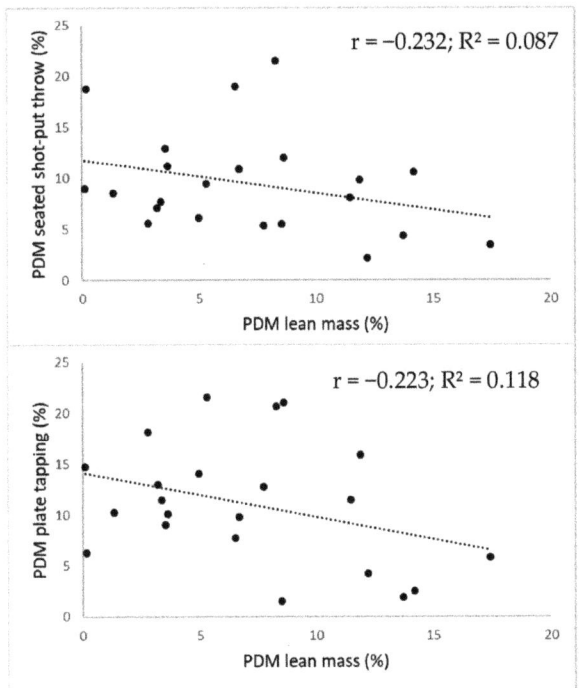

Figure 1. Scatter plot illustrating the relationship between the magnitude of upper extremity lean mass asymmetry (x-axis) and the magnitude of upper extremity functional asymmetry (y-axis) for the high-level female tennis players (N = 22). Note: The dotted line represents the linear trend line; PDM = percentage difference method; r = correlation coefficient; R^2 = R squared value.

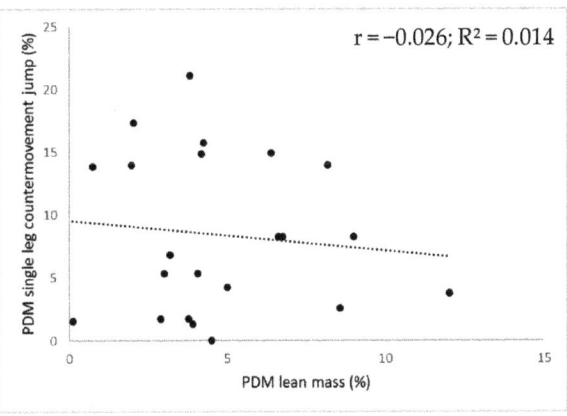

Figure 2. *Cont.*

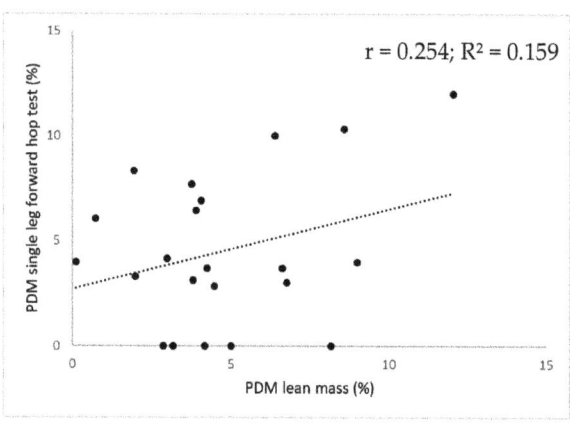
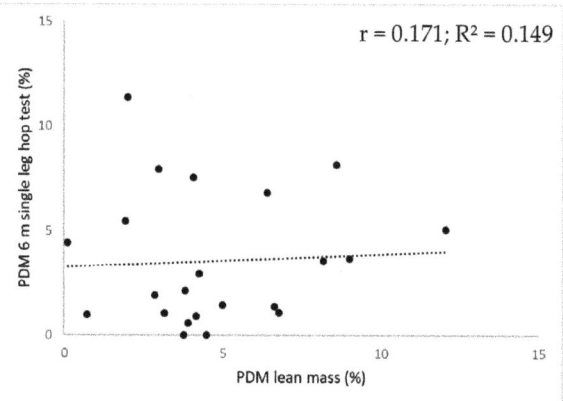
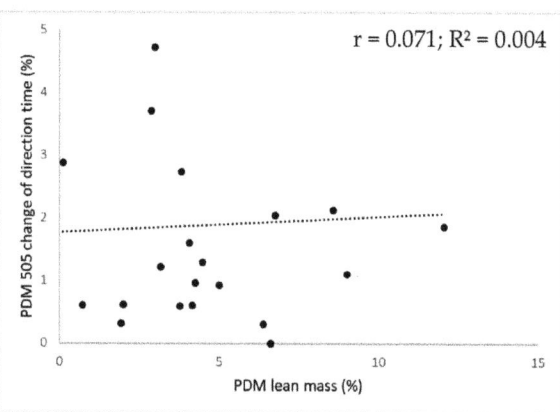

Figure 2. *Cont.*

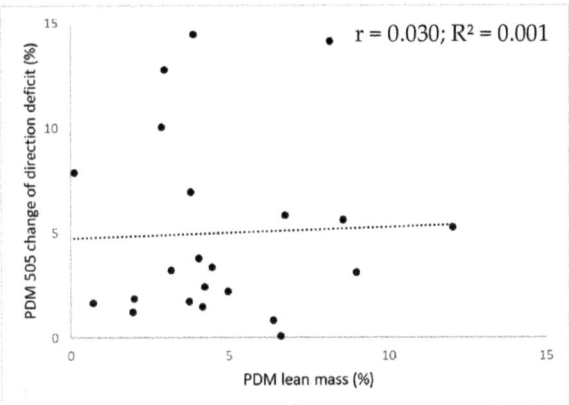

Figure 2. Scatter plot illustrating the relationship between the magnitude of lower extremity lean mass asymmetry (x-axis) and the magnitude of lower extremity functional asymmetry (y-axis) for the high-level female tennis players (N = 22). Note: The dotted line represents the linear trend line; PDM = percentage difference method; r = correlation coefficient; R^2 = R squared value.

Table 4. Kappa coefficients indicating the consistency in direction between the dominant lean mass value and the dominant performance value across unilateral tests for the high-level female tennis players (N = 22).

	Kappa	Description
Upper extremity lean mass		
Handgrip strength	1.00	Perfect
Seated shot-put throw	1.00	Perfect
Plate tapping	1.00	Perfect
Lower extremity lean mass		
Single leg countermovement jump	0.18	Slight
Single leg forward hop test	0.00	Poor
6 m Single leg hop test	0.18	Slight
505 Change of direction time/deficit	0.21	Fair

Note: Kappa coefficients are classified as poor (≤0), slight (0.01–0.20), fair (0.21–0.40), moderate (0.41–0.60), substantial (0.61–0.80), almost perfect (0.81–0.99) and perfect (1.00).

The consistency in direction between the upper extremity displaying the dominant lean mass value and the upper extremity performing dominantly on the tests of the functional test battery was classified as perfect. For the lower extremity, the consistency between the lower extremity displaying the dominant lean mass value and the lower extremity performing dominantly across tests was classified from poor to fair, depending on the field test at hand (Table 4).

4. Discussion

This observational cross-sectional study aimed to examine the relationship between lean mass and functional asymmetry in terms of their magnitude and direction in high-level female tennis players. The results of our study indicated no meaningful relationships between the magnitude of lean mass asymmetry and functional asymmetry in either the upper or the lower extremities. Additionally, consistency in the direction of asymmetry between the extremity displaying the highest lean mass value and the extremity displaying the dominant performance value for the functional tests across body sides was perfect for the upper extremity, whereas this consistency in dominance for both types of asymmetry ranged from poor to fair as regards to the lower extremity.

The significant magnitude of upper extremity lean mass asymmetry found in this study (i.e., 7.1%) can be largely attributed to the mechanical loading imposed to the preferred upper extremity associated with the repetitive performance of tennis strokes [4]. Interestingly, the preferred upper extremity of all high-level female tennis players included in the present always displayed the highest lean mass value. In agreement with the results of the upper extremity, significant lower extremity lean mass asymmetries (i.e., 4.8%) were found in our sample of Belgian high-level female tennis players. Even though most of them were right-handed (i.e., 21 out of 22 players), the majority displayed a higher lean mass of the left leg compared to the right leg (i.e., 18 out of 22 players). This could be explained by the previously reported occurrence of cross-asymmetry where the contralateral leg (i.e., the leg opposed to the preferred upper extremity) plays an important role in counterbalancing the torques of the upper extremity performing the various tennis strokes [6,8,9]. It is important to consider that the present study compared the dominant versus the non-dominant value to examine and report lower extremity lean mass asymmetries as opposed to using the values of the self-reported preferred lower extremity by asking, for example, on which leg participants prefer to perform a single leg hop [24]. The latter could lead to an incorrect calculation of the asymmetry magnitude as a percentage should be calculated with respect to the highest value [24,30].

The magnitude of upper extremity functional asymmetry ranged from 9.5 to 13.2% in our study, which is indicative of significant inter-limb asymmetries. Again, these significant inter-limb asymmetries can be principally attributed to the predominantly unilateral nature of tennis [3]. It is important to note that the preferred upper extremity of the included high-level female tennis players always performed dominantly across all upper extremity tests. Although lower than the magnitude of upper extremity functional asymmetry, the overall magnitude of functional asymmetry at the lower extremity level ranged from 1.9 to 8.4%, indicating significant functional asymmetries for all lower extremity performance tests. However, due to the task specificity of lower extremity functional asymmetries, there was no occurrence of cross-asymmetry across the functional tests for the lower extremity, as also mentioned in earlier research [12]. The highest asymmetry magnitude was found for the single leg countermovement jump (i.e., 8.4%). This result is in agreement with previous studies that have reported jump height from the single leg countermovement jump as being a sensitive physical performance test to examine functional asymmetries, especially when compared to jumping in a forward direction [31,32]. Nevertheless, it can be argued that it is surprising to find significant lower extremity functional asymmetries in a study sample of high-level female tennis players because being equally physically skilled on both lower extremities could be advantageous from a performance perspective [13].

As indicated by the results of this study, lean mass asymmetry and functional asymmetry do not seem to be related in terms of their magnitude given that lean mass asymmetry magnitude could only explain between 0.1 and 15.9% of the functional asymmetry magnitude. This is surprising because lean mass (which also encompasses muscle mass) has been reported to be a key determinant of functional strength and power [16], although it has been reported that other factors such as neuromuscular control and joint coordination also contribute to strength and power development [15,33]. Therefore, it is recommended that practitioners examine lean mass and functional asymmetries independently from one another. Additionally, the non-existent relationship between lean mass and functional asymmetry may have implications when designing targeted training programmes to counteract the reported negative influences of asymmetry (as it is unclear whether practitioners should focus on lean mass and/or functional parameters) [13–15]. Regarding the direction of asymmetry, there was a poor to slight consistency between the lower extremity displaying the dominant lean mass value and the lower extremity performing dominantly across the functional tests. This result was in contrast to the upper extremity, which displayed perfect levels of agreement. Consequently, the reported lower extremity results in this respect highlight the task and direction specific nature of asymmetry during the execution of different tasks, with Kappa values of the present study being comparable to those in previous research [20,32]. Because the extremity displaying the highest lean mass value does not consistently perform dominantly at lower limb level, it is recommended that practitioners examine and interpret both lean mass and functional asymmetry in an independent manner. Additionally, the assessment of asymmetries should be performed regularly and on an individual player basis, so that an asymmetry profile can be made to closely monitor each tennis player [20,34].

This is the first study to examine and report both lean and functional asymmetry of the upper and the lower extremity in high-level female tennis players using individual data. It can be argued that high-level tennis players are well suited to examine asymmetries because reaching such a level requires a high training volume and given the reported association between a high training volume and the occurrence of asymmetry [10]. Additionally, all players included in our study sample started to play tennis before the onset of puberty, which has been reported to result in greater asymmetry magnitudes [4]. Furthermore, functional asymmetry was examined using a valid, reliable and elaborated field-based test battery, as opposed to isolated testing, which is important given that asymmetries are reported to be movement or task-specific [34], as clearly demonstrated by our findings at the level of the lower limb. However, some limitations to our research are apparent. The present study implemented a cross-sectional design, which included a small sample size (although a post hoc power analysis revealed that the statistical power of this study was 91%). However, a control group was not included and the association between lean mass and functional asymmetry with decreased sport-specific performance, and injury incidence, was not examined. Therefore, future research is needed to examine the influence of lean mass and functional asymmetry on sports-specific performance and injury incidence using a longitudinal design. Additionally, more precise tools (e.g., force plates or isokinetic dynamometry) and outcome measures (e.g., leg stiffness, ground contact time or force) could be used when examining functional asymmetries [35].

5. Conclusions

To conclude, the significant lean mass and functional asymmetries of both the upper and lower extremity were not related in terms of their magnitude among high-level female tennis players. Additionally, the consistency between the extremity displaying the dominant lean mass value and the extremity displaying the dominant performance value across the functional tests was perfect for the upper extremity, whereas this consistency ranged from poor to fair for the lower extremity. When examining asymmetries in tennis players, it is recommended that both the magnitude and direction thereof should be considered and interpreted independently of one another in view of asymmetry profiling because no mutual relationship between both constructs could be demonstrated. It is also essential to examine and monitor both upper and lower extremity asymmetries on an individual player basis and to examine functional asymmetries using an elaborated field-based test battery. Future more in-depth research is also needed to investigate the impact of lean mass and functional asymmetries on female players' sports-specific performance and injury incidence using longitudinal (and/or experimental) study designs.

Author Contributions: L.C. recruited the participants, collected all data and also took responsibility for data analysis and drafting the manuscript. C.B., P.C. and E.D. substantially contributed to the conception of the study design, the interpretation of the data and critically revised the manuscript's drafting. All authors have read and agreed to the published version of the manuscript.

Funding: This research received no external funding.

Institutional Review Board Statement: The study was conducted according to the guidelines of the Declaration of Helsinki and approved by the Ethics Committee of the Vrije Universiteit Brussel (B.U.N. 143201836107).

Informed Consent Statement: Informed consent was obtained from all participants involved in the study before data collection took place.

Data Availability Statement: The data that support the findings of this study are available from the corresponding author upon request.

Conflicts of Interest: The authors declare no conflict of interest.

References

1. Fernandez-Fernandez, J.; Ulbricht, A.C.; Ferrauti, A. Fitness testing of tennis players: How valuable is it? *Br. J. Sports Med.* **2014**, *48*, i22–i31. [CrossRef]
2. Kovacs, M.S. Applied physiology of tennis performance. *Br. J. Sports Med.* **2006**, *40*, 381–386. [CrossRef]
3. Elliott, B.; Fleisig, G.; Nicholls, R.; Escamilia, R. Technique effects on upper limb loading in the tennis serve. *J. Sci. Med. Sport* **2003**, *6*, 76–87. [CrossRef]
4. Sanchis-Moysi, J.; Dorado, C.; Idoate, F.; Henríquez, J.J.G.; Serrano-Sanchez, J.A.; Calbet, J.A. The asymmetry of pectoralis muscles is greater in male prepubertal than in professional tennis players. *Eur. J. Sport Sci.* **2016**, *16*, 780–786. [CrossRef]
5. Ireland, A.; Degens, H.; Maffulli, N.; Rittweger, J. Tennis Service Stroke Benefits Humerus Bone: Is Torsion the Cause? *Calcif. Tissue Int.* **2015**, *97*, 193–198. [CrossRef]
6. Chapelle, L.; Rommers, N.; Clarys, P.; D'Hondt, E. Whole-body morphological asymmetries in high-level female tennis players: A cross-sectional study. *J. Sports Sci.* **2020**, *39*, 777–782. [CrossRef] [PubMed]
7. Ducher, G.; Courteix, D.; Même, S.; Magni, C.; Viala, J.; Benhamou, C. Bone geometry in response to long-term tennis playing and its relationship with muscle volume: A quantitative magnetic resonance imaging study in tennis players. *Bone* **2005**, *37*, 457–466. [CrossRef] [PubMed]
8. Elliott, B. Biomechanics and tennis. *Br. J. Sports Med.* **2006**, *40*, 392–396. [CrossRef]
9. Akutagawa, S.; Kojima, T. Trunk rotation torques through the hip joints during the one- and two-handed backhand tennis strokes. *J. Sports Sci.* **2005**, *23*, 781–793. [CrossRef]
10. Sanchis-Moysi, J.; Dorado, C.; Olmedillas, H.; Sánchez, J.A.S.; Calbet, J.A. Bone and lean mass inter-arm asymmetries in young male tennis players depend on training frequency. *Eur. J. Appl. Physiol.* **2010**, *110*, 83–90. [CrossRef] [PubMed]
11. Calbet, J.A.L.; Moysi, J.S.; Dorado, C.; Rodríguez, L.P. Bone Mineral Content and Density in Professional Tennis Players. *Calcif. Tissue Int.* **1998**, *62*, 491–496. [CrossRef]
12. Chapelle, L.; Bishop, C.; Clarys, P.; D'Hondt, E. International vs. National female tennis players: A comparison of upper and lower extremity functional asymmetries. *J. Sports Med. Phys. Fit.* **2021**. online ahead of print. [CrossRef]
13. Bishop, C.; Turner, A.; Read, P. Effects of inter-limb asymmetries on physical and sports performance: A systematic review. *J. Sports Sci.* **2017**, *36*, 1135–1144. [CrossRef]
14. Sannicandro, I.; Cofano, G.; Rosa, R.A.; Piccinno, A. Balance Training Exercises Decrease Lower-Limb Strength Asymmetry in Young Tennis Players. *J. Sports Sci. Med.* **2014**, *13*, 397–402.
15. Bell, D.R.; Sanfilippo, J.L.; Binkley, N.; Heiderscheit, B.C. Lean Mass Asymmetry Influences Force and Power Asymmetry During Jumping in Collegiate Athletes. *J. Strength Cond. Res.* **2014**, *28*, 884–891. [CrossRef] [PubMed]
16. Balshaw, T.G.; Maden-Wilkinson, T.M.; Massey, G.J.; Folland, J.P. The Human Muscle Size and Strength Relationship: Effects of Architecture, Muscle Force, and Measurement Location. *Med. Sci. Sports Exerc.* **2021**, *53*, 2140–2151. [CrossRef]
17. Roberts, H.C.; Denison, H.J.; Martin, H.J.; Patel, H.P.; Syddall, H.; Cooper, C.; Sayer, A.A. A review of the measurement of grip strength in clinical and epidemiological studies: Towards a standardised approach. *Age Ageing* **2011**, *40*, 423–429. [CrossRef] [PubMed]
18. Negrete, R.J.; Hanney, W.J.; Kolber, M.J.; Davies, G.J.; Ansley, M.K.; McBride, A.B.; Overstreet, A.L. Reliability, Minimal Detectable Change, and Normative Values for Tests of Upper Extremity Function and Power. *J. Strength Cond. Res.* **2010**, *24*, 3318–3325. [CrossRef] [PubMed]
19. Tsigilis, N.; Douda, H.; Tokmakidis, S. Test-Retest Reliability of the Eurofit Test Battery Administered to University Students. *Percept. Mot. Ski.* **2002**, *95*, 1295–1300. [CrossRef] [PubMed]
20. Bishop, C.; Turner, A.; Jarvis, P.; Chavda, S.; Read, P. Considerations for Selecting Field-Based Strength and Power Fitness Tests to Measure Asymmetries. *J. Strength Cond. Res.* **2017**, *31*, 2635–2644. [CrossRef] [PubMed]
21. Hoog, P.; Warren, M.; Smith, C.A.; Chimera, N.J. Functional hop tests and tuck jump assessment scores between female division I collegiate athletes participating in high versus low acl injury prone sports: A cross sectional analysis. *Int. J. Sports Phys. Ther.* **2016**, *11*, 945–953.
22. Nimphius, S.; Callaghan, S.J.; Spiteri, T.; Lockie, R.G. Change of Direction Deficit: A More Isolated Measure of Change of Direction Performance Than Total 505 Time. *J. Strength Cond. Res.* **2016**, *30*, 3024–3032. [CrossRef] [PubMed]
23. Newton, R.U.; Gerber, A.; Nimphius, S.; Shim, J.K.; Doan, B.K.; Robertson, M.; Pearson, D.R.; Craig, B.W.; Häkkinen, K.; Kraemer, W.J. Determination of Functional Strength Imbalance of the Lower Extremities. *J. Strength Cond. Res.* **2006**, *20*, 971–977. [CrossRef] [PubMed]
24. Bishop, C.; Read, P.; Chavda, S.; Turner, A. Asymmetries of the Lower Limb: The Calculation Conundrum in Strength Training and Conditioning. *Strength Cond. J.* **2016**, *38*, 27–32. [CrossRef]
25. Cormack, S.; Newton, R.U.; McGuigan, M.R.; Doyle, T.L. Reliability of Measures Obtained During Single and Repeated Countermovement Jumps. *Int. J. Sports Physiol. Perform.* **2008**, *3*, 131–144. [CrossRef]

26. Koo, T.K.; Li, M.Y. A Guideline of Selecting and Reporting Intraclass Correlation Coefficients for Reliability Research. *J. Chiropr. Med.* **2016**, *15*, 155–163. [CrossRef]
27. Durlak, J.A. How to Select, Calculate, and Interpret Effect Sizes. *J. Pediatr. Psychol.* **2009**, *34*, 917–928. [CrossRef] [PubMed]
28. Marill, K.A. Advanced statistics: Linear regression, part I: Simple linear regression. *Acad Emerg. Med.* **2004**, *11*, 87–93. [CrossRef]
29. Viera, A.J.; Garrett, J.M. Understanding interobserver agreement: The kappa statistic. *Fam. Med.* **2005**, *37*, 360–363.
30. Virgile, A.; Bishop, C. A Narrative Review of Limb Dominance: Task Specificity and the Importance of Fitness Testing. *J. Strength Cond. Res.* **2021**, *35*, 846–858. [CrossRef] [PubMed]
31. Fort-Vanmeerhaeghe, A.; Bishop, C.; Buscà, B.; Aguilera-Castells, J.; Vicens-Bordas, J.; Gonzalo-Skok, O. Inter-limb asymmetries are associated with decrements in physical performance in youth elite team sports athletes. *PLoS ONE* **2020**, *15*, e0229440. [CrossRef] [PubMed]
32. Madruga-Parera, M.; Romero-Rodríguez, D.; Bishop, C.; Beltran-Valls, M.R.; Latinjak, A.T.; Beato, M.; Fort-Vanmeerhaeghe, A. Effects of Maturation on Lower Limb Neuromuscular Asymmetries in Elite Youth Tennis Players. *Sports* **2019**, *7*, 106. [CrossRef] [PubMed]
33. Walsh, M.; Boling, M.C.; McGrath, M.; Blackburn, J.T.; Padua, D.A. Lower Extremity Muscle Activation and Knee Flexion During a Jump-Landing Task. *J. Athl. Train.* **2012**, *47*, 406–413. [CrossRef]
34. Bishop, C.; Lake, J.; Loturco, I.; Papadopoulos, K.; Turner, A.; Read, P. Interlimb Asymmetries: The Need for an Individual Approach to Data Analysis. *J. Strength Cond. Res.* **2021**, *35*, 695–701. [CrossRef]
35. Kotsifaki, A.; Korakakis, V.; Whiteley, R.; Van Rossom, S.; Jonkers, I. Measuring only hop distance during single leg hop testing is insufficient to detect deficits in knee function after ACL reconstruction: A systematic review and meta-analysis. *Br. J. Sports Med.* **2019**, *54*, 139–153. [CrossRef] [PubMed]

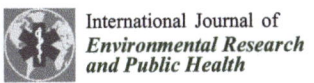

International Journal of Environmental Research and Public Health

Article

The Effects of Running Compared with Functional High-Intensity Interval Training on Body Composition and Aerobic Fitness in Female University Students

Yining Lu [1], Huw D. Wiltshire [1], Julien S. Baker [2] and Qiaojun Wang [3,*]

1. Cardiff School of Sport and Health Sciences, Cardiff Metropolitan University, Cardiff CF5 2YB, UK; st20184530@outlook.cardiffmet.ac.uk (Y.L.); hwiltshire@cardiffmet.ac.uk (H.D.W.)
2. Department of Sport, Physical Education and Health, Hong Kong Baptist University, Kowloon Tong, Hong Kong; jsbaker@hkbu.edu.hk
3. Faculty of Sport Science, Ningbo University, Ningbo 315000, China
* Correspondence: wangqiaojun@nbu.edu.cn; Tel.: +86-138-0588-5586

Abstract: High-intensity interval running (HIIT-R) and high-intensity functional training (HIFT) are two forms of HIIT exercise that are commonly used. The purpose of this study was to determine the effects of HIFT on aerobic capacity and body composition when compared to HIIT-R in females. Twenty healthy, untrained female university students (age 20.5 ± 0.7 year) were randomly assigned to a 12-week HIIT-R or HIFT intervention. The HIIT-R group involved a 30 s maximal shuttle run with a 30 s recovery period, whereas the HIFT involved multiple functional exercises with a 2:1 work-active recovery ratio. Body composition, VO_2max, and muscle performance were measured before and post intervention. As a result, HIIT-R and HIIT-F stimulated similar improvements in VO_2max (17.1% ± 5.6% and 12.7% ± 6.7%, respectively, $p > 0.05$). Only the HIIT-F group revealed significant improvements in muscle performance (sit-ups, 16.5% ± 3.1%, standing broad jump 5.1% ± 2.2%, $p < 0.05$). Body fat percentage decreased (17.1% ± 7.4% and 12.6% ± 5.1%, respectively, $p < 0.05$) in both HIIT-R and HIIT-F with no between-group differences. We concluded that HIFT was equally effective in promoting body composition and aerobic fitness compared to HIIT-R. HIFT resulted in improved muscle performance, whereas the HIIT-R protocol demonstrated no gains.

Keywords: high-intensity interval training; high-intensity functional training; body composition; aerobic fitness; muscle performance

1. Introduction

Regular physical activity (PA) is beneficial for health [1–3]. Despite the well documented benefits of moderate- to vigorous-intensity PA, 31% of adults worldwide do not engage in sufficient PA for health benefits as recommended by the World Health Organization (WHO) and the American College of Sports Medicine (ACSM) [4–6]. Frequently reported barriers to physical activity are physical exertion, time, and financial expenditure [7,8]. Thus, compared to traditional continuous training, which is characterized by long-duration, continuous aerobic exercises, and moderate-intensities, high-intensity interval training (HIIT) appears to be an efficient pathway to enhance PA and improve health [9].

HIIT involves repeated bouts of high-intensity exercises separated by a recovery using low-intensity activities or inactivity [10]. Recent studies had indicated that HIIT has a similar, or even greater positive, effect on physical fitness, especially on body composition and cardiorespiratory health [11–14]. From a time/benefit perspective, HIIT appears to help physically inactive individuals overcome a major time and participation barrier to maintaining a healthier lifestyle [15].

Originally, HIIT was used to improve the performance of endurance athletes [16]. Cycling, running, and rowing are traditional exercise modalities that adopted the use of HIIT protocols, while for individuals who perform exercise for health and recreation, these traditional modalities seem boring and do not engage individuals because of the repetitive nature of the exercise combined with repetition. This is considered as a negative impact for maintaining regular exercise and has been cited as "lack of enjoyment" when investigating barriers to exercise [17].

The intrinsic factors of participants are also important when considering exercise adherence [18,19]. Several studies have revealed that adherence is affected by exercise intensity, especially among inactive individuals [20,21].

High-intensity functional training (HIFT) has become a relatively popular training modality in recent years and is an alternative to traditional aerobic activities. The HIFT protocol consists of a variety of functional movements that are executed at a high intensity [22,23]). Recently, several investigators have studied the effects of HIFT on physical fitness promotion. After engaging in HIFT protocols, participants show significant improvements in cardiorespiratory fitness [24,25] and body composition [25,26]. Providing similar or greater health promotions compared to moderate-intensity continuous training, HIFT demonstrates further improvements in muscle fitness [27,28]. Additionally, participants perceive this type of activity to be more enjoyable when engaging in HIFT compared to those individuals performing traditional HIIT [29,30]. Moreover, most HIFT protocols are executed using the participant's own body weight, allowing the participant to control the exercise intensity. This helps to improve exercise adherence [7,19,20].

Although studies have shown that HIFT has similar or superior benefits for physical fitness compared to moderate-intensity continuous training and have indicated more enjoyment compared to HIIT, the question remains as to whether HIFT is as efficient as HIIT for improving health-related fitness.

While HIFT is not synonymous with HIIT, they share an important conceptual commonality in the modality of both being of a high intensity. The current study was undertaken to clarify how a functional exercise based on HIIT would improve fitness parameters such as fat mass, blood pressure, VO_2max, and muscle endurance following a 12-week intervention compared to changes achieved using a running-based HIIT. The purpose of this study was to investigate the effects of different kinds of training on fitness parameters in untrained female university students. It was hypothesized that (a) aerobic fitness would be increased in both the HIIT-F and HIIT-R groups; (b) that fat mass would be decreased in both the HIIT-F and HIIT-R groups; and (c) that muscular strength and endurance would be improved in the HIIT-F group.

2. Materials and Methods

2.1. Participants

Twenty untrained healthy females who were physical inactive volunteered to participate the study. Participants who did not exercise for more than 2 h weekly for at least 12 months were considered as physically inactive [31]. All of the participants were in their second year of a non-physical education-related degree at Ningbo University. Similar self-reported menstrual cycles were required, ensuring the simultaneity of testing and training. Interventions were suspended for 1 week during menstruation, and the normal menstruation period lasted for 3 to 10 days [32,33]. A randomized controlled research design was utilized, and participants were randomly assigned into a running-based HIIT (HIIT-R) (n = 10) or a functional training-based HIIT (HIIT-F) (n = 10). The participants were nonsmokers and were instructed to maintain their normal dietary intake and lifestyle habits (sleep, sit, and physical activity) throughout the intervention. Nutritional supplements and intense exercise beyond their usual exercise habits were forbidden during the intervention period [31]. All of the participants were fully familiarized with the test procedures and data collection methods prior to the intervention. Written informed consent was provided by all participants. The study was approved by the Ningbo University ethics committee. The characteristics of the participants at baseline are detailed in Table 1.

Table 1. Baseline characteristics of HIIT-R and HIIT-F group.

Parameter	HIIT-R Group ($n = 10$)	HIIT-F Group ($n = 10$)	p-Value
Age (yrs)	20.7 ± 0.6	20.2 ± 0.7	$p = 0.14$
Height (m)	161.1 ± 3.1	160.7 ± 2.8	$p = 0.76$
Weight (kg)	56.6 ± 6.7	57.8 ± 6.7	$p = 0.69$
Lean muscle mass (kg)	36.5 ± 1.7	36.0 ± 2.1	$p = 0.53$
BMI (kg/m^2)	21.9 ± 3.1	22.4 ± 2.2	$p = 0.70$
WHR	0.80 ± 0.0	0.80 ± 0.0	$p = 0.79$
Body fat (%)	31.6 ± 4.1	32.3 ± 3.6	$p = 0.71$
HR resting (bpm)	70.8 ± 13.9	72.5 ± 11.2	$p = 0.77$
HR max (bpm)	188.2 ± 9.7	189.1 ± 10.4	$p = 0.18$
VO2max (mL/kg/min)	31.3 ± 7.0	32.8 ± 5.4	$p = 0.61$

Notes: BMI, body mass index; bpm, beats per minute, HIIT-F, functional exercise-based high-intensity interval training; HIIT-R, running-based high-intensity interval training; HR resting, resting heart rate; HR max, maximal heart rate; VO$_2$max, maximal oxygen uptake; WHR, waist to hip ratio; yrs, years old.

2.2. Procedures

A randomized controlled trial was used in this study. Each participant completed twelve weeks of 36 sessions of HIIT-R or HIIT-F intervention (three sessions per week) comprising a total of 19 min per session (10 min warm-up, 4 min work-out, and 5 min cool-down). All sessions were conducted and monitored at the same indoor stadium and at the same time of day between 9:00–10:00 a.m. Heart rates (HR) were collected with an activity wristband (Mi Smart Band 5, Xiaomi, Beijing, China) during each session to ensure that the required high intensity was achieved. The reliability and validity of the heart rate index and distance index were reported in a previous study [34]. The activity wristband was required to be worn tightly on the participant's wrist. The HR index was measured based on changes in the light transmittance caused by blood flow density using optical sensing technology, and the distance index was measured by a triaxial acceleration sensor. Two measurement time points (pre- and post-intervention) were included. The participants were instructed to abstain from drugs, alcohol, and intense exercise two days prior to the baseline and post-intervention measurements. On the first measurement day, the participants presented themselves at 8:00 a.m. and underwent a body composition analysis, physical, and physiology measures as well as resting heart rate (HRresting) and blood pressure (BP) measurements under standardized conditions. The aerobic fitness assessment was conducted using a 12 min running test, which was completed on two days, with 24 h observed between each test. The first running test was scheduled on the first measurement day following the completion of all of the other tests, and the second trial was 24 h later. The average of the two data sets was used to assess aerobic fitness. After resting for a week [35], both groups began the training intervention. Post-intervention measurements were performed using the same methodologies as at baseline and were undertaken two days following all of the training sessions [11]. During the intervention period, additional exercises including habitual training were suspended.

2.3. Physical, Physiological and Body Composition Assessment

Participants were instructed to arrive at the laboratory 9:00 a.m. after a normal breakfast. Before the measurements were taken, participants were asked to empty their bladder to minimize measurement errors caused by "electrically silent" [36]. Under the guidance of two skilled operators and while wearing normal PE clothing, the participants stood on a bioelectrical impedance analysis device (BIA) (MC-180, TANITA CO., Dongguan, China) and data were presented from the device's associated software and included height, weight, waist and hip circumference, lean muscle mass, and body fat percentage. Body mass index

(BMI) was obtained by dividing weight (kg) by height (m) squared. Waist-to-hip ratio (WHR) was obtained by dividing waist (cm) by hip (cm). Blood pressure and resting HR were measured using an automatic upper arm blood pressure monitor (HEM-1000, Omron, Dalian, China). The average of the two data sets was used for analysis.

2.4. Aerobic Fitness Test

The most reliable and effective way to measure aerobic capacity is to record each individual subject's VO_2max [37]. Although maximal-effort tests are commonly used to measure VO_2max, for untrained participants, submaximal exercises can be used as a reliable measure to estimate this value. Cooper's 12 min running test was used to assess aerobic fitness in this study. All of the participants completed two trials of the running test separated by 24 h of rest. After a 5 min warm up, the participants were required to wear an activity wristband (Mi Smart Band 5, Xiaomi, China) and commenced running on a standard 400-metre running track. Subjects were instructed to run as many laps as possible on a standard outdoor track during the 12 min test period. All of the participants were encouraged verbally and were instructed to focus on their own pace throughout the test. The experimenter verbally provided the elapsed time at 3, 6, and 9 min. At the end of the 12 min period, the experimenter called "stop". All of the participants ceased running and stood still, until the distance achieved, and maximal heart rate (HRmax) were recorded. The HRmax displayed on the activity wristband was recorded immediately upon the cessation of exercise, and the higher value of the two trials was used for analysis. The total distance run was determined by measures obtained from the activity band. An estimated VO_2max was calculated using Cooper's standardized equation [38]. The calculated VO_2max was highly correlated with the laboratory-determined one and had acceptable reliability and validity ($r = 0.897$) [38]. The average of the two data sets was used to determine the VO_2max.

2.5. Muscle Performance Test

Muscle performance was assessed using a field-based muscle fitness test battery. Timed sit-ups, push-ups with flexed knee (modified for females), and standing broad jump were recommended by previous studies to assess muscle performance [26,39–41]. All of the participants were instructed to perform the tests under supervision, and the data were recorded by the same experimenter. To assess abdominal muscular performance, the participants were asked to perform as many sit-ups as possible during a one-minute test period. The number of sit-ups that were completed correctly were recorded. A sit-up that met the following criteria was recorded: the participant lay supine on the mat with their hands crossed behind their head, elbows pointed straight forward, and knees bent at 90 degrees. The ankles were firmly held by the experimenter. During the execution of the test, the participants sat up with their heads clasped in their hands, and then their elbows touched or went over the knees, and the participant went back with their shoulders touching the mat [42]. To assess upper body strength and endurance, the flexed knee push-up option was used as a gender modification [39]. A correct flexed knee push-up met the following criteria: participants knelt on the mat with their knees bent to the mat with their arms propped on the mat slightly wider than the shoulders. When the test began, the participants were instructed to lower their body by bending their arms until their elbows were bent at a 90-degree angle and their chest was placed within 2 inches of the mat, subjects then pushed up to the starting position [43,44]. The number of correctly completed push-ups during a one-minute test period was recorded as upper body strength and endurance. Finally, the standing broad jump test was used to assess the muscle power of the lower limbs. The participants wore sneakers and stood behind the starting line with their feet placed naturally at a shoulder width apart. When testing began, the participants were instructed to bend the knees, swing the arms, and jump with both feet at the same time [45]. The jumping distance measured in centimeters was recorded, and the best of three jumps was used to determine lower limb performance. All scores were compared for statistical analysis.

2.6. Intervention

Exercise interventions commenced one week after the last measurement day. Both the HIIT-R and HIIT-F interventions were conducted three days per week on Mondays, Wednesdays, and Saturdays for twelve weeks. If the participants were unable to attend a scheduled exercise day, the exercise was performed on the next day and was monitored by the same researcher.

Participants in the HIIT-R group were required to complete 144 repetitions of maximal shuttle running for a total exercise time of 72 min. Each bout included a 30 s maximal shuttle run between cones placed 20 m apart with a 30 s recovery period between runs. The validity and reliability of 40 m maximal shuttle run as a measure of anaerobic performance has been reported previously [46]. The participants completed 4 bouts per session over three sessions per week. Prior to the intervention, a familiarization trial was provided to acquaint the participants with the training procedure. Running and recovery times were recorded manually using a digital stopwatch by the same experimenter. Participants were encouraged to run at their individual maximal speed for each bout.

Participants in the HIIT-F group performed multiple functional exercises using their own body weight based on Tabata training [47]. According to a recent study [48], eight movements were implemented in each session (Table 2). Participants were motivated to complete as many repetitions of a given movement as possible over 20 s followed by a 10 s recovery in the form of low intensity stepping. There was no rest period between each movement. The total training time for each session was 4 min.

Table 2. Details of the functional high-intensity interval training intervention.

Duration	Frequency	Exercises	Exercise Bout/ Recovery Duration
12 weeks	3 sessions/week	Jumping Jacks	20 s
		Stepping	10 s
		High knees	20 s
		Stepping	10 s
		Side to side squat	20 s
		Stepping	10 s
		Mountain climbers	20 s
		Stepping	10 s
		Forearm plank to high plank	20 s
		Stepping	10 s
		Burpees	20 s
		Stepping	10 s
		Deep squat jumps	20 s
		Stepping	10 s
		Butt kickers	20 s
		Stepping	10 s

The training frequency was the same as the HIIT-R group. All training exercises were recorded by video, which was provided to the HIIT-F participants prior to intervention to ensure that they were familiar with the movements and procedures. This video was played on a screen during the training intervention to ensure that the participants kept up with the rhythm of each movement.

To ensure that the interventions were performed at adequate exercise intensity, participants' HRs were recorded throughout the session with an activity wristband. The peak heart rate (HR peak) of each session was considered to be 75% or more of the HRmax that had been recorded during Cooper's 12 min running test. All of the sessions began with a standardized 10 min low-to-moderate running and stretching followed by maximal shuttle run or functional training and ended with a 5 min cool-down and stretching.

2.7. Statistical Analyses

Statistical analyses were performed using SPSS, version 23.0 (Chicago, IL, USA). Data were presented as means x± SD. A two-factor analysis of variance with repeated measures was used to analyze differences in body composition, muscle performance, and aerobic capacity, with intervention (pretraining and post training) as a within-group factor and group (HIIT-R and HIIT-F) as a between-group factor. A significant intervention x group interaction was used to identify training-induced changes in body composition, muscle performance and aerobic capacity. Data were subsequently checked by Tukey's post hoc test if a significant interaction was revealed. Furthermore, paired t-tests were used to estimate within-group effects, and independent t-tests were conducted to examine differences between groups. The significance level was established as $p < 0.05$.

3. Results

All of the participants completed all of the sessions over the twelve-week period. There were no significant between-group differences in the variables measured at baseline (Table 1).

- Body Composition

Body composition data are presented in Table 3. There was a significant decrease (17.4% ± 7.4% for HIIT-R and 12.6% ± 5.1% for HIIT-F, $p < 0.05$) in the percent body fat for both groups (Figure 1a), with no interaction effect between HIIT-R and HIIT-F ($p > 0.05$). Body mass index (BMI) (Figure 1b) and waist hip ratio (WHR) (Figure 1c) did not change in either intervention ($p > 0.05$). Lean muscle mass increased in both groups (1.8% ± 1.4% for HIIT-R and 1.2% ± 1.2% for HIIT-F, $p < 0.05$).

- Resting Heart Rate and Blood Pressure

Resting HR ($p < 0.05$) was improved compared to baseline in both intervention groups, while no interaction effect was observed. Resting systolic BP and diastolic BP remained unchanged ($p > 0.05$) after training in both the HIIT-R and HIIT-F groups.

- Aerobic Capacity

VO₂max data was calculated from the following Cooper's equation: VO_2max (mL/kg/min) = (distance(m)-506)/45. VO_2max data for all participants are presented in Table 3. A significant increase ($p < 0.05$) in the VO_2max was demonstrated in both training groups compared to baseline measures, while no significant intervention x group interaction was revealed between HIIT-R and HIIT-F after intervention compared to baseline (Figure 1c). ($p > 0.05$). The extent of the change in VO_2max was 17.1% ± 5.6% and 12.7% ± 6.7% in the HIIT-R and HIIT-F groups, respectively.

- Muscle Performance

A significant intervention x group interaction displayed significant changes in the HIIT-R and HIIT-F groups in terms of measures of abdominal and lower limb strength (Figure 1d). In the HIIT-F group, repetitions completed during the one-minute sit-up test increased ($p < 0.05$) by 16.5% ± 3.1% and the distance obtained in the stand broad jumping test improved ($p < 0.05$) by 5.1% ± 2.2%, whereas these variables were unaltered ($p > 0.05$) in the HIIT-R group. Flexed push-ups were unaltered in both the HIIT-R and HIIT-F groups (Table 4).

Table 3. Body composition and aerobic capacity data from HIIT-R and HIIT-F groups.

Parameter	HIIT-R Group (n = 10)				HIIT-F Group (n = 10)				Interaction Effect	
	Baseline	Post	Δ	p-Value	Baseline	Post	Δ	p-Value	p-Value	η²
Weight (kg)	56.6 ± 6.7	55.8 ± 6.5	−1.3% ± 2.1%	ns	57.8 ± 6.7	56.6 ± 6.4	−1.9% ± 3.0%	ns	ns	0.020
Lean muscle mass (kg)	36.5 ± 1.7	37.2 ± 1.8	1.8% ± 1.4%	p < 0.05	36.0 ± 2.1	36.4 ± 2.1	1.2% ± 1.2%	p < 0.05	ns	0.056
BMI (kg/m²)	21.9 ± 3.1	21.6 ± 3.1	−1.3% ± 2.1%	ns	22.4 ± 2.2	21.9 ± 2.1	−1.9% ± 3.0%	ns	ns	0.018
WHR	0.8 ± 0.0	0.8 ± 0.0	−0.6% ± 0.9%	ns	0.8 ± 0.0	0.8 ± 0.0	−0.3% ± 0.5%	ns	ns	0.032
Body fat (%)	31.6 ± 4.1	26.3 ± 4.8	−17.1% ± 7.4%	p < 0.01	32.3 ± 3.6	28.3 ± 3.9	−12.6% ± 5.1%	p < 0.01	ns	0.118
HR resting (bpm)	76.5 ± 10.1	74.2 ± 7.4	−2.5% ± 5.5%	ns	77.8 ± 9.1	75.3 ± 8.6	−3.1% ± 5.3%	ns	ns	0.001
HR max (bpm)	188.7 ± 6.7	185.8 ± 6.0	−1.5% ± 1.1%	p < 0.05	183.7 ± 9.3	181.8 ± 7.8	−1.0% ± 1.3%	p < 0.05	ns	0.050
VO2max (mL/kg/min)	31.3 ± 7.0	36.7 ± 8.8	17.1 ± 5.6%	p < 0.01	32.8 ± 5.4	36.9 ± 6.4	12.7% ± 6.7%	p < 0.01	ns	0.075

Note: Δ (post-baseline)/baseline; ns, no significance; partial η^2 value for effect size.

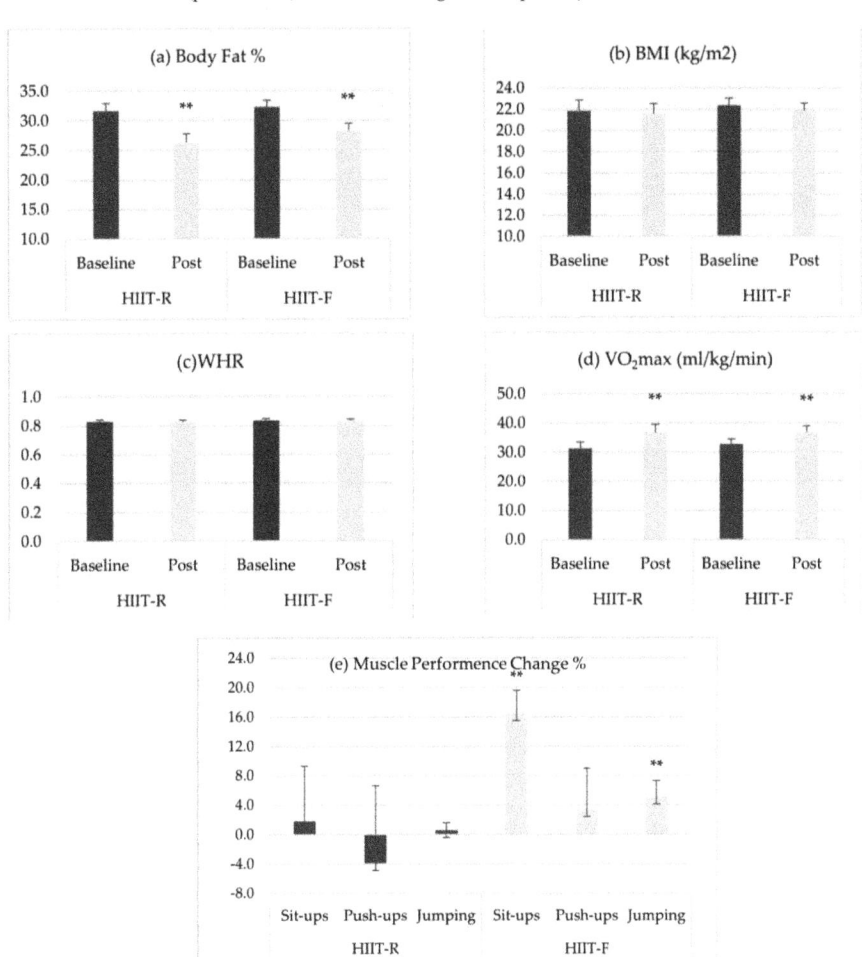

Figure 1. Changes in (**a**) BMI, (**b**) body fat%, (**c**) WHR, (**d**) VO2max, and (**e**) muscle performance change. Note: ** significantly different from baseline at $p < 0.01$.

Table 4. Muscle performance data from HIIT-R and HIIT-F groups.

Parameter	HIIT-R Group (n = 10)				HIIT-F Group (n = 10)				Interaction Effect	
	Baseline	Post-Training	Δ	p-Value	Baseline	Post-Training	Δ	p-Value	p-Value	η^2
Sit-ups (reps)	35.3 ± 6.7	35.7 ± 5.9	1.8% ± 7.5%	ns	37.3 ± 4.8	43.4 ± 5.3	16.5% ± 3.1%	$p < 0.01$	$p < 0.01$	0.760
Flexed push-ups (reps)	7.7 ± 1.3	7.4 ± 1.6	−3.9% ± 10.5%	ns	8.0 ± 1.4	8.3 ± 1.7	3.4% ± 5.6%	ns	ns	0.180
Standing broad jump (cm)	176.0 ± 5.8	177.1 ± 5.5	0.6% ± 1.0%	ns	178.0 ± 6.1	187.0 ± 5.5	5.1% ± 2.2%	$p < 0.01$	$p < 0.01$	0.686

Note: Δ (post-baseline)/baseline; ns, no significance; partial η^2 value for effect size.

4. Discussion

The present study aimed to investigate the effects of running and functional high-intensity training on body composition, aerobic capacity, and muscle fitness. The primary finding was that high-intensity functional training was as effective as high-intensity interval running for aerobic capacity and body composition promotion in healthy inactive females, and moreover, it induced a significant improvement in muscle fitness. The validity of this finding is supported by the fact that the mean heart rate of all of the participants reached 75% VO$_2$max or above throughout the intervention. Increases in resting heart rate were also detected after training in both groups.

4.1. Body Composition

Our findings that HIIT-R and HIIT-F had positive effects on body composition promotion regarding the reduction of the body fat percentage were consistent with other researchers. A previous study [49] showed improved body mass, BMI, and percent body fat among obese females after a total of 108 min HIIT-R. Similarly, previous research [50] found that HIIT-R was effective in reducing BMI and body fat percentage in overweight adults. Additionally, for individuals with normal BMI, body composition improved by decreasing fat mass and increasing lean mass after a 6-week HIIT-R intervention [51].

Not surprisingly, body composition benefits were also found in other studies investigating HIFT. Improved body fat percentage was reported after a 5-week, thrice weekly HIFT intervention [25], and further studies have also indicated a beneficial influence of HIFT on body composition [52].

However, current research has indicated that body fat percentage was significantly improved after an eight-week HIFT, while body mass was unaltered [31]. Likewise, after 16 weeks of HIFT, a significant decrease in body fat percentage was observed with no changes in the body mass [26]. Previous HIIT-R studies have provided similar results [53,54]. These results are consistent with our findings that although body fat percentage was improved, body mass and BMI were not affected by the intervention. The improved body fat percentage may be explained by the significant increase in lean muscle mass ($p = 0.001$ for HIIT-R and $p = 0.006$ HIIT-F) without significant changes in the body mass ($p = 0.064$ for HIIT-R and $p = 0.051$ for HIIT-F). The non-significant change in BMI may be due to the following reasons: the insufficient exercise duration per session (2 min vs. 6–10 min); the uncontrolled dietary intake during the intervention; and the characteristics of the participants regarding body weight. This suggestion has been highlighted in a recent systematic review [55] that indicated that for normal weight populations, low-volume HIIT is inefficient for body composition improvement. Furthermore, several studies have indicated that HIIT-R and HIFT have a more significant effect on weight loss or body fat loss among obese individuals [41,48–50].

Finally, no significant interaction effect was revealed for any body composition variables. This suggests that HIIT-R and HIIT-F were equally effective in the modulation of body fat percentage.

4.2. Aerobic Fitness

VO_2max was assessed in the present study to estimate the effects of HIIT-R and HIIT-F protocols on aerobic fitness. Running-based HIIT has been shown to increase aerobic capacity in numerous previous investigations. Several studies have reported significant increases in VO_2max after HIIT [11,12,55]. Furthermore, a systematic review also showed that HIIT was beneficial for aerobic fitness improvements among healthy young people [56]. Nevertheless, there has been no consensus on the effect of HIFT on aerobic capacity. Some studies investigating HIFT have shown an improvement in VO_2max [35,52,57]. On the contrary, recent research has only found aerobic capacity improvement in underweight and overweight boys, with no changes being found among normal weight people [39]. Similarly, no significant changes in VO_2max were found after a 6-week HIFT protocol [58,59].

In our study, participants from both the HIIT-R and HIIT-F groups experienced improvements in VO_2max (17.1% ± 5.6% and 12.7% ± 6.7%, respectively). In line with the magnitude of our results, an increase of 8% in the VO_2max was found after a low-volume HIFT [28]. It should be noted that in the current study, the enhanced VO_2max observed in the HIFT group was significantly higher than values recorded in previous studies. VO_2max has been reported to improve by 5% after a HIFT with no aerobic exercise [60]. Another study showed a moderate improvement in the VO_2max of 6.3% [31]. In our study, the greater response of VO_2max to HIFT could be explained by the following reasons: firstly, improvements in VO_2max were related to the testing modality [61]; Cooper's 12 min run test demonstrated a systematic bias in favor of higher-scoring individuals [62]; secondly, this study used a longer duration (12 weeks vs. 6–8 weeks) for the implementation of functional exercises. Short or low-volume training reported no improvements in aerobic capacity, which was shown to require continuous training [14,63]. However, other investigations reported that the extent of improvement was not clearly related to training duration but to training intensity [56,64]. Therefore, further studies are required to investigate the effectiveness of the duration (work bouts/total work duration) and intensity on training-induced aerobic capacity improvement; finally, the magnitude of the improvement in VO_2max can be attributed to the fatigue index, which was not measured in our study [11].

Although high-intensity running and functional training were both beneficial for aerobic capacity promotion, few studies have compared the effectiveness of these two exercise modalities in terms of aerobic capacity enhancement. In the current study, we controlled for the same intervention intensity and duration and found that surprisingly, there was no significant difference in terms of the changes in VO_2max between the HIIT-R and HIIT-F groups. It is worth noting that running showed higher oxygen consumption for the same intensity compared to other modalities [65]. Our findings were partially in line with a previous study [66] that indicated no significant differences in VO_2max promotion between high-intensity cycling and HIFT. The results from the present study illustrate that functional training is as effective as running for aerobic fitness improvement when performed at high intensity with the same volume and intensity.

4.3. Muscle Performance

Importantly, the repetition of sit-ups and the distance of the standing broad jump were significantly increased after HIIT-F, whereas both parameters remained unaltered in the HIIT-R group. Moreover, significant interaction effects were observed in terms of the effects on abdominal and lower limb strength and duration. Our finding is consistent with other HIFT studies. A significant increase in muscle performance after 6 weeks of HIFT was reported, whereas no increase was found in HIIT group using rowing as the exercise modality [27]. Significant improvements in lower body strength and power among patients and Army personnel were also evident [24,25]. Likewise, a study with female participants compared the effects of HIFT and endurance treadmill training on muscle fitness and demonstrated that sit-ups, chest presses, and push-ups improved by 64%, 207% and 135%, respectively, in the HIFT group after 4 weeks of intervention [24].

It is worth noting that the number of flexed push-ups that was completed in the repetition exercise was unchanged in both groups. The unchanged results are in contrast with findings from other investigations. Findings from recent studies revealed increased upper body strength and endurance after functional training executed at a high intensity [24,26–28]. It was possible that the observed unvaried parameters were the consequence of insufficient movements during our functional training, which lacked upper body adaptations [26]. Additionally, the assessment methods used in the present study could have also induced unaltered results. Although the flexed push-ups had been modified for females and even though the participants were familiarized with testing procedures, the participants in the present study had no or little experience and were not familiar with this movement. Furthermore, they had no knowledge of specific strategies that could be used to maximize their performance.

The effects of HIFT on muscle performance varies across exercise design and test methods. HIIT significantly increases the proportion of type I fibers [67], while muscle adaptions are specific to the exercise modality. A previous study revealed that compared to high-intensity interval running, strength training with functional movements resulted in type I muscle fibers increasing in size and a higher percentage of type IIA muscle fibers [68]. In the present study, functional exercise was more effective in strengthening muscle power than running when both were performed at relatively the same high intensity and for the same duration. However, further studies are required to investigate the training-induced individual changes in the type and size of muscle fibers between participants. Additionally, the functional exercise design should consider the fitness of the participants to reduce muscle soreness, and a previous study reported no injuries using this methodology [31].

A general limitation in the HIFT investigation was the different types of functional exercises that were included. The results might be dissimilar if HIFT was performed with other combinations of movements. Furthermore, the results of our study came from a small sample size and a non-exercising control group was not used. Finally, dietary intake was not controlled during the intervention, and the total calories consumed were not calculated. In addition, the fatigue index was not measured during the aerobic test.

5. Conclusions

Twelve weeks of high-intensity training based on running or functional exercises were both effective in reducing body fat percentage and improving aerobic capacity among healthy inactive females. Relative to running-based high-intensity training, HIFT shows an equally effective alternative with more exercise enjoyment and much stronger adherence regarding body composition and aerobic fitness promotion. Additionally, HIFT resulted in greater muscle performance increases than running-based high-intensity training, after which no gains were observed in terms of muscle fitness.

HIFT with self-selected intensity represents an alternative to high-intensity interval running for eliminating exercise barriers for physical exertion. Furthermore, HIFT can be performed anywhere at any time, which limits the barriers of lacking time/money. Finally, HIFT reveals strong exercise adherence and more enjoyment among females. It may be helpful for individuals to promote physical activity and the associated benefits of a prolonged healthy lifestyle.

Author Contributions: Conceptualization, Y.L., H.D.W. and J.S.B.; methodology, H.D.W. and J.S.B.; software, Y.L.; validation, Y.L., H.D.W. and J.S.B.; formal analysis, Y.L.; investigation, Y.L.; resources, Y.L. and Q.W.; data curation, Y.L.; writing—original draft preparation, Y.L.; writing—review and editing, H.D.W. and J.S.B.; visualization, Y.L.; supervision, H.D.W. and J.S.B.; project administration, Y.L.; funding acquisition, Q.W. All authors have read and agreed to the published version of the manuscript.

Funding: This research received no external funding.

Institutional Review Board Statement: The study was conducted according to the guidelines of the Declaration of Helsinki and was approved by the Institutional Review Board (or Ethics Committee) of Ningbo University (RAGH202103150366.8; 15 March 2021).

Informed Consent Statement: Informed consent was obtained from all subjects involved in the study.

Data Availability Statement: The data presented in this study are available upon request from the corresponding author. The data are not publicly available due to student privacy.

Acknowledgments: I would like to show my deepest gratitude to my supervisory team, Wiltshire and Professor Baker; they are respectable, responsible and resourceful scholars. They have provided me with valuable guidance in every stage of my research. Additionally, I would like to thank the researchers from Faculty of Sport Science, Ningbo University, for helping me to complete the assessment. Finally, many thanks to the participants who continued to exercise for their health.

Conflicts of Interest: The authors declare no conflict of interest.

References

1. Bermejo-Cantarero, A.; Álvarez-Bueno, C.; Martinez-Vizcaino, V.; García-Hermoso, A.; Torres-Costoso, A.I.; Sánchez-López, M. Association between physical activity, sedentary behavior, and fitness with health related quality of life in healthy children and adolescents: A protocol for a systematic review and meta-analysis. *Medicine* **2017**, *96*, e6407. [CrossRef]
2. Biddle, S.J.; Gorely, T.; Stensel, D.J. Health-enhancing physical activity and sedentary behaviour in children and adolescents. *J. Sports Sci.* **2004**, *22*, 679–701. [CrossRef]
3. Hallal, P.C.; Victora, C.G.; Azevedo, M.R.; Wells, J.C. Adolescent physical activity and health: A systematic review. *Sports Med.* **2006**, *36*, 1019–1030. [CrossRef]
4. Bull, F.C.; Al-Ansari, S.S.; Biddle, S.; Borodulin, K.; Buman, M.P.; Cardon, G.; Carty, C.; Chaput, J.P.; Chastin, S.; Chou, R.; et al. World Health Organization 2020 guidelines on physical activity and sedentary behaviour. *Br. J. Sports Med.* **2020**, *54*, 1451–1462. [CrossRef]
5. Liguori, G.; Feito, Y.; Fountaine, C.; Roy, B. *ACSM's Guidelines for Exercise Testing and Prescription*, 11th ed.; Wolters Kluwer: Philadelphia, PA, USA, 2021.
6. Hallal, P.C.; Andersen, L.B.; Bull, F.C.; Guthold, R.; Haskell, W.; Ekelund, U. Global physical activity levels: Surveillance progress, pitfalls, and prospects. *Lancet* **2012**, *380*, 247–257. [CrossRef]
7. Lovell, G.P.; El Ansari, W.; Parker, J.K. Perceived exercise benefits and barriers of non-exercising female university students in the United Kingdom. *Int. J. Environ. Res. Public Health* **2010**, *7*, 784–798. [CrossRef]
8. Reichert, F.F.; Barros, A.J.; Domingues, M.R.; Hallal, P.C. The role of perceived personal barriers to engagement in leisure-time physical activity. *Am. J. Public Health* **2007**, *97*, 515–519. [CrossRef]
9. Gillen, J.B.; Gibala, M.J. Is high-intensity interval training a time-efficient exercise strategy to improve health and fitness? *Appl. Physiol. Nutr. Metab.* **2014**, *39*, 409–412. [CrossRef]
10. Laursen, P.B.; Jenkins, D.G. The scientific basis for high-intensity interval training: Optimising training programmes and maximising performance in highly trained endurance athletes. *Sports Med.* **2002**, *32*, 53–73. [CrossRef] [PubMed]
11. Astorino, T.A.; Allen, R.P.; Roberson, D.W.; Jurancich, M. Effect of high-intensity interval training on cardiovascular function, VO2max, and muscular force. *J. Strength Cond. Res.* **2012**, *26*, 138–145. [CrossRef] [PubMed]
12. Dias, K.A.; Ingul, C.B.; Tjønna, A.E.; Keating, S.E.; Gomersall, S.R.; Follestad, T.; Hosseini, M.S.; Hollekim-Strand, S.M.; Ro, T.B.; Haram, M.; et al. Effect of High-Intensity Interval Training on Fitness, Fat Mass and Cardiometabolic Biomarkers in Children with Obesity: A Randomised Controlled Trial. *Sports Med.* **2018**, *48*, 733–746. [CrossRef]
13. Milanović, Z.; Sporiš, G.; Weston, M. Effectiveness of High-Intensity Interval Training (HIT) and Continuous Endurance Training for VO2max Improvements: A Systematic Review and Meta-Analysis of Controlled Trials. *Sports Med.* **2015**, *45*, 1469–1481. [CrossRef]
14. Sultana, R.N.; Sabag, A.; Keating, S.E.; Johnson, N.A. The Effect of Low-Volume High-Intensity Interval Training on Body Composition and Cardiorespiratory Fitness: A Systematic Review and Meta-Analysis. *Sports Med.* **2019**, *49*, 1687–1721. [CrossRef]
15. Gaesser, G.A.; Angadi, S.S. High-intensity interval training for health and fitness: Can less be more? *J. Appl. Physiol.* **2011**, *111*, 1540–1541. [CrossRef] [PubMed]
16. Billat, L.V. Interval training for performance: A scientific and empirical practice. Special recommendations for middle- and long-distance running. Part I: Aerobic interval training. *Sports Med.* **2001**, *31*, 13–31. [CrossRef] [PubMed]
17. Bartlett, J.D.; Close, G.L.; MacLaren, D.P.; Gregson, W.; Drust, B.; Morton, J.P. High-intensity interval running is perceived to be more enjoyable than moderate-intensity continuous exercise: Implications for exercise adherence. *J. Sports Sci.* **2011**, *29*, 547–553. [CrossRef]

18. Aaltonen, S.; Rottensteiner, M.; Kaprio, J.; Kujala, U.M. Motives for physical activity among active and inactive persons in their mid-30s. *Scand. J. Med. Sci. Sports* **2014**, *24*, 727–735. [CrossRef] [PubMed]
19. Parfitt, G.; Rose, E.A.; Burgess, W.M. The psychological and physiological responses of sedentary individuals to prescribed and preferred intensity exercise. *Br. J. Health Psychol.* **2006**, *11*, 39–53. [CrossRef]
20. Ekkekakis, P.; Parfitt, G.; Petruzzello, S.J. The pleasure and displeasure people feel when they exercise at different intensities: Decennial update and progress towards a tripartite rationale for exercise intensity prescription. *Sports Med.* **2011**, *41*, 641–671. [CrossRef] [PubMed]
21. Ekkekakis, P.; Hall, E.E.; Petruzzello, S.J. The relationship between exercise intensity and affective responses demystified: To crack the 40-year-old nut, replace the 40-year-old nutcracker! *Ann. Behav. Med.* **2008**, *35*, 136–149. [CrossRef]
22. Feito, Y.; Heinrich, K.M.; Butcher, S.J.; Poston, W.S.C. High-Intensity Functional Training (HIFT): Definition and Research Implications for Improved Fitness. *Sports* **2018**, *6*, 76. [CrossRef]
23. Haddock, C.K.; Poston, W.S.; Heinrich, K.M.; Jahnke, S.A.; Jitnarin, N. The Benefits of High-Intensity Functional Training Fitness Programs for Military Personnel. *Mil. Med.* **2016**, *181*, e1508–e1514. [CrossRef]
24. Heinrich, K.M.; Spencer, V.; Fehl, N.; Poston, W.S. Mission essential fitness: Comparison of functional circuit training to traditional Army physical training for active duty military. *Mil. Med.* **2012**, *177*, 1125–1130. [CrossRef] [PubMed]
25. Heinrich, K.M.; Becker, C.; Carlisle, T.; Gilmore, K.; Hauser, J.; Frye, J.; Harms, C.A. High-intensity functional training improves functional movement and body composition among cancer survivors: A pilot study. *Eur. J. Cancer Care* **2015**, *24*, 812–817. [CrossRef] [PubMed]
26. Feito, Y.; Hoffstetter, W.; Serafini, P.; Mangine, G. Changes in body composition, bone metabolism, strength, and skill-specific performance resulting from 16-weeks of HIFT. *PLoS ONE* **2018**, *13*, e0198324. [CrossRef] [PubMed]
27. Buckley, S.; Knapp, K.; Lackie, A.; Lewry, C.; Horvey, K.; Benko, C.; Trinh, J.; Butcher, S. Multimodal high-intensity interval training increases muscle function and metabolic performance in females. *Appl. Physiol. Nutr. Metab.* **2015**, *40*, 1157–1162. [CrossRef] [PubMed]
28. McRae, G.; Payne, A.; Zelt, J.G.; Scribbans, T.D.; Jung, M.E.; Little, J.P.; Gurd, B.J. Extremely low volume, whole-body aerobic-resistance training improves aerobic fitness and muscular endurance in females. *Appl. Physiol. Nutr. Metab.* **2012**, *37*, 1124–1131. [CrossRef] [PubMed]
29. Fisher, J.; Sales, A.; Carlson, L.; Steele, J. A comparison of the motivational factors between CrossFit participants and other resistance exercise modalities: A pilot study. *J. Sports Med. Phys. Fitness* **2017**, *57*, 1227–1234. [CrossRef]
30. Heinrich, K.M.; Patel, P.M.; O'Neal, J.L.; Heinrich, B.S. High-intensity compared to moderate-intensity training for exercise initiation, enjoyment, adherence, and intentions: An intervention study. *BMC Public Health* **2014**, *14*, 789. [CrossRef]
31. Brisebois, M.F.; Rigby, B.R.; Nichols, D.L. Physiological and Fitness Adaptations after Eight Weeks of High-Intensity Functional Training in Physically Inactive Adults. *Sports* **2018**, *6*, 146. [CrossRef]
32. Armour, M.; Ee, C.C.; Naidoo, D.; Ayati, Z.; Chalmers, K.J.; Steel, K.A.; de Manincor, M.J.; Delshad, E. Exercise for dysmenorrhoea. *Cochrane Database Syst. Rev.* **2019**, *9*, Cd004142. [CrossRef]
33. Motahari-Tabari, N.; Shirvani, M.A.; Alipour, A. Comparison of the Effect of Stretching Exercises and Mefenamic Acid on the Reduction of Pain and Menstruation Characteristics in Primary Dysmenorrhea: A Randomized Clinical Trial. *Oman Med. J.* **2017**, *32*, 47–53. [CrossRef] [PubMed]
34. Li, H. Reliability and Validity of Three Wristbands in Running with Change of Direction. Master's Thesis, Shanghai University of Sports, Shanghai, China, 2021.
35. Menz, V.; Marterer, N.; Amin, S.B.; Faulhaber, M.; Hansen, A.B.; Lawley, J.S. Functional vs. Running Low-Volume High-Intensity Interval Training: Effects on VO(2)max and Muscular Endurance. *J. Sports Sci. Med.* **2019**, *18*, 497–504.
36. Kushner, R.F.; Gudivaka, R.; Schoeller, D.A. Clinical characteristics influencing bioelectrical impedance analysis measurements. *Am. J. Clin. Nutr* **1996**, *64*, 423s–427s. [CrossRef] [PubMed]
37. Safrit, M.J.; Glaucia Costa, M.; Hooper, L.M.; Patterson, P.; Ehlert, S.A. The validity generalization of distance run tests. *Can. J. Sport Sci.* **1988**, *13*, 188–196. [PubMed]
38. Cooper, K.H. A means of assessing maximal oxygen intake. Correlation between field and treadmill testing. *Jama* **1968**, *203*, 201–204. [CrossRef] [PubMed]
39. Laughlin, N.T.; Busk, P.L. Relationships between selected muscle endurance tasks and gender. *J. Strength Cond. Res.* **2007**, *21*, 400–404. [CrossRef] [PubMed]
40. Ruiz, J.R.; Castro-Pinero, J.; Espana-Romero, V.; Artero, E.G.; Ortega, F.B.; Cuenca, M.M.; Jimenez-Pavon, D.; Chillon, P.; Girela-Rejon, M.J.; Mora, J.; et al. Field-based fitness assessment in young people: The ALPHA health-related fitness test battery for children and adolescents. *Br. J. Sports Med.* **2011**, *45*, 518–524. [CrossRef]
41. Sperlich, B.; Wallmann-Sperlich, B.; Zinner, C.; Von Stauffenberg, V.; Losert, H.; Holmberg, H.C. Functional High-Intensity Circuit Training Improves Body Composition, Peak Oxygen Uptake, Strength, and Alters Certain Dimensions of Quality of Life in Overweight Women. *Front. Physiol.* **2017**, *8*, 172. [CrossRef]
42. Bianco, A.; Lupo, C.; Alesi, M.; Spina, S.; Raccuglia, M.; Thomas, E.; Paoli, A.; Palma, A. The sit up test to exhaustion as a test for muscular endurance evaluation. *Springerplus* **2015**, *4*, 309. [CrossRef]

43. Snarr, R.L.; Esco, M.R. Electromyographic comparison of traditional and suspension push-ups. *J. Hum. Kinet* **2013**, *39*, 75–83. [CrossRef]
44. Chen, W.; Hammond-Bennett, A.; Hypnar, A.; Mason, S. Health-related physical fitness and physical activity in elementary school students. *BMC Public Health* **2018**, *18*, 195. [CrossRef] [PubMed]
45. Krishnan, A.; Sharma, D.; Bhatt, M.; Dixit, A.; Pradeep, P. Comparison between Standing Broad Jump test and Wingate test for assessing lower limb anaerobic power in elite sportsmen. *Med. J. Armed Forces India* **2017**, *73*, 140–145. [CrossRef]
46. Baker, J.; Ramsbottom, R.; Hazeldine, R. Maximal shuttle running over 40 m as a measure of anaerobic performance. *Br. J. Sports Med.* **1993**, *27*, 228–232. [CrossRef] [PubMed]
47. Tabata, I.; Nishimura, K.; Kouzaki, M.; Hirai, Y.; Ogita, F.; Miyachi, M.; Yamamoto, K. Effects of moderate-intensity endurance and high-intensity intermittent training on anaerobic capacity and VO2max. *Med. Sci. Sports Exerc.* **1996**, *28*, 1327–1330. [CrossRef]
48. Domaradzki, J.; Cichy, I.; Rokita, A.; Popowczak, M. Effects of Tabata Training During Physical Education Classes on Body Composition, Aerobic Capacity, and Anaerobic Performance of Under-, Normal- and Overweight Adolescents. *Int. J. Environ. Res. Public Health* **2020**, *17*, 876. [CrossRef]
49. Racil, G.; Coquart, J.B.; Elmontassar, W.; Haddad, M.; Goebel, R.; Chaouachi, A.; Amri, M.; Chamari, K. Greater effects of high- compared with moderate-intensity interval training on cardio-metabolic variables, blood leptin concentration and ratings of perceived exertion in obese adolescent females. *Biol. Sport* **2016**, *33*, 145–152. [CrossRef]
50. Tjønna, A.E.; Stølen, T.O.; Bye, A.; Volden, M.; Slørdahl, S.A.; Odegård, R.; Skogvoll, E.; Wisløff, U. Aerobic interval training reduces cardiovascular risk factors more than a multitreatment approach in overweight adolescents. *Clin. Sci.* **2009**, *116*, 317–326. [CrossRef] [PubMed]
51. Macpherson, R.E.; Hazell, T.J.; Olver, T.D.; Paterson, D.H.; Lemon, P.W. Run sprint interval training improves aerobic performance but not maximal cardiac output. *Med. Sci. Sports Exerc.* **2011**, *43*, 115–122. [CrossRef] [PubMed]
52. Murawska-Cialowicz, E.; Wojna, J.; Zuwala-Jagiello, J. Crossfit training changes brain-derived neurotrophic factor and irisin levels at rest, after wingate and progressive tests, and improves aerobic capacity and body composition of young physically active men and women. *J. Physiol. Pharmacol.* **2015**, *66*, 811–821.
53. Buchan, D.S.; Ollis, S.; Young, J.D.; Cooper, S.M.; Shield, J.P.; Baker, J.S. High intensity interval running enhances measures of physical fitness but not metabolic measures of cardiovascular disease risk in healthy adolescents. *BMC Public Health* **2013**, *13*, 498. [CrossRef] [PubMed]
54. Weston, K.L.; Azevedo, L.B.; Bock, S.; Weston, M.; George, K.P.; Batterham, A.M. Effect of Novel, School-Based High-Intensity Interval Training (HIT) on Cardiometabolic Health in Adolescents: Project FFAB (Fun Fast Activity Blasts)—An Exploratory Controlled Before-And-After Trial. *PLoS ONE* **2016**, *11*, e0159116. [CrossRef]
55. Batacan, R.B., Jr.; Duncan, M.J.; Dalbo, V.J.; Tucker, P.S.; Fenning, A.S. Effects of high-intensity interval training on cardiometabolic health: A systematic review and meta-analysis of intervention studies. *Br. J. Sports Med.* **2017**, *51*, 494–503. [CrossRef]
56. Gist, N.H.; Fedewa, M.V.; Dishman, R.K.; Cureton, K.J. Sprint interval training effects on aerobic capacity: A systematic review and meta-analysis. *Sports Med.* **2014**, *44*, 269–279. [CrossRef]
57. Nieuwoudt, S.; Fealy, C.E.; Foucher, J.A.; Scelsi, A.R.; Malin, S.K.; Pagadala, M.; Rocco, M.; Burguera, B.; Kirwan, J.P. Functional high-intensity training improves pancreatic β-cell function in adults with type 2 diabetes. *Am. J. Physiol. Endocrinol. Metab.* **2017**, *313*, E314–E320. [CrossRef]
58. Crawford, D.A.; Drake, N.B.; Carper, M.J.; DeBlauw, J.; Heinrich, K.M. Are Changes in Physical Work Capacity Induced by High-Intensity Functional Training Related to Changes in Associated Physiologic Measures? *Sports* **2018**, *6*, 26. [CrossRef]
59. Sobrero, G.; Arnett, S.; Schafer, M.; Stone, W.; Tolbert, T.A.; Salyer-Funk, A.; Crandall, J.; Farley, L.B.; Brown, J.; Lyons, S.; et al. A Comparison of High Intensity Functional Training and Circuit Training on Health and Performance Variables in Women: A Pilot Study. *Women Sport Phys. Act. J.* **2017**, *25*, 1–10. [CrossRef]
60. Gettman, L.R.; Pollock, M.L. Circuit Weight Training: A Critical Review of Its Physiological Benefits. *Phys. Sportsmed.* **1981**, *9*, 44–60. [CrossRef] [PubMed]
61. Magel, J.R.; Foglia, G.F.; McArdle, W.D.; Gutin, B.; Pechar, G.S.; Katch, F.I. Specificity of swim training on maximum oxygen uptake. *J. Appl. Physiol.* **1975**, *38*, 151–155. [CrossRef] [PubMed]
62. Penry, J.T.; Wilcox, A.R.; Yun, J. Validity and reliability analysis of Cooper's 12-minute run and the multistage shuttle run in healthy adults. *J. Strength Cond. Res.* **2011**, *25*, 597–605. [CrossRef] [PubMed]
63. Rodas, G.; Ventura, J.L.; Cadefau, J.A.; Cussó, R.; Parra, J. A short training programme for the rapid improvement of both aerobic and anaerobic metabolism. *Eur. J. Appl. Physiol.* **2000**, *82*, 480–486. [CrossRef]
64. Sloth, M.; Sloth, D.; Overgaard, K.; Dalgas, U. Effects of sprint interval training on VO2max and aerobic exercise performance: A systematic review and meta-analysis. *Scand. J. Med. Sci. Sports* **2013**, *23*, e341–e352. [CrossRef] [PubMed]
65. Viana, R.B.; de Lira, C.A.B.; Naves, J.P.A.; Coswig, V.S.; Del Vecchio, F.B.; Gentil, P. Tabata protocol: A review of its application, variations and outcomes. *Clin. Physiol. Funct. Imaging* **2019**, *39*, 1–8. [CrossRef] [PubMed]
66. Gist, N.H.; Freese, E.C.; Cureton, K.J. Comparison of responses to two high-intensity intermittent exercise protocols. *J. Strength Cond. Res.* **2014**, *28*, 3033–3040. [CrossRef] [PubMed]

67. Simoneau, J.A.; Lortie, G.; Boulay, M.R.; Marcotte, M.; Thibault, M.C.; Bouchard, C. Human skeletal muscle fiber type alteration with high-intensity intermittent training. *Eur. J. Appl. Physiol. Occup. Physiol.* **1985**, *54*, 250–253. [CrossRef]
68. Jakobsen, M.D.; Sundstrup, E.; Randers, M.B.; Kjær, M.; Andersen, L.L.; Krustrup, P.; Aagaard, P. The effect of strength training, recreational soccer and running exercise on stretch-shortening cycle muscle performance during countermovement jumping. *Hum. Mov. Sci.* **2012**, *31*, 970–986. [CrossRef] [PubMed]

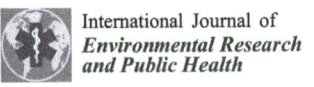

Article

Associations between Physical Status and Training Load in Women Soccer Players

Lillian Gonçalves [1,*], Filipe Manuel Clemente [2,3,*], Joel Ignacio Barrera [4,5], Hugo Sarmento [4,5], Gibson Moreira Praça [6], André Gustavo Pereira de Andrade [6], António José Figueiredo [4,5], Rui Silva [2], Ana Filipa Silva [2,7] and José María Cancela Carral [1]

1. Faculty of Educational Sciences and Sports Sciences, University of Vigo, 36005 Pontevedra, Spain; chemacc@uvigo.es
2. Escola Superior Desporto e Lazer, Instituto Politécnico de Viana do Castelo, Rua Escola Industrial e Comercial de Nun'Álvares, 4900-347 Viana do Castelo, Portugal; rui.s@ipvc.pt (R.S.); anafilsilva@gmail.com (A.F.S.)
3. Instituto de Telecomunicações, Delegação da Covilhã, 1049-001 Lisboa, Portugal
4. Faculty of Sport Sciences and Physical Education, University of Coimbra, 3000-248 Coimbra, Portugal; jibarrera@outlook.es (J.I.B.); hg.sarmento@gmail.com (H.S.); afigueiredo@fcdef.uc.pt (A.J.F.)
5. Research Unit for Sport and Physical Activity (CIDAF), 3000-248 Coimbra, Portugal
6. Sports Department, Universidade Federal de Minas Gerais, Belo Horizonte 31270-901, Brazil; gibson_moreira@yahoo.com.br (G.M.P.); andreguto@yahoo.com.br (A.G.P.d.A.)
7. The Research Centre in Sports Sciences, Health Sciences and Human Development (CIDESD), 5001-801 Vila Real, Portugal
* Correspondence: lilliangoncalves@ipvc.pt (L.G.); filipe.clemente5@gmail.com (F.M.C.)

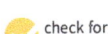

Citation: Gonçalves, L.; Clemente, F.M.; Barrera, J.I.; Sarmento, H.; Praça, G.M.; Andrade, A.G.P.d.; Figueiredo, A.J.; Silva, R.; Silva, A.F.; Carral, J.M.C. Associations between Physical Status and Training Load in Women Soccer Players. *Int. J. Environ. Res. Public Health* **2021**, *18*, 10015. https://doi.org/10.3390/ijerph181910015

Academic Editors: Cristina Cortis and Paul B. Tchounwou

Received: 20 August 2021
Accepted: 22 September 2021
Published: 23 September 2021

Publisher's Note: MDPI stays neutral with regard to jurisdictional claims in published maps and institutional affiliations.

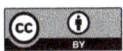

Copyright: © 2021 by the authors. Licensee MDPI, Basel, Switzerland. This article is an open access article distributed under the terms and conditions of the Creative Commons Attribution (CC BY) license (https://creativecommons.org/licenses/by/4.0/).

Abstract: This study aimed to analyze the variations of fitness status, as well as test the relationships between accumulated training load and fitness changes in women soccer players. This study followed an observational analytic cohort design. Observations were conducted over 23 consecutive weeks (from the preseason to the midseason). Twenty-two women soccer players from the same first Portuguese league team (22.7 ± 5.21 years old) took part in the study. The fitness assessment included anthropometry, hip adductor and abductor strength, vertical jump, change of direction, linear speed, repeated sprint ability, and the Yo-Yo intermittent recovery test. The training load was monitored daily using session rating of perceived exertion (s-RPE). A one-way repeated ANOVA revealed no significant differences for any of the variables analyzed across the three moments of fitness assessments ($p > 0.05$). The t-test also revealed no differences in the training load across the moments of the season ($t = 1.216$; $p = 0.235$). No significant correlations were found between fitness levels and accumulated training load (range: $r = 0.023$ to -0.447; $p > 0.05$). This study revealed no differences in the fitness status during the analyzed season, and the fitness status had no significant relationship with accumulated training load.

Keywords: football; athletic performance; training load; sports training; physical fitness

1. Introduction

Soccer is a high-intensity intermittent sport that recruits different energetic systems based on the intermittence of the match [1,2]. Among other factors, soccer performance requires technical skills, tactical awareness, and physical fitness [1,3]. In women's soccer, players may cover 9–12 km in total in a single match, with 1.5–2.5 km covered during high-intensity runs [4–6]. Moreover, throughout a women's soccer match, the average heart rate can reach up to 167 beats per minute (bpm), and the maximum heart rate (HRmax) can reach up to 193 bpm [7]. Therefore, to be successful, women soccer players should possess well-developed aerobic and anaerobic capacities, as well as good neuromuscular properties [2].

Well-developed physical fitness can help ensure overall success to the same extent as other important factors such as technical and tactical skills [1,8]. Accordingly, seeking an improvement in fitness status, it is necessary to understand the status of players, thus making the assessment a determinant factor for individualization of the training and controlling the development of the players [1,9]. Regarding the control of evolution, it is also expectable that some fitness variations may occur across a season, specifically considering the three main periods of training and competition: (i) preseason, (ii) early-season, and (iii) end-season [1,10,11].

For example, body fat is usually lower after the preseason training period than at the start of the preseason [10,12]. Additionally, significant changes occur in the biomarkers of physiological stress [1,13]. Considering the physical fitness of female soccer players, it was found that countermovement jump scores seem to improve during the season [1]. Furthermore, the linear speed at 15 m improves during the preseason before stabilizing until the end of the season, whereas the linear speed at 25 m starts to decrease at the end of the season [11]. Naturally, considering seasonal variations, most of the fitness changes occur during the preseason because the training sessions during this phase are focused on establishing the players' fitness [3,14,15]. In contrast, during the season, more focus is placed on tactical and technical skills [16], with some efforts to stabilize players' fitness.

Even though no perfectly related variations were observed across the season, physical/physiological adaptations could be related to the training load and stimuli imposed on the players [17]. Therefore, a dose–response relationship is expected to arise between the training load and changes in fitness that may occur in soccer players [18]. However, such a relationship can vary on the basis of the training load measures and fitness parameters used; moreover, the relationship might not be as obvious or straightforward as expected [18,19]. As an example, in a study conducted on professional soccer players, relationships were found between accumulated perceived exertion and the speed achieved in the 30–15 Intermittent Fitness Test by professional players [20]. However, in another study (also on soccer players), such a relationship was not meaningful [21].

As mentioned above, the magnitude of the relationship between load and adaptations can vary as a function of the measures used. In the case of training load monitoring, one of the most commonly used measures is the rating of perceived exertion (RPE) [22,23]. This measure has been confirmed as valid and reliable, based on different scales (e.g., CR-10, CR-100), to estimate the intensity of a training session. According to the score provided by the player, RPE can be used to calculate the session RPE (s-RPE), which is the multiplication of the RPE score by the duration of the session (in minutes) [23,24]. Since this measure (s-RPE) has been highly correlated with internal load markers (e.g., heart rate measures) and external load markers (e.g., total distance, player load) [25,26], it seems to be a good measure to test relationships with fitness adaptations across the season.

Adaptions in soccer players take time and are influenced by multiple factors, such as age, gender, training history, psychological factors, and the duration, intensity, and frequency of training [18,27]. Therefore, it is difficult to understand which factors promote changes in players in women's soccer. In the particular case of women's soccer, dose–response relationships have not been explored' for that reason, there is a need to test whether such a relationship exists.

Testing the possibility of relationships between accumulated training load and the changes in fitness status would help to identify whether training load is a determinant of these changes or if there are other factors that coaches should be aware of. For that reason, the aims of this study were to analyze variations in the fitness status of women soccer players over time (repeated measures) and test the relationships between accumulated training load and fitness variations.

2. Materials and Methods

2.1. Experimental Approach

This study followed an observational analytic cohort design. Observations were made across 23 consecutive weeks (from the preseason to midseason). Fitness assessments of the players were performed three times: (i) at the beginning of the preseason, (ii) at the end of the preseason, and (iii) during the middle of the season. Internal loads were collected daily in all training sessions between August and January (Figure 1).

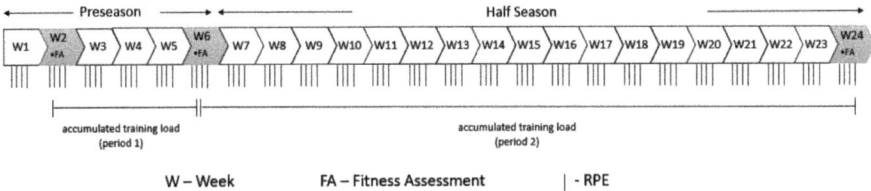

Figure 1. Timeline of the study.

2.2. Participants

The cohort included 22 female soccer players (age: 22.7 ± 5.21 years; height: 162 ± 6.84 cm; weight: 57.6 ± 4.9 kg) competing in the first Portuguese League. The team had four weekly training sessions and one official match per week. The eligibility criteria for being considered in the analysis were as follows: (i) participation in at least 85% of the training sessions during the study, (ii) participants were present in all three assessments, (iii) absence of injuries or illness in the last four consecutive weeks, and (iv) players had at least 2 years of experience. Three players were excluded because they did not participate in all physical assessments. Before the assessments, all players were informed about the study procedures and signed an informed consent. The study was approved by the local university and followed the ethical standards of the Declaration of Helsinki for the study of humans.

2.3. Fitness Assessment

Fitness assessments were conducted between August and January. All tests were performed during the same day of the week, following the same order, and at the same time of the day (7:30 p.m.) to limit data bias. During the three periods of assessments, all tests were distributed across three sessions, interspersed by 24 h of recovery. We acknowledge the fact that a testing battery can be carried out in a single day [28]. However, it can ideally be distributed over 2–3 days [29]. Regardless of the days, it is important that the sequence is designed with the aim of ensuring the most adequate conditions of absence of fatigue in tests with a greater need for neuromuscular recruitment, leaving the tests with greater metabolic stress to the end [29]. Bioenergetic and neuromuscular considerations resulted in the applied test sequencing in the present study. Regarding the warm-up protocol, it was out of the scope of the authors to intervene as it was always the team staff (physical trainer) conducting the warm-ups. The warm-ups consisted of low and self-paced running, followed by calisthenic exercises in which players performed two sets of 10 repetitions of walking lunges, single-leg deadlifts, and fontal and lateral high knee movements. These warm-ups were based on proposed strategies, highlighting the post-activation potentiation (PAP) exercises, as previously recommended and used [30,31].

The first assessments comprised anthropometry and hip adductor and abductor strength tests. The second assessments comprised lower-body power, change-of-direction (COD), and linear speed tests. The third assessments comprised repeated sprint ability (RSA) and Yo-Yo intermittent recovery (YYIR) tests. All indoor tests were performed in a room with a stable temperature of 23 °C and relative humidity of 55%. All field tests were conducted on a synthetic turf with a mean temperature of 19.5 ± 3.4 °C and a relative humidity of 63% ± 4%.

A measuring tape (SECA 206, Hamburg, Germany) and a digital scale (SECA 874, Hamburg, Germany) were used to measure the participants' height and body weight, measured to the nearest 0.1 kg. During both assessments, all participants were in a vertical position and had no shoes and unnecessary accessories. To measure hip strength, the squeeze test was conducted using a dynamometer (Smart Groin Trainer, Neuro excellence, Portugal), as in a previously recommended protocol [32]. For lower-body power performance, the squat jump (SJ) and countermovement jump (CMJ) with both hands on hips were assessed, using the Optojump system (Optojump, Microgate, Bolzano, Italia [33]. The jump height was used for analysis. The 20 m zig-zag test was conducted to measure the participants' COD performance, using photocell timing gates (Photocells, Brower Timing System, USA) with a protocol described elsewhere [34]. The best time in seconds was used for further analysis. A 30 m linear sprint test was executed using three pairs of photocell timing gates (Photocells, Brower Timing System, UT, USA). Three maximal trials were performed, and the best time was used for analysis. Furthermore, an RSA protocol was conducted using two pairs of photocell timing gates (Photocells, Brower Timing System, UT, USA). The running anaerobic sprint test (RAST) test was conducted. This test consisted of six 35 m linear sprints, interspersed by 10 s of recovery. The best time to complete the test, peak power, and fatigue index measures were used for analysis [35]. The minimum and maximum peak power and the fatigue index were determined using the following equations [36]:

$$\text{Power} = \frac{\text{Weight} \times \text{Distance}^2}{\text{Time}^3} \text{ and Fatigue Index} = \frac{\text{Max}_{\text{Power}} - \text{Min}_{\text{Power}}}{\text{Sum of 6 sprints (s)}}.$$

Lastly, the participants completed the YYIR test to measure the VO_2max. All player had to run 20 m from cone A to cone B and return to cone A (total: 40 m). After every 40 m covered, a 10 s recovery period was ensured. The speed started at 10 km/h, following progressive increases in velocity throughout the test. The YYIR ended when the player achieved total exhaustion or did not reach one of the 20 m cones at the beep timing. The number of completed shuttles and the total distance covered were recorded [37]. Additionally, during the YYIR test, all players used individual Bluetooth HRsensors for heart rate monitor (Polar H10, Polar-Electro, Kempele, Finland, recorded in 5 s intervals) to quantify each athlete's heart rate maximum (HRmax).

2.4. Training Load Monitoring

For measuring the internal load, 10 to 30 min after each training session, all players were asked about how hard the training session was, scored from 1–10, were 1 corresponds to "very light activity" and 10 corresponds to "maximal exertion" [38]. These scores were based on the CR-10 Borg scale [23]. All players were previously familiarized with this daily practice. The collected scores were then multiplied by the total duration in minutes of each training session, to obtain the session RPE [23]. The session RPE for each training session was used as the final outcome for further analysis.

2.5. Statistical Analysis

Subjects' characteristics are presented as means and standard deviations of the variables. For the variables of fitness assessment, a one-way repeated-measure analysis of variance (ANOVA) was performed to clarify the differences among the three assessments. If there was a significant effect, we used the Bonferroni multiple comparison test to determine significant differences among the three conditions for each variable. Eta squared (η^2) values were used as an indicator of effect size. An η^2 value of 0.00–0.19 was considered trivial, 0.20–0.49 was small, 0.50–0.79 was moderate, and ≥ 0.80 was large [39]. The strength of the relationship between the variables of the fitness assessment and accumulated training load was determined using a Pearson product moment linear correlation coefficient (r). A paired t-test was used to compare the training load between the periods (preseason and midseason). Statistical analyses were conducted using the Statistical Package for the Social Sciences (SPSS version 22.0; Chicago, IL, USA), with a significance level of 0.05.

3. Results

The one-way repeated ANOVA revealed no significant differences for any of the variables analyzed at the three moments of fitness assessment (Table 1). As there were no significant changes in the three moments observed, we chose to use the mean as a representative measure of physical status. The *t*-test revealed no differences in the training load between the periods of the season ($t = 1.216$; $p = 0.235$).

Table 1. Descriptions, F-statistics, and *p*-values of the fitness variables analyzed at the three moments of fitness assessment.

Variable	M1 (Mean ± SD)	M2 (Mean ± SD)	M3 (Mean ± SD)	Mean ± SD	*p*	η²
HRmax (beats/min)	198.2 ± 3.57	201.41 ± 12.80	202.34 ± 8.68	200.65 ± 9.48	0.961	0.03
VO2max mL/(kg·min)	41.21 ± 1.57	43.72 ± 1.57	43.96 ± 1.57	42.96 ± 1.57	0.833	0.07
V10 (m/s)	1.91 ± 0.04	1.84 ± 0.07	1.91 ± 0.15	1.89 ± 0.09	0.564	0.13
V30 (m/s)	4.83 ± 0.09	4.69 ± 0.17	4.81 ± 0.39	4.78 ± 0.20	0.633	0.11
COD20 (s)	5.75 ± 0.09	5.70 ± 0.16	5.83 ± 0.32	5.76 ± 0.20	0.496	0.15
p.max (W)	423.66 ± 50.95	405.12 ± 68.29	403.10 ± 92.00	410.62 ± 64.16	0.365	0.13
p.min (W)	271.43 ± 34.30	266.83 ± 33.77	246.76 ± 50.92	264.87 ± 37.79	0.219	0.13
FI (%)	4.91 ± 1.40	4.03 ± 1.48	5.12 ± 1.81	4.68 ± 1.49	0.768	0.04
SJ (cm)	24.01 ± 2.14	25.03 ± 4.49	25.56 ± 3.68	24.85 ± 3.29	0.684	0.21
CMJ (cm)	25.20 ± 2.43	26.22 ± 4.29	26.29 ±3.39	25.89 ± 3.29	0.179	0.23
YYIR (m)	687.40± 168.93	943.33± 138.33	714.2 ± 163.17	781.67± 210.1	0.095	0.27
Addu (kg)	35.95 ± 7.07	33.51± 7.81	32.69± 6.10	34.03 ± 7.45	0.220	0.15
Abdu (kg)	34.32 ± 5.71	30.92 ± 5.32	32.1 ± 6.16	32.45 ± 6.16	0.561	0.12

M1, M2, and M3: three measurement moments; *p*: *p*-value of F-statistic; η²: eta squared values; HRmax: heart rate maximum; VO₂max: maximum oxygen volume; V10: 10 m sprint; V30: 30 m sprint; COD20: 20 m zig-zag test; p.max: maximum power; p.min: minimum power; FI: fatigue index; SJ: squat jump; CMJ: countermovement jump; YYIR: Yo-Yo intermittent recovery test; Addu: adductors; Abdu: abductors.

The time-course of the training load accumulated in the different microcycles is shown in Figure 2.

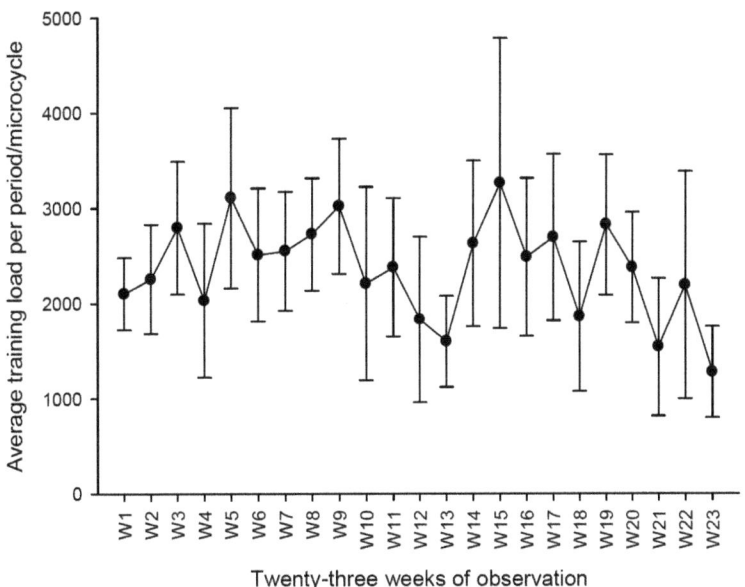

Figure 2. Average training load in the 23 weeks of observation.

Correlations between fitness variables and average training load can be observed in Table 2.

Table 2. Correlations between mean values fitness and average training load.

Variable	r	p-Value	r	p-Value
HRmax	−0.126	0.585	−0.447	0.048
VO$_2$max	−0.042	0.850	−0.157	0.486
V10	−0.187	0.417	0.056	0.816
V30	−0.123	0.596	0.023	0.922
COD20	−0.091	0.695	−0.225	0.341
p.max	0.249	0.276	0.058	0.808
p.min	0.351	0.119	0.256	0.276
FI	0.080	0.731	−0.104	0.662
SJ	0.314	0.166	0.330	0.156
CMJ	0.351	0.119	0.441	0.052
YYIR	−0.059	0.811	−0.261	0.295

HRmax: heart rate maximum; VO$_2$max: maximum oxygen volume; V10: 10 m sprint; V30: 30 m sprint; COD20: 20 m zig-zag test; p.max: maximum power; p.min: minimum power; FI: fatigue index; SJ: squat jump; CMJ: countermovement jump; YYIR: Yo-Yo intermittent recovery test.

4. Discussion

The current study aimed to analyze the variations of fitness status in women soccer players over time (repeated measures) and test the relationships between accumulated training load and fitness variations. To the best of our knowledge, this is the first study to simultaneously analyze variations in fitness status and training load from the beginning of preseason to the end of midseason, in the context of women's soccer. Concerning the first aim, there were no differences in fitness status during the analyzed period, contrary to our original hypothesis. Furthermore, no significant relationships were observed between the fitness status and the accumulated training load, which is also contrary to our hypothesis.

The literature has shown that athletes generally change their fitness status over the season, although this is not so straightforward. For example, a study showed that players' aerobic capacity was higher in the midseason than in the pre- and postseason, indicating that the participants tend to reach a peak performance in this variable in the middle of the competitive schedule before it decreases over the subsequent weeks [17]. However, another study revealed that these changes can be very different from season to season [40]. Furthermore, physical performance changes throughout a soccer season can be dependent on the fitness status observed at the beginning of the preseason period [41]. Furthermore, the abovementioned study revealed a lack of positive changes after a preseason period [41].

Similar results were observed regarding VO$_2$max, 15 m sprint, and agility tests in another study [10]. On the other hand, [1] found no differences in performance in the countermovement jump with arm-swing and sprint performance over a season, similar to the current results. In addition, previous studies showed that training loads can vary between the different periods of a season [14,15], which suggests that variations in fitness status could be related to the training loads that the players experience.

However, in the current study, there were no significant differences in the training load when comparing the preseason and the midseason, which might justify the absence of differences in players' fitness status. In fact, there is a need to respect the training principles, such as progressive overload, individualization, and variation for ensuring training adaptations [42]. Indeed, training variation assumes an important role for avoiding a monotonous training cycle and allowing supercompensation to occur [43,44]. For those reasons, the lack of differences in training load during the period observed in the present study may be related to poor management of training loads, as well as poor micro- and mesocycle planning [41]. Therefore, a dose–response relationship between training load variations and fitness status changes in the season could be suggested, although additional studies are required to confirm such an assumption. Specifically, studies in which the training load is consciously manipulated to generate different magnitudes of changes are welcome.

Concerning the associations between physical status and training load, no significant values were reported. The literature suggests that a higher accumulated match time during the season is linked to better speed and CMJ performance, while a higher total exposure time is related to decreased power performances [19]. Therefore, it appears that both training and competitions define soccer players' physical status. However, another study showed significant negative associations between sRPE and physical fitness changes after a 9 week training period [21]. In fact, corroborating the abovementioned statement regarding the progressive overload training principle need for adaptations to occur, a study conducted on 34 junior male soccer players revealed that elite players with higher perceived training loads throughout a training period presented greater improvements in aerobic performance, when compared with their nonelite counterparts [45]. These facts reinforce the need for a better load management, respecting the training principles and biologic individuality for ensuring positive fitness changes after a training intervention.

At this point, sRPE is postulated as a consistent method of measuring internal training load among sessions for an entire season for youth soccer players [46]. However, sRPE is weakly related to independent high-intensity external load measures [47], indicating that this measure might not capture the complexity of training loads in soccer. Therefore, we suggest that future studies investigate the correlations between fitness status and external training loads in soccer, which could shed light on this topic.

Studies in women's soccer are still scarce, which justifies one of the strengths of the current research. Moreover, we monitored the players over half a soccer season, which indicates the relevance of the current results to understanding the complexity of the relationship between training loads and fitness status in women's soccer. However, there is a need for future studies to analyze an entire season, for a greater perception of such relationships.

Nevertheless, caution is required when interpreting the data. First, all athletes in this study belonged to the same team, which reduces the study's external validity. Additionally, no measures of external training load were taken, which limits the comprehension of the phenomenon. Lastly, we were unable to collect measures of fitness status during the midseason period (just after this stage). For this reason, changes might have occurred that were not captured by our measurements. For those reasons, we recommend future studies to expand the current findings by investigating athletes from a larger sample, collecting external load measures (i.e., high-intensity data), and including more intermediate assessments of fitness status.

5. Conclusions

This study revealed no differences in the fitness status of women soccer players during the analyzed season. Moreover, fitness status had no significant relationship with accumulated training load. Further studies should be conducted to identify other possible relationships and eventually determine how specific elements of fitness status are associated with specific efforts exerted during training drills.

Author Contributions: L.G., F.M.C. and J.M.C.C. led the project, established the protocol, and wrote and revised the original manuscript; J.I.B. and H.S. collected the data, and wrote and revised the original manuscript; G.M.P., A.G.P.d.A., A.F.S., A.J.F. and R.S. wrote and revised the original manuscript. All authors have read and agreed to the published version of the manuscript.

Funding: This research received no external funding.

Institutional Review Board Statement: The study was conducted according to the guidelines of the Declaration of Helsinki and approved by the Institutional Review Board (or Ethics Committee) of the Polytechnic Institute of Viana do Castelo School of Sport and Leisure (code: CTC-ESDL-CE001-2021).

Informed Consent Statement: Informed consent was obtained from all subjects involved in the study.

Acknowledgments: This work was funded by Fundação para a Ciência e Tecnologia/Ministério da Ciência, Tecnologia e Ensino Superior through national funds and, when applicable, co-funded EU funds under the project UIDB/50008/2020 to Filipe Manuel Clemente. Hugo Sarmento gratefully acknowledges the support of a Spanish government subproject 'Integration ways between qualitative and quantitative data, multiple case development, and synthesis review as the main axis for an innovative future in physical activity and sports research' [PGC2018-098742-B-C31] (Ministerio de Economía y Competitividad, Programa Estatal de Generación de Conocimiento y Fortalecimiento Científico y Tecnológico del Sistema I + D + i), which is part of the coordinated project 'New approach of research in physical activity and sport from a mixed methods perspective' (NARPAS_MM) [SPGC201800x098742CV0].

Conflicts of Interest: The authors declare no conflict of interest.

References

1. Stepinski, M.; Ceylan, H.I.; Zwierko, T. Seasonal Variation of Speed, Agility and Power Performance in Elite Female Soccer Players: Effect of Functional Fitness. *Phys. Act. Rev.* **2020**, *8*, 16–25. [CrossRef]
2. McCormack, W.; Stout, J.; Wells, A.; Gonzalez, A.; Mangine, G.; Hoffman, J. Predictors of High-Intensity Running Capacity in Collegiate Women during a Soccer Game. *J. Stregth Cond. Res.* **2014**, *28*, 964–970. [CrossRef] [PubMed]
3. Bangsbo, J.; Mohr, M.; Krustrup, P. Physical and Metabolic Demands of Training and Match-Play in the Elite Foot- Ball Player. *J. Sports Sci.* **2006**, *24*, 665–674. [CrossRef]
4. Datson, N.; Drust, B.; Weston, M.; Jarman, I.; Lisboa, P.; Gregson, W. Match Physical Performance of Elite Female Soccer Player during International Competition. *J. Stregth Cond. Res.* **2017**, *31*, 2379–2387. [CrossRef] [PubMed]
5. Andersson, H.; Randers, M.; Heiner-Moller, A.; Krustrup, P.; Mohr, M. Elite Female Soccer Players Perform More High-Intensity Running When Playing in International Games Compared with Domestic League Games. *J. Stregth Cond. Res.* **2010**, *24*, 912–919. [CrossRef]
6. Doyle, B.; Browne, D.; Horan, D. The Relationship of Aerobic Endurance and Linear Speed on Repeat Sprint Ability Performance in Female International Footballers. *Int. J. Hum. Mov. Sports Sci.* **2020**, *8*, 147–153. [CrossRef]
7. Krustrup, P.; Mohr, M.; Ellingsgaard, H.; Bangsbo, J. Physical Demands during an Elite Female Soccer Game: Importance of Training Status. *Med. Sci. Sports Exerc.* **2005**, *37*, 1242–1248. [CrossRef] [PubMed]
8. Sánchez, J.; Carretero, M.; Casamichana, D.; Arcos, A.L. Effects of Man-Marking on Heart Rate, Perceived Exertion and Technical-Tactical Demands on Youth Soccer Players. *RICYDE. Rev. Int. Cienc. Deport.* **2016**, 281–296. [CrossRef]
9. Gravina, L.; Gil, S.; Ruiz, F.; Zubero, J.; Gil, J.; Irazusa, J. Anthropometric and Physiological Differences Betweem First Team and Reverse Soccer Players Aged 10-14 Years at the Beginning and End of the Season. *J. Strength Cond. Res.* **2008**, *22*, 1308–1314. [CrossRef]
10. Caldwell, B.; Peters, D. Seasonal Variation in Physiological Fitness of a Semiprofessional Soccer Team. *J. Strength Cond. Res.* **2009**, *23*, 1370–1377. [CrossRef]
11. Mara, J.; Thompson, K.; Pumpa, K.; Ball, N. Periodisation and Physical Performance in Elite Female Soccer Players. *Int. J. Sports Physiol. Perform.* **2015**, *10*, 664–669. [CrossRef]
12. Ostojic, S.M. Seasonal Alterations in Body Composition and Sprint Performance of Elite Soccer Players. *J. Exer. Physiol.* **2003**, *6*, 24–27.
13. Silva, J.R. Biochemical Impact of Soccer: An Analysis of Hormonal, Muscle Damage, and Redox Markers during the Season. *Appl. Physiol. Nutr. Metab.* **2014**, *39*, 432–438. [CrossRef] [PubMed]
14. Jeong, T.S.; Reilly, T.; Morton, J.; Bae, S.W.; Drust, B. Quantification of the Physiological Loading of One Week of "Pre-Season" and One Week of "in-Season" Training in Professional Soccer Players. *J. Sports Sci.* **2011**, *29*, 1161–1166. [CrossRef]
15. Fessi, M.S.; Nouira, S.; Dellal, A.; Owen, A.; Elloumi, M.; Moalla, W. Changes of the Psychophysical State and Feeling of Wellness of Professional Soccer Players during Pre-Season and in-Season Periods. *Res. Sport. Med.* **2016**, *24*, 375–386. [CrossRef] [PubMed]
16. Dupont, G. The Effect of in Season High Intensity Interval. *J. Strength Cond. Res.* **2004**, *18*, 584–589. [PubMed]
17. Purdom, T.M.; Levers, K.S.; McPherson, C.S.; Giles, J.; Brown, L. A Longitudinal Prospective Study: The Effect of Annual Seasonal Transition and Coaching Influence on Aerobic Capacity and Body Composition in Division I Female Soccer Players. *Sports* **2020**, *8*, 107. [CrossRef]
18. Clemente, F.; Clark, C.; Castillo, D.; Sarmento, H.; Nikolaidis, P.T.; Rosemann, T.; Knechtle, B. Variations of Training Load, Monotony, and Strain and Dose-Response Relationships with Maximal Aerobic Speed, Maximal Oxygen Uptake, and Isokinetic Strength in Professional Soccer Players. *PLoS ONE* **2019**, *14*, e0225522. [CrossRef]
19. Jaspers, A.; Brink, M.S.; Probst, S.G.M.; Frencken, W.G.P.; Helsen, W.F. Relationships Between Training Load Indicators and Training Outcomes in Professional Soccer. *Sport. Med.* **2017**, *47*, 533–544. [CrossRef]
20. Campos-Vazquez, M.A.; Toscano-Bendala, F.J.; Mora-Ferrera, J.C.; Suarez-Arrones, L.J. Relationship between Internal Load Indicators and Changes on Intermittent Performance after the Preseason in Professional Soccer Players. *J. Strength Cond. Res.* **2017**, *31*, 1477–1485. [CrossRef]

21. Arcos, A.; Martínez-Santos, R.; Yanci, J.; Mendiguchia, J.; Méndez-Villanueva, A. Negative Associations between Perceived Training Load, Volume and Changes in Physical Fitness in Professional Soccer Players. *J. Sport. Sci. Med.* **2015**, *14*, 394–401.
22. Borg, G. *Perceived Exertion and Pain Scales*; Human Kinetics: Champaign, IL, USA, 1998.
23. Foster, C.; Florhaug, J.A.; Franklin, J.; Gottschall, L.; Hrovatin, L.A.; Parker, S.; Doleshal, P.; Dodge, C. A New Approach to Monitoring Exercise Training. *J. Strength Cond. Res.* **2001**, *15*, 109–115. [CrossRef]
24. Haddad, M.; Stylianides, G.; Djaoui, L.; Dellal, A.; Chamari, K. Session-RPE Method for Training Load Monitoring: Validity, Ecological Usefulness, and Influencing Factors. *Front. Neurosci.* **2017**, *11*, 612. [CrossRef]
25. Casamichana, D.; Castellano, J.; Calleja-Gonzalez, J.; RomaN, J.S.; Castagna, C. Relationship between Indicators of Training Load in Soccer Players. *J. Strength Cond. Res.* **2013**, *27*, 369–374. [CrossRef] [PubMed]
26. McLaren, S.J.; Macpherson, T.W.; Coutts, A.J.; Hurst, C.; Spears, I.R.; Weston, M. The Relationships Between Internal and External Measures of Training Load and Intensity in Team Sports: A Meta-Analysis. *Sport. Med.* **2018**, *48*, 641–658. [CrossRef] [PubMed]
27. Avalos, M.; Hellard, P.; Chatard, J.-C. Modeling the Training-Performance Relatioship Using a Mixed Model in Elite Swimmers. *Med. Sci. Sport. Exerc. Sci. Sport Exerc.* **2003**, *35*, 838–846. [CrossRef] [PubMed]
28. Walker, S.; Turner, A. A One-Day Dield Test Battery for the Assessment of Aerobic Capacity, Anaerobic Capacity, Speed, and Agility of Soccer Players. *Strength Cond. J.* **2009**, *31*, 52–60. [CrossRef]
29. Turner, A.; Walker, S.; Stembridge, M.; Coneyworth, P.; Reed, G.; Birdsey, L.; Barter, P.; Moody, J. A Testing Battery for the Assessment of Fitness in Soccer Players. *Strength Cond. J.* **2011**, *33*, 29–39. [CrossRef]
30. Gonçalves, L.; Clemente, F.M.; Barrera, J.I.; Sarmento, H.; González-Fernández, F.T.; Vieira, L.H.P.; Figueiredo, A.J.; Clark, C.C.T.; Carral, J.M.C. Relationships between Fitness Status and Match Running Performance in Adult Women Soccer Players: A Cohort Study. *Medicina* **2021**, *57*, 617. [CrossRef] [PubMed]
31. McGowan, C.J.; Pyne, D.B.; Thompson, K.G.; Rattray, B. Warm-Up Strategies for Sport and Exercise: Mechanisms and Applications. *Sport. Med.* **2015**, *45*, 1523–1546. [CrossRef] [PubMed]
32. Delahunt, E.; Kennelly, C.; McEntee, B.L.; Coughlan, G.F.; Green, B.S. The Thigh Adductor Squeeze Test: 45° of Hip Flexion as the Optimal Test Position for Eliciting Adductor Muscle Activity and Maximum Pressure Values. *Man. Ther.* **2011**, *16*, 476–480. [CrossRef] [PubMed]
33. Glatthorn, J.; Gouge, S.; Nussbaumer, S.; Stauffacher, S.; Impellizzeri, F.M.; Maffiuletti, N. Validity and Reliability of Optojump Photoelectric Cells for Estimating Vertical Jump Height. *J. Strength* **2011**, *25*, 556–560. [CrossRef]
34. Little, T.; Williams, A.G. Specificity of Acceleration, Maximum Speed, and Agility in Professional Soccer Players. *J. Strength Cond. Res.* **2005**, *19*, 76–78. [CrossRef] [PubMed]
35. MacKenzie, B. *101 Performance Evaluation Tests*; Electric Word Plc.: London, UK, 2005.
36. Cipryan, L.; Gajda, V. The Influence of Aerobic Power on Repeated Anaerobic Exercise in Junior Soccer Players. *J. Hum. Kinet.* **2011**, *28*, 63–71. [CrossRef] [PubMed]
37. Bangsbo, J.; Iaia, F.M.; Krustrup, P. The Yo-Yo Intermittent Recovery Test. *Sport. Med.* **2008**, *38*, 37–51. [CrossRef] [PubMed]
38. Foster, C. Monitoring Training in Athletes with Reference to Overtraining Syndrome. *Med. Sci. Sports Exerc.* **1998**, *30*, 1164–1168. [CrossRef]
39. Cohen, J. *Statistical Power Analysis for the Behavioral Sciences*, 2nd ed.; Routledge: New York, NY, USA, 1988.
40. Los Arcos, A.; Castillo, D.; Martínez-Santos, R. Influence of Initial Performance Level and Tactical Position on the Aerobic Fitness in Soccer Players after Preseason Period. *Sci. Med. Footb.* **2018**, *2*, 294–298. [CrossRef]
41. Silva, R.; Lima, R.; Camões, M.; Leão, C.; Matos, S.; Pereira, J.; Bezerra, P.; Clemente, F.M. Physical Fitness Changes among Amateur Soccer Players: Effects of the Pre-Season Period. *Biomed. Hum. Kinet.* **2021**, *13*, 63–72. [CrossRef]
42. Kasper, K. Sports Training Principles. *Curr. Sports Med. Rep.* **2019**, *18*, 95–96. [CrossRef]
43. Marrier, B.; Robineau, J.; Piscione, J.; Lacome, M.; Peeters, A.; Hausswirth, C.; Morin, J.-B.; Le Meur, Y. Supercompensation Kinetics of Physical Qualities During a Taper in Team-Sport Athletes. *Int. J. Sports Physiol. Perform.* **2017**, *12*, 1163–1169. [CrossRef]
44. Gabbett, T.; Nassis, G.P.; Oetter, E.; Pretorius, J.; Johnston, N.; Medina, D.; Rodas, G.; Myslinski, T.; Howells, D.; Beard, A.; et al. The Athlete Monitoring Cycle: A Practical Guide to Interpreting and Applying Training Monitoring Data. *Br. J. Sports Med.* **2017**, *51*, 1451–1452. [CrossRef] [PubMed]
45. Gil-Rey, E.; Lezaun, A.; Los Arcos, A. Quantification of the Perceived Training Load and Its Relationship with Changes in Physical Fitness Performance in Junior Soccer Players. *J. Sports Sci.* **2015**, *33*, 2125–2132. [CrossRef] [PubMed]
46. Vahia, D.; Kelly, A.; Knapman, H.; Williams, C.A. Variation in the Correlation Between Heart Rate and Session Rating of Perceived Exertion-Based Estimations of Internal Training Load in Youth Soccer Players. *Pediatr. Exerc. Sci.* **2019**, *31*, 91–98. [CrossRef]
47. Gaudino, P.; Iaia, F.M.; Strudwick, A.J.; Hawkins, R.D.; Alberti, G.; Atkinson, G.; Gregson, W. Factors Influencing Perception of Effort (Session Rating of Perceived Exertion) during Elite Soccer Training. *Int. J. Sports Physiol. Perform.* **2015**, *10*, 860–864. [CrossRef] [PubMed]

Article

Quantifying Coordination between Agonist and Antagonist Elbow Muscles during Backhand Crosscourt Shots in Adult Female Squash Players

Abdel-Rahman Akl [1], Amr Hassan [2], Helal Elgizawy [1] and Markus Tilp [3,*]

1. Faculty of Physical Education-Abo Qir, Alexandria University, Alexandria 21913, Egypt; abdelrahman.akl@alexu.edu.eg (A.-R.A.); helal.elgizawy@alexu.edu.eg (H.E.)
2. Department of Sports Training, Faculty of Sports Education, Mansoura University, Mansoura 35516, Egypt; amrahh@mans.edu.eg
3. Institute of Human Movement Science, Sport and Health, University of Graz, A-8010 Graz, Austria
* Correspondence: markus.tilp@uni-graz.at

Abstract: The purpose of this study was to quantify the coordination between agonist and antagonist elbow muscles during squash backhand crosscourt shots in adult female players. Ten right-handed, international-level, female squash players participated in the study. The electrical muscle activity of two right elbow agonist/antagonist muscles, the biceps brachii and triceps brachii, were recorded using a surface EMG system, and processed using the integrated EMG to calculate a co-activation index (CoI) for the preparation phase, the execution phase, and the follow-through phase. A significant effect of the phases on the CoI was observed. Co-activation was significantly different between the follow-through and the execution phase (45.93 ± 6.00% and 30.14 ± 4.11%, $p < 0.001$), and also between the preparation and the execution phase (44.74 ± 9.88% and 30.14 ± 4.11%, $p < 0.01$). No significant difference was found between the preparation and the follow-through phase ($p = 0.953$). In conclusion, the co-activation of the elbow muscles varies within the squash backhand crosscourt shots. The highest level of co-activation was observed in the preparation phase and the lowest level of co-activation was observed during the execution. The co-activation index could be a useful method for the interpretation of elbow muscle co-activity during a squash backhand crosscourt shot.

Keywords: racket sport; injury; elbow; electromyography; co-activation

1. Introduction

The popularity of squash is increasing and now it is one of the racket sports that is played in most countries in the world. Similarly, the number of squash studies is growing, together with the interest of scientists who have analyzed various aspects of the game [1–4].

Modern squash is a fast-performing sport including complex and multidirectional movement patterns with a high density and intermittent rhythm. Therefore, it is multifaceted in its motor skills and its physiological, kinetic, and cognitive requirements. Performance success depends to a large extent on the interaction and complementarity of these factors [3,5–7].

Previous studies analyzed the effect of upper extremity movement and racquet speed during skill performance in squash [8], examined the electromyographical activity during strokes [9], and performed three-dimensional kinematic analyses of the forehand [10] and backhand strokes [11].

In their study, Hong, Chang, and Chan [10] reported interesting differences in the types of skills used during a squash game, among them the fact that the backhand was played more frequently (63.1%) than the forehand (36.9%), which underlines the importance of the backhand stroke in squash. Others investigated the association between the rotating motion of the upper extremities and racket speed when playing squash., The rate of performance of the forehand and backhand stroke was similar in other studies [8,9,12].

The backhand in squash is different from other strokes because the player must control the racket to fully control the angle of the hit without losing control of the swing speed while controlling the angular displacements of the elbow, torso, and shoulder joints [12].

Seoung Eun, Seung Nam, and Murali [12] used a 3D motion analysis system to analyze the backhand stroke performance of both elite and novice players. The study aimed to compare the displacement and velocity of the trunk and racquet, and the angular displacements and the velocities of the elbow and shoulder joints. The significant differences observed between novice and expert players underline the importance of studying the muscular activity during the backhand stroke. Vukovic et al. [13] measured the trajectory and velocity of movement using a tracking system to determine whether there were significant differences between winners and losers. They analysed the used skills, the time patterns, and the position of the squash players during their performance. Subsequently, they compared the dynamic movements of players of different technical abilities and related them to the tactics adopted by different players in 24 competitive matches with elite male squash players [14]. McGarry [15] examined the space–time patterns of squash players as they move around the squash court in the context of a dynamical system using movements analysis of forty-eight squash rallies—twelve from each quarter-final match in a high-level knock-out competition.

Besides the analysis of performance, squash injuries have also been a focus for researchers. Finch and Eime [7] conducted a review on retrospective studies of squash injuries that analyzed records of hospitalized, injured, or emergency patients, and surveys from squash players. The studies included data from 2232 domestic league players and university teams from the USA, UK, New Zealand, Germany, and the Netherlands and concluded that better-controlled studies are needed, particularly to determine the risk of injuries associated with squash.

In recent years, there have been steady increases in the duration of the game, perhaps due to the improvement in the physical and technical abilities of squash players. In addition, it should be noted that in 2009 squash underwent changes in the rules (e.g., changing the scoring system in squash to 'Point-A-Rally' (PAR) to 11 points per game) according to which players have less time to perform shots, which increases the workload of the players [14]. Both developments may cause high loads leading to injury.

Therefore, an important research aim in sports medicine has been to understand the relationship between the intensity or volume of training and the type and grade of injuries mainly due to overuse, particularly following stroke training [16–18]. During the last few years, some researchers have focused on injuries in squash [18]. Horsley et al. [19] studied the diversity of injuries suffered by professional squash players in both training and competition through a survey of injury records between 2004–2015. However, this study only looked at injuries of the lower limbs because of the mechanical loading of the players during strokes in racket games. Habitual participation in racquet games over years often results in specific strength and flexibility imbalances [20]. Previous studies have reported that the ratio of upper-limb injuries is around 36% of all squash injuries, making the elbow the most commonly injured body region [3,5,7]. Despite this, little is known about injury mechanisms, exhaustion, recovery, and performance in training and competition [21–23].

Previous studies have indicated the relationship between muscular co-activation and injury. Hirokawa, et al. [24] reported that increased quadriceps–hamstring muscle co-activation at the knee may reduce the risk of anterior cruciate ligament (ACL) injury.

Lehman [25] reported that there is a relationship between muscle extensor endurance with decreases in injury risk. The aberrant flexor/extensor endurance ratios have also been correlated with a history of injury. From this perspective, adequate joint stability is related to the amount of muscle co-activation [26,27]. Elbow stability is not provided by one specific muscle but rather via the coordinated efforts of agonist and antagonists muscles. These muscles are active throughout the whole backhand crosscourt movement in squash. Due to the muscular demands of the backhand crosscourt shot and the prevalence of injury in the elbow, training the agonist and antagonist musculature may improve performance and decrease injury risk.

Surprisingly, so far, no study has investigated the electrical activity of the muscles during the backhand stroke, which has been identified as the skill with the highest frequency and also the highest cause of injury rate [3,7].

Given the importance of the coordination between the muscles working on the elbow joint with regards to performance and injury prevention, especially among female athletes, this study aims to investigate the coordination between agonist and antagonist elbow muscles during the backhand crosscourt stroke in adult female squash players.

2. Materials and Methods

2.1. Participants

Female, right-handed elite squash players ($n = 10$) participated in the present study (age: 18.4 ± 0.8 years; body mass: 60.8 ± 1.8 kg; height: 165.2 ± 1.6 cm; training age: 9.1 ± 0.9 years). The subjects were officially ranked between 4 and 20 in the Egyptian squash federation and were currently competing in professional squash tournaments (national and international). Written informed consent of the players was obtained, and the study was approved by the institutional ethics committee of studies and research.

2.2. Experiment Protocol

After a 15 min warm-up including general, elbow-, and shoulder-specific mobility exercises, as well as stretching and familiarization with the protocol, participants performed Squash backhand crosscourt strokes. A total of three successful attempts were recorded for each player, with a one-minute rest between attempts. The Squash backhand crosscourt skill was broken into three phases: the preparation phase, the execution phase, and the follow-through phase.

2.3. Data Recording

The electrical muscle activity of two right elbow agonist/antagonist muscles, the biceps brachii (BB) and triceps brachii (TB) were recorded using surface EMG system (Myon m320RX; Myon, Switzerland). The skin over the muscles of the dominant arm was shaved and cleaned with alcohol and bipolar, circular 10 mm diameter silver chloride surface electrodes (SKINTACT FS-RG1/10, Leonhard Lang GmbH, Archenweg 56, 6020 Innsbruck, Austria) were secured on the selected muscles. Electrodes were attached over each muscle following the SENIAM guidelines maintaining a 2 cm center to center inter-electrode spacing [28]. The EMG signals were stored at a sampling frequency of 1000 Hz and digitized using a 16-bit analog to digital (A/D) converter. EMG data was processed using Visual 3D software (C-Motion, Germantown, MD, USA). Raw EMG data were band-pass filtered (20 Hz–450 Hz) applying a Butterworth filter. The signals were preprocessed using full wave rectifier and a linear envelope obtained using the root mean square (RMS) approach with a window size of 100 ms. Data were normalized to an isometric maximum voluntary contraction (MVC), which was recorded after each subject finished the experimental tasks. To obtain the MVC values, subjects performed three repetitions for 5 s, with 60 s rest in between while sitting in a stable chair with forearm resistance. Peak muscle activity over the three repetitions for each muscle was taken as the MVC value.

2.4. Co-Activation Index

Muscle co-activation was estimated by the calculation of a co-activation index (CoI) using the following equation adapted from Kellis et al. [29]

$$CoI = \frac{iEMG_{anta}}{(iEMG_{anta} + iEMG_{ago})} \times 100$$

where *iEMGanta* and *iEMGago*, respectively, refer to iEMG of antagonist and agonist muscle in different movement phases. The preparation phase was defined from the beginning of the movement to the end of the elbow flexion, the execution phase was defined from the beginning of the elbow extension until the shot, and the follow-through phase was defined from the instant of the shot until the end of the movement, see Figure 1. The phases were defined by video analysis using 3D simi motion capture, which was synchronized with EMG.

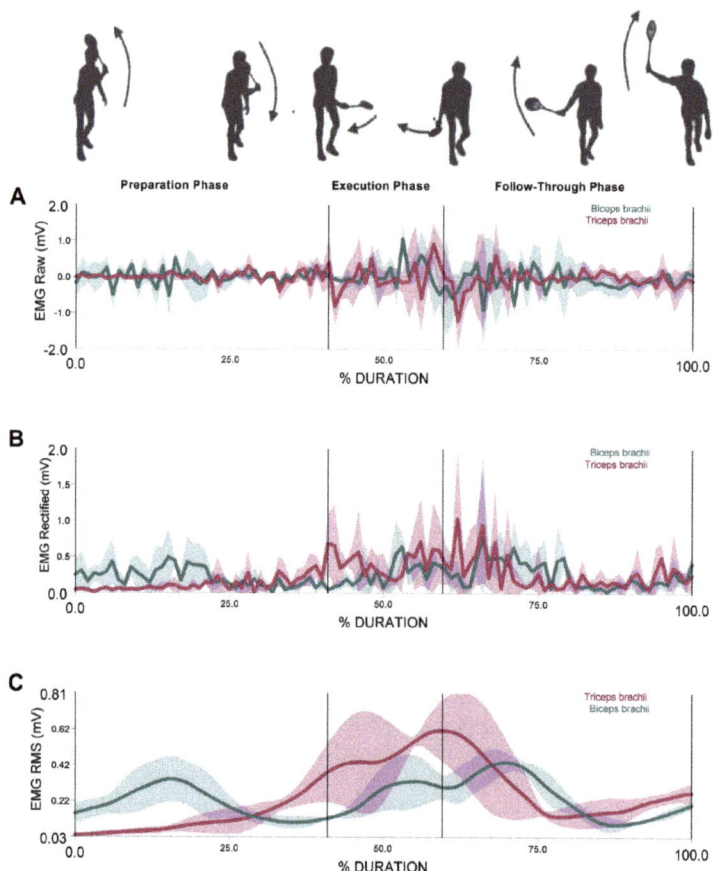

Figure 1. Backhand crosscourt phases (Preparation phase, Execution phase, Follow-Through phase) of the Biceps brachii (BB) and Triceps brachii (TB). (**A**) EMG raw data, (**B**) EMG rectified data, and (**C**) EMG RMS. Means (solid lines) and standard deviation (shaded areas) of three stroke attempts from a representative subject.

2.5. Statistical Analysis

Descriptive statistics were reported as means and standard deviations (mean ± SD). The normality of the data was analyzed using the Shapiro–Wilk test and all data were found to be suitable for parametric analysis. Repeated Measures Analysis of Variance (ANOVA) with Sidak post hoc tests were used to detect significant differences and compare the mean of each variable during the three phases (preparation, execution, and follow-through). Partial eta squared ($\eta^2 p$) was calculated to assess the effect size. The statistical analysis was performed using IBM SPSS software Statistics v21 (IBM® Corporation, Armonk, NY, USA).

3. Results

3.1. Muscular Activity

Average values and standard deviations for the normalized RMS for the BB are presented in Figure 2, and the TB in Figure 3, during the three analyzed phases (the preparation, the execution, and the follow-through phase). The highest activities of the BB were observed during the follow-through phase, followed by the execution phase, and the preparation phase, with values of $13.80 \pm 2.97\%$, $11.57 \pm 1.45\%$, and $8.32 \pm 3.47\%$, respectively. There was a significant difference between the BB activity during the preparation compared to the follow-through phases ($p < 0.05$; $\eta^2 p = 0.50$, Figure 2). For TB, the highest activities were observed during the execution phase, followed by the follow-through phase and the preparation phase, with values of $27.02 \pm 3.43\%$, $16.14 \pm 2.32\%$, and $6.38 \pm 1.86\%$, respectively, while high significant differences for the TB were observed among the three phases ($p < 0.001$; $\eta^2 p = 0.97$, Figure 3).

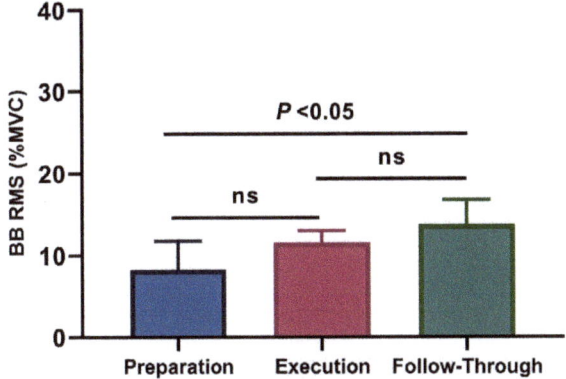

Figure 2. Average values and standard deviations for the normalized EMG (%MVC) per phase of the biceps brachii ($\eta^2 p = 0.50$).

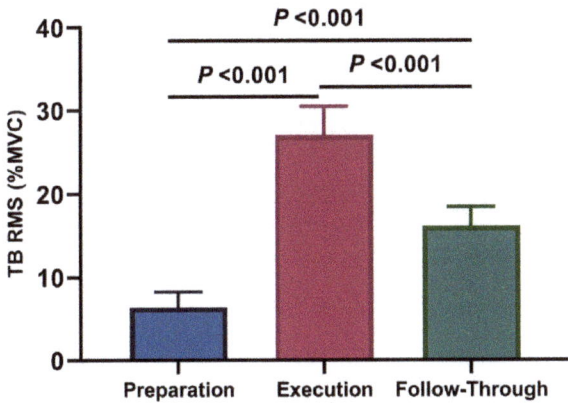

Figure 3. Average values and standard deviations for the normalized EMG (%MVC) per phase of the Triceps brachii ($\eta^2 p = 0.97$).

3.2. Co-Activation Index

A significant effect ($p < 0.01$, $\eta^2 p = 0.73$) of the phases on the CoI was observed (Figure 4). Post hoc analyses showed that the co-activation was significantly higher in the follow-through phase compared to the execution phase (45.93 ± 6.00% and 30.14 ± 4.11%, $p < 0.001$), and also between the preparation phase and the execution phase (44.74 ± 9.88% and 30.14 ± 4.11%, $p < 0.01$). No significant difference was found between the preparation and follow-through phases ($p = 0.95$).

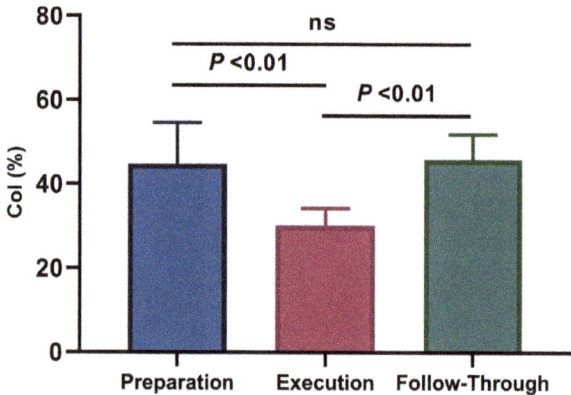

Figure 4. Average values and standard deviations for the co-activation index (CoI) (%) per phase ($\eta^2 p = 0.73$). The agonist/antagonist muscle of each phase was BB/TB, TB/BB, and TB/BB, respectively.

4. Discussion

The main aim of this study was to determine muscle co-activation of elbow muscles as an indicator of coordination between agonist and antagonist muscle activity during three phases of the squash backhand crosscourt shots in adult female players. While we observed similar co-activation in the preparation and follow-through phase, the co-activation was significantly decreased during the execution phase.

The main activities for the BB and the TB were observed during three phases in which they acted as a prime mover (agonist), BB during the preparation phase and TB during the execution and follow-through phases.

Low values of muscle activity were observed in the preparation phase where both BB and TB showed activations less than 10% of MVC (BB: 8.3% MVC and TB 6.4% MVC). This can be explained by the fact that the elbow flexion includes muscle synergies (e.g., brachioradialis and anterior deltoid muscle) [30,31]. However, the relative muscle activity of BB was greater than that of TB muscle activity because the BB is the prime mover during elbow flexion.

Greater TB activation was observed during the execution phase with 27.02% MVC (BB: 11.57% MVC). Despite substantial activation differences between TB and BB during the execution phase, the observed BB activation was still greater when compared with the preparation phase. This is somewhat surprising, since the BB is an agonist muscle in the preparation phase but an antagonist muscle in the execution phase. The reason for this result may be the variation in movement muscle activity amplitude. While the agonist muscle activity increased during the execution phase to accelerate the movement, the antagonist initiated an increase in muscle activity, possibly to prevent an elbow joint injury due to overextension of the elbow joint in the follow-through phase [32].

Previous studies [33–38] indicate that experienced athletes could have a distinct muscle activation pattern with less antagonist muscle activation, implying that antagonistic muscle coupling might be altered by specialized activity. As a result, top athletes may have lower muscle co-activation than non-athletes, particularly during fast movements [39].

According to the observed results, muscle co-activation was greater in the preparation and the follow-through phases compared to the execution phase. Both Bazzucchi et al. [40]

and Rouard and Clarys [31] reported greater co-activation values of the arm muscles during fast compared to slow movements, increasing at the preparation phase, decreasing at execution to allow faster acceleration, and increasing at the end of the movement to provide dynamic braking, which is similar to the elbow extension in the backhand crosscourt shot. In addition, Darainy and Ostry [41] and Bazzucchi, Sbriccoli, Marzattinocci, and Felici [40] underlined that greater antagonist activity could make the motor task controllable and also increases the stiffness and stability of the joint.

Wagner et al. [42] reported that overarm movements are essential skills in different types of sports. Hence, strong elbow extension might be considered as one of the determinants of efficiency in the squash backhand crosscourt shot. Bazzucchi, Riccio, and Felici [39] observed that muscle co-activation decreased during the execution phase for generating higher forces to increase performance. This is in accordance with our findings where the TB as the agonist muscle showed a strong activity during the execution phase, with low values of the BB as the antagonist muscle. This led to a low value of co-activation during the execution phase with values around 30%.

Muscle co-activation increased again in the follow-through phase to inhibit end range elbow extensions. The high value of co-activation in the follow-through phase with values of 45.93% increased joint stiffness and, therefore, stability [40]. This result was expected as increased co-activation is considered a determinant for preventing injury of the elbow joint.

Thus, an initial decreased co-activation allows a faster acceleration in the execution phase, while an increase at the end of the movement range provides dynamic braking of the movement. Furthermore, the high co-activation at the end of the movement allows players to better prepare the arm for the next response during the game [30,40].

Whereas most previous research has concentrated on antagonist muscle co-activation during maximal isometric efforts or as a function of isokinetic velocity, our research focused on sports movements including both concentric and eccentric contractions [43].

5. Conclusions

In summary, the co-activation of the elbow muscles varies within the squash backhand crosscourt stroke. The highest level of co-activation was observed in the preparation phase to control the forearm velocity before the execution phase, and in the follow-through phase to stabilize the elbow joint to prevent injuries and slow down the arm at the end of the movement. The lowest level of co-activation was observed in the execution phase for generating the appropriate force from the prime mover muscle to increase the efficiency of the backhand crosscourt shot.

Author Contributions: Conceptualization, A.-R.A. and H.E.; methodology, A.-R.A. and H.E.; software, A.-R.A.; validation, A.-R.A., A.H. and M.T.; formal analysis, A.-R.A., A.H. and M.T.; investigation, A.-R.A.; resources, A.-R.A.; data curation, A.-R.A., A.H. and M.T.; writing—original draft preparation, A.-R.A., H.E., A.H. and M.T.; writing—review and editing, A.-R.A., A.H. and M.T.; visualization, A.-R.A., A.H. and M.T.; supervision, A.-R.A.; project administration, A.-R.A. All authors have read and agreed to the published version of the manuscript.

Funding: This research received no external funding.

Institutional Review Board Statement: The study was conducted according to the guidelines of the Declaration of Helsinki and approved by the Ethics Committee of the Alexandria University.

Informed Consent Statement: Informed consent was freely obtained, and the study was approved by the institutional ethics committee of studies and research.

Data Availability Statement: The data presented in this study are available on request from the first author.

Acknowledgments: Open Access Funding by the University of Graz.

Conflicts of Interest: The authors declare no conflict of interest.

References

1. Williams, B.K.; Sanders, R.H.; Ryu, J.H.; Graham-Smith, P.; Sinclair, P.J. The kinematic differences between skill levels in the squash forehand drive, volley and drop strokes. *J. Sports Sci.* **2020**, *38*, 1550–1559. [CrossRef]
2. Murray, S.; James, N.; Pers, J.; Mandeljc, R.; Vuckovic, G. Using a Situation Awareness Approach to Identify Differences in the Performance Profiles of the World's Top Two Squash Players and Their Opponents. *Front. Psychol.* **2019**, *10*, 1036. [CrossRef] [PubMed]
3. Horobeanu, C.; Johnson, A.; Pullinger, S.A. The Prevalence of Musculoskeletal Injuries in Junior Elite Squash Players. *Asian J. Sports Med.* **2019**, *10*, 1–8. [CrossRef]
4. Gamal, T.; Akl, A.-R. Electromyographic comparison of squash forehand shot after midcourt and frontcourt traditional movement patterns. *Sport Sci. Pract. Asp.* **2016**, *13*, 19–25.
5. Okhovatian, F.; Ezatolahi, A. Sport injuries in squash. *Pak. J. Med Sci.* **2009**, *25*, 413–417.
6. Lees, A. Technique analysis in sports: A critical review. *J. Sports Sci.* **2002**, *20*, 813–828. [CrossRef] [PubMed]
7. Finch, C.F.; Eime, R.M. The epidemiology of squash injuries. *Int. SportMed J.* **2001**, *2*, 1–11.
8. Elliott, B.; Marshall, R.; Noffal, G. The role of upper limb segment rotations in the development of racket-head speed in the squash forehand. *J. Sports Sci.* **1996**, *14*, 159–165. [CrossRef]
9. Cho, K.-K.; Kim, Y.-S. The kinematic analysis and the study of muscle activities during backhand drive in squash. *Korean J. Sport Biomech.* **2007**, *17*, 11–21.
10. Hong, Y.; Chang, T.C.-M.; Chan, D. A comparison of the game strategies employed by national and international squash players in competitive situation by notational analysis. *J. Hum. Mov. Stud.* **1996**, *31*, 89–104.
11. An, Y.-H.; Ryu, J.-S.; Ryu, H.-Y.; Soo, J.-M.; Lim, Y.-T. The kinematic analysis of the upper extremity during backhand stroke in squash. *Korean J. Sport Biomech.* **2007**, *17*, 145–156.
12. Seoung Eun, K.; Seung Nam, M.; Murali, S. Motion analysis of squash backhand drop shot—A kinematic analysis study. In *Proceedings of 2nd International conference on Advances in Mechanical Engineering (ICAME 2018)*; IOP Publishing Ltd.: Kattankulathur, India, 2018.
13. Vuckovic, G.; Dezman, B.; Erculj, F.; Kovacic, S.; Pers, J. Comparative movement analysis of winning and losing players in men's elite squash. *Kinesiol. Slov.* **2003**, *9*, 74–84.
14. Jones, T.W.; Williams, B.K.; Kilgallen, C.; Horobeanu, C.; Shillabeer, B.C.; Murray, A.; Cardinale, M. A review of the performance requirements of squash. *Int. J. Sports Sci. Coach.* **2018**, *13*, 1223–1232. [CrossRef]
15. McGarry, T. Identifying patterns in squash contests using dynamical analysis and human perception. *Int. J. Perform. Anal. Sport* **2017**, *6*, 134–147. [CrossRef]
16. Vanrenterghem, J.; Nedergaard, N.J.; Robinson, M.A.; Drust, B. Training Load Monitoring in Team Sports: A Novel Framework Separating Physiological and Biomechanical Load-Adaptation Pathways. *Sports Med.* **2017**, *47*, 2135–2142. [CrossRef] [PubMed]
17. Drew, M.K.; Finch, C.F. The Relationship Between Training Load and Injury, Illness and Soreness: A Systematic and Literature Review. *Sports Med.* **2016**, *46*, 861–883. [CrossRef]
18. Gibson, N.; Gibbon, K.; Bell, P.; Clyne, A.; Lobban, G.; Aitken, L. Physical preparation for elite-level squash players: Monitoring, assessment, and training practices for the strength and conditioning coach. *Strength Cond. J.* **2019**, *41*, 51–62. [CrossRef]
19. Horsley, I.G.; O'Donnell, V.; Leeder, J. The epidemiology of injuries in English professional squash; A retrospective analysis between 2004 and 2015. *Phys. Ther. Sport* **2020**, *46*, 1–6. [CrossRef]
20. Nutt, C.; Mirkovic, M.; Hill, R.; Ranson, C.; Cooper, S.M. Reference Values for Glenohumeral Joint Rotational Range of Motion in Elite Tennis Players. *Int. J. Sports Phys. Ther.* **2018**, *13*, 501–510. [CrossRef]
21. Pallis, J.M.; McNitt-Gray, J.L.; Hung, G.K. *Biomechanical Principles and Applications in Sports*; Springer: Heidelberg, Germany, 2019.
22. Perri, T.; Norton, K.I.; Bellenger, C.R.; Murphy, A.P. Training loads in typical junior-elite tennis training and competition: Implications for transition periods in a high-performance pathway. *Int. J. Perform. Anal. Sport* **2018**, *18*, 327–338. [CrossRef]
23. Gescheit, D.T.; Cormack, S.J.; Reid, M.; Duffield, R. Consecutive days of prolonged tennis match play: Performance, physical, and perceptual responses in trained players. *Int. J. Sports Physiol. Perform.* **2015**, *10*, 913–920. [CrossRef]
24. Hirokawa, S.; Solomonow, M.; Luo, Z.; Lu, Y.; D'Ambrosia, R. Muscular co-contraction and control of knee stability. *J. Electromyogr. Kinesiol.* **1991**, *1*, 199–208. [CrossRef]
25. Lehman, G.J. Resistance training for performance and injury prevention in golf. *J. Can. Chiropr. Assoc.* **2006**, *50*, 27–42. [PubMed]
26. Salem, A.; Hassan, A.; Tilp, M.; Akl, A.-R. Antagonist Muscle Co-Activation during Kettlebell Single Arm Swing Exercise. *Appl. Sci.* **2021**, *11*, 4033. [CrossRef]
27. Akl, A.R.; Goncalves, P.; Fonseca, P.; Hassan, A.; Vilas-Boas, J.P.; Conceicao, F. Muscle Co-Activation around the Knee during Different Walking Speeds in Healthy Females. *Sensors* **2021**, *21*, 677. [CrossRef]
28. Hermens, H.J.; Freriks, B.; Disselhorst-Klug, C.; Rau, G. Development of recommendations for SEMG sensors and sensor placement procedures. *J. Electromyogr. Kinesiol.* **2000**, *10*, 361–374. [CrossRef]
29. Kellis, E.; Arabatzi, F.; Papadopoulos, C. Muscle co-activation around the knee in drop jumping using the co-contraction index. *J. Electromyogr. Kinesiol.* **2003**, *13*, 229–238. [CrossRef]
30. Lauer, J.; Figueiredo, P.; Vilas-Boas, J.P.; Fernandes, R.J.; Rouard, A.H. Phase-dependence of elbow muscle coactivation in front crawl swimming. *J. Electromyogr. Kinesiol.* **2013**, *23*, 820–825. [CrossRef] [PubMed]

31. Rouard, A.H.; Clarys, J.P. Cocontraction in the elbow and shoulder muscles during rapid cyclic movements in an aquatic environment. *J. Electromyogr. Kinesiol.* **1995**, *5*, 177–183. [CrossRef]
32. Gribble, P.L.; Ostry, D.J. Independent coactivation of shoulder and elbow muscles. *Exp. Brain Res.* **1998**, *123*, 355–360. [CrossRef]
33. Wang, L.; Niu, W.; Wang, K.; Zhang, S.; Li, L.; Lu, T.; SpringerLink. Badminton players show a lower coactivation and higher beta band intermuscular interactions of ankle antagonist muscles during isokinetic exercise. *Med. Biol. Eng. Comput.* **2019**, *57*, 2407–2415. [CrossRef] [PubMed]
34. Pizzamiglio, S.; De Lillo, M.; Naeem, U.; Abdalla, H.; Turner, D.L. High-Frequency Intermuscular Coherence between Arm Muscles during Robot-Mediated Motor Adaptation. *Front. Physiol. Front. Physiol.* **2017**, *7*, 668. [CrossRef] [PubMed]
35. Wang, L.; Lu, A.; Zhang, S.; Niu, W.; Zheng, F.; Gong, M. Fatigue-related electromyographic coherence and phase synchronization analysis between antagonistic elbow muscles. *Exp. Brain Res.* **2015**, *233*, 971–982. [CrossRef]
36. van Asseldonk, E.H.; Campfens, S.F.; Verwer, S.J.; van Putten, M.J.; Stegeman, D.F. Reliability and agreement of intramuscular coherence in tibialis anterior muscle. *PLoS ONE* **2014**, *9*, e88428. [CrossRef] [PubMed]
37. Masakado, Y.; Ushiyama, J.; Katsu, M.; Kimura, A.; Liu, M.; Ushiba, J.; Yokohama, J. Muscle fatigue-induced enhancement of corticomuscular coherence following sustained submaximal isometric contraction of the tibialis anterior muscle. *NSR Neurosci. Res.* **2011**, *71*, e347. [CrossRef]
38. Mima, T.; Steger, J.; Schulman, A.E.; Gerloff, C.; Hallett, M. Electroencephalographic measurement of motor cortex control of muscle activity in humans. *Clin. Neurophysiol.* **2000**, *111*, 326–337. [CrossRef]
39. Bazzucchi, I.; Riccio, M.E.; Felici, F. Tennis players show a lower coactivation of the elbow antagonist muscles during isokinetic exercises. *J. Electromyogr. Kinesiol.* **2008**, *18*, 752–759. [CrossRef]
40. Bazzucchi, I.; Sbriccoli, P.; Marzattinocci, G.; Felici, F. Coactivation of the elbow antagonist muscles is not affected by the speed of movement in isokinetic exercise. *Muscle Nerve Off. J. Am. Assoc. Electrodiagn. Med.* **2006**, *33*, 191–199. [CrossRef]
41. Darainy, M.; Ostry, D.J. Muscle cocontraction following dynamics learning. *Exp. Brain Res.* **2008**, *190*, 153–163. [CrossRef]
42. Wagner, H.; Pfusterschmied, J.; Tilp, M.; Landlinger, J.; von Duvillard, S.P.; Muller, E. Upper-body kinematics in team-handball throw, tennis serve, and volleyball spike. *Scand. J. Med. Sci. Sports* **2014**, *24*, 345–354. [CrossRef] [PubMed]
43. Pincivero, D.M.; Polen, R.R.; Byrd, B.N. Contraction mode and intensity effects on elbow antagonist muscle co-activation. *J. Electromyogr. Kinesiol.* **2019**, *44*, 101–107. [CrossRef] [PubMed]

Article

The Impact of Physical Performance on Functional Movement Screen Scores and Asymmetries in Female University Physical Education Students

Dawid Koźlenia *[ID] and Jarosław Domaradzki [ID]

Department of Biostructure, Faculty of Physical Education & Sport, University School of Physical Education in Wroclaw, al. I.J. Paderewskiego 35, 51-612 Wroclaw, Poland; jaroslaw.domaradzki@awf.wroc.pl
* Correspondence: dawid.kozlenia@awf.wroc.pl

Abstract: Association between physical performance and movement quality remains ambiguous. However, both affect injury risk. Furthermore, existing research rarely regards women. Therefore, this study aimed to assess the impact of physical performance components on FMS scores and asymmetries among young women—University Physical Education Students. The study sample was 101 women, 21.72 ± 1.57 years, body mass index 21.52 ± 2.49 [kg/m^2]. The FMS test was conducted to assess the movement patterns quality. Physical performance tests were done to evaluate strength, power, flexibility. Flexibility has the strongest correlation with FMS overall (r = 0.25, p = 0.0130) and single tasks scores. A higher level of flexibility and strength of abdominal muscles are associated with fewer asymmetries (r = −0.31, p = 0.0018; r = −0.27, p = 0.0057, respectively). However, the main findings determine that flexibility has the strongest and statistically significant impact on FMS overall (ß = 0.25, p = 0.0106) and asymmetries (ß = −0.30, p = 0.0014). Additionally, a significant effect of abdominal muscles strength on FMS asymmetries were observed (ß = −0.29, p = 0.0027). Flexibility and abdominal muscles strength have the most decisive impact on movement patterns quality. These results suggest possibilities for shaping FMS scores in young women.

Keywords: movement quality; physical performance; strength; power; flexibility; women; physical activity

1. Introduction

The physical performance and movement patterns quality affect injury risk [1,2]. Physical performance is defined as a body function that an appropriate test can objectively measure. It is a multidimensional concept which involves musculoskeletal system function, cardiorespiratory and nervous system. Physical performance is expressed by a level of single components such as strength, flexibility, speed, or endurance. [3,4]. Movement patterns quality is mainly examined by the FMS test, which detects dysfunctional movement patterns [5]. The relationships between the quality of movement patterns and physical performance components have been investigated. However, these associations have not been clearly defined. The studies published so far have focused mainly on men and mixed groups. Therefore, it is needed to establish these associations among women.

The tool for assessing the quality of the movement patterns is the Functional Movement Screen (FMS), which allows for a comprehensive evaluation of the functional state of the movement apparatus and to identify dysfunctional movement and differences in paired tests to identify asymmetries [5]. Numerous studies have indicated associations of low FMS scores with more injuries among men and women as well [6–9] and the possibility of injury prediction based on FMS score [10]. Mokha et al. [9] and Chalmers et al. [11] also demonstrated the relationship between asymmetries in the FMS test and injuries, studying young athletes. However, these results should be treated with some caution. In a replication study by Chalmers et al. [12], no similar links were observed.

The attempts to determine the relationship between the quality of movement patterns and physical performance components indicate their existence [13]. However, the direction and strength of these relationships are unclear. Especially possible associations remain ambiguous among women due to a low number of studies regarding females. Parchmann and McBridge [14], in a mixed group, and Lockie et al. [15] among female team sports athletes, did not show any links between the quality of the movement patterns, speed, and agility. These reports are opposed to Koźlenia et al. [16], who showed that better quality of the movement patterns is associated with better speed and agility tests outcomes among men. Support for these results can be found in the studies by Campa et al. [17]. Chang et al. [18] indicated the relationship between a trunk stability push-up with agility t-test result. Sannicandro et al. [19] showed a connection between the FMS score and the power of the lower limbs among professional footballers, showing that better quality of movement patterns was associated with greater power of the lower limbs. Chimera et al. [20] established strong relationships between flexibility and the trunk muscles' strength with movement patterns quality. Similar observations also provide studies by Silva et al. [21,22] which showed the strength of the trunk muscles as a factor determining the quality of the movement patterns. However, the studies mentioned above [14,16–22] regard men and mixed groups, not focusing only on women and possible sex differences in associations between FMS score and asymmetries with physical performance components. However, Kibler et al. [23] proved that women are characterized by greater flexibility compared to men, who, in turn, have greater strength than women. The above observations could translate into relationships between the results of physical performance tests and the movement patterns quality and cause the sex differences in the single motor tasks scores in the FMS test described by Schneiders et al. [24]. They showed that men performed better than women in the trunk stability push-up (TSPU) and rotary stability (RS). Miller and Susa [25] noted a similar observation.

In the light of this observation, there is a need to keep in mind that physical performance and movement quality have an influence on injury risk [1,2]. Therefore, their interconnectedness should be explored. However, published studies mostly regard men and mixed groups in the literature, not only on women. Thus, this study aims to assess the impact of physical performance components on FMS scores and FMS asymmetries among young women—University Physical Education Students. Specifically, it was also examined the simple association between physical performance tests and FMS scores. These observations let to described which physical performance components are crucial to improving the quality of movement patterns, what can positively affect physical fitness and reduce injury risk.

2. Materials and Methods

2.1. Study Sample

The study sample consisted of 101 young adult women whose average age was 21.72 ± 1.57 years. All subjects were volunteers recruited from students at the University School of Physical Education in Wroclaw, Faculty of Physical Education and Sport. The average body weight was 60.54 ± 9.05 [kg], body height 1.68 ± 0.07 [m], and body mass index 21.52 ± 2.49 [kg/m^2]. Subjects averagely declared 5.04 ± 3.56 h per week of physical activity. The inclusion criteria were no injuries before six weeks of the start of the study and no other medical contradiction for physical activity. All participants were fully informed about the purpose, type, research methodology, and participation conditions. They could withdraw from the research at any time without giving any reason.

2.2. Measurements

We followed the methods described in the study by Koźlenia and Domaradzki [2]. Participants were informed to avoid any physical activity directly before the measurements and tests. The measurements were performed in the Biokinetics Research Laboratory of the University School of Physical Education in Wroclaw (Quality Management System Certificate PN-EN ISO 9001: 2009; No. PW-48606-10E).

A SECA model 764 height and weight measuring device (SECA manufactured, Hamburg, Germany. Quality control number C-2070) was used to measure body height and weight. Based on the obtained values, the index of relative body mass BMI (kg/m^2) was calculated according to the formula: BMI = body weight [kg]/body height [m^2].

The quality of the movement patterns was assessed using the Functional Movement Screen (FMS). The FMS test is a battery of seven movement tasks that make up the entire test: Deep Squat (DS), Hurdle Step (HS), (In-Line Lunge (IN-L), Shoulder Mobility (SM), Active Straight Leg Raise (ASLR), Trunk Stability Push-up (TSPU), Rotary Stability (RS). The tests were performed with a standard FMS kit (Functional Movement Systems, Inc, Chatham, MA, USA). According to Cook et al. [5], no warm-up directly before the test was performed. Single motor tasks are rated on a scale of 0 to 3 according to clear guidelines described for each test [5]. The maximum score is 21 points. From 14 points and below, the risk of injury increases significantly [26].

Handgrip strength of the upper limbs was examined using a hydraulic dynamometer with an adjustable handle SAEHAN SH5001 (Saehan Corporation, Masan, South Korea). The measurements were done with an accuracy of 1 kg. The subject keeps his arm lowered so that the upper limb does not touch the body. Holding the dynamometer tightly their hand, hand clenching was performed with maximum force for about 2 s. Two attempts were made for each limb. The best result on both limbs was considered.

A long jump test was used to assess lower limbs power. From two made attempts, the better result was considered. Jump length was measured from the back of the heels. The measurement was performed with an accuracy of 0.5 cm. The subject performed the test from the established line, made a jump from both lower limbs with a swing of the upper limbs landing on both legs.

The strength of the abdominal muscles was tested with the sit-ups test. The test consists of making as many sit-ups as possible within 30 s. One attempt was made. The subject was laid down with the lower limbs bent at the knee joints at an angle of 90°. The feet were blocked. The subject began the test by lying down with her hands clasped behind the nape of her neck, performing torso bends and touching knees with elbows.

Flexibility was measured using the sit-and-reach test. The measurement was performed with an accuracy of 0.5 cm. The examined person sat down with the lower limbs straightened in the knee joints by placing feet against the sidewall of the table. While maintaining the extension in the knee joints, the subject bent forward and tried to move the ruler on the table as far as possible along the scale. The tests scores were measured from the 0 cm point. The measurement was performed with an accuracy of 0.5 cm. Of the two trials, the better result was considered.

2.3. Statistics

The means, standard deviations, and confidence intervals were calculated for the data meeting the assumptions of normality of the distribution or the median, and standard errors for the data that did not meet the assumptions of the normal distribution. Spearman's rank correlation was calculated to investigate the strength and direction of relationships between the quality of the movement patterns (FMS scores) and physical performance tests. Multiple regression was used to determine the impact of the physical performance components on FMS overall and asymmetries. The significance level $\alpha = 0.05$. Statistica v13.3 from Statsoft Polska (Cracow, Poland) was used for statistical analyses.

3. Results

Table 1 includes descriptive statistics for physical performance tests results.

Table 1. Physical performance tests results.

Variable	Mean	SD	CI −95%	CI +95%
Hand grip (N/kg)	36.11	5.93	34.94	37.28
Long jump (cm)	179.42	31.08	173.28	185.55
Sit-ups (reps/30 s)	24.23	4.66	23.31	25.15
Sit and reach (cm)	13.67	7.37	12.21	15.12

Table 2 shows the FMS overall score, single tasks score, and asymmetries numbers in the bilateral test. The mean FMS overall score is 14.96 ± 2.21, and a median of 15 points indicates the study sample has high-quality movement patterns.

Table 2. Characteristics of the FMS scores.

Variable	Median	SE
FMS	15	0.22
DS	2	0.07
HS	2	0.06
IN-L	2	0.07
SM	3	0.09
ASLR	3	0.06
TSPU	2	0.08
RS	2	0.05
HS A	0	0.04
IN-L A	0	0.04
SM A	0	0.05
ASLR A	0	0.04
RS A	0	0.02
FMS Asymmetries	1	0.09

Abbreviations: FMS—overall score; DS—deep squat; HS—hurdle step; HS A—hurdle step-asymmetry; IN-L—in-line lunge; IN-L A—in-line lunge-asymmetry; SM—shoulder mobility; SM A—shoulder mobility-asymmetry; ASLR—active straight leg raise; ASLR—active straight leg raise-asymmetry; TSPU—trunk stability push-up; RS—rotary stability—overall; RS A—rotary stability-asymmetry.

Spearman's correlation for FMS overall, single tasks score, and asymmetries number revealed the higher sit-and-reach test result is associated with the better FMS overall r = 0.25, p = 0.2130 and lower number of FMS asymmetries r = −0.31, p = 0.0018, better hurdle step score (HS) r = 0.21, p = 0.0357, shoulder mobility score (SM) r = 0.34, p = 0.0133, and asymmetries r = −0.23, p = 0.2010, active straight leg raise score r = 0.50, p > 0.0001 and asymmetries r = −0.27, p = 0.0055. Additionally, the higher sit-ups test results were associated with the lower number of FMS asymmetries r = −0.27, p = 0.0057, and in-line lunge asymmetries r−0.25, p = 0.0126. No other statistically significant correlation was observed.

The multiple regression model for FMS overall is presented in Figure 1. The model is statistically significant, p < 0.0406.

Multiple regression results for FMS overall score are included in Table 3. Flexibility had the strongest statistically significant impact on FMS overall ß = 0.25, p = 0.0206. An increase in the sit-and-reach test score by 1 cm is associated with improving FMS overall score by 0.08 points.

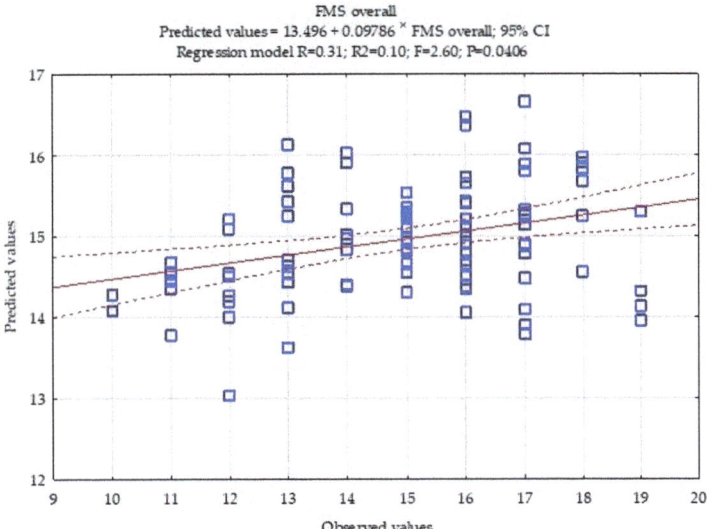

Figure 1. Multiple regression model for FMS overall score.

Table 3. Multiple regression results for FMS overall score.

Dependent Variable	Independent Variables	ß	ß SE	B	b SE	t	p
FMS overall	Hand grip (N/kg)	0.11	0.10	0.04	0.04	1.08	0.2811
	Long jump (cm)	0.09	0.10	0.01	0.01	0.89	0.3781
	Sit-ups (reps/30 s)	0.15	0.10	0.07	0.05	1.49	0.1395
	Sit and reach (cm)	0.25	0.10	0.08	0.03	2.61	0.0106

The multiple regression model for FMS asymmetries is presented in Figure 2. The model is statistically significant, $p < 0.0005$.

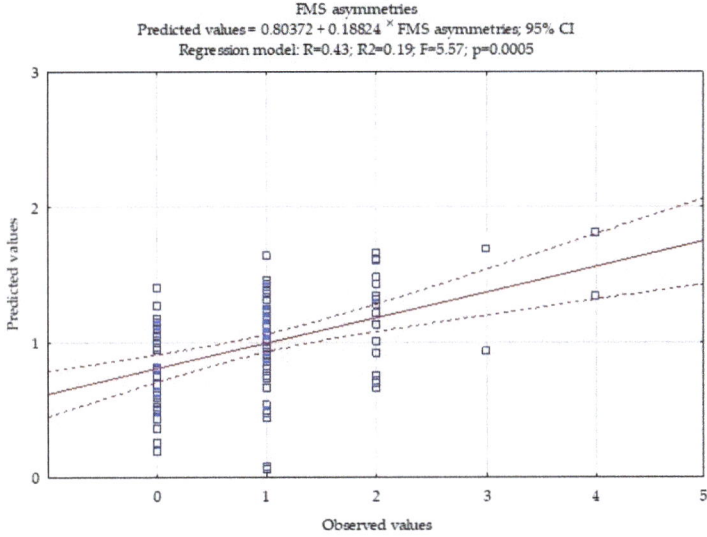

Figure 2. Multiple regression model for FMS asymmetries number.

Multiple regression results for FMS asymmetries numbers are included in Table 4. Flexibility had the strongest statistically significant impact on FMS asymmetries ß = −0.30, $p = 0.0014$. Additionally, FMS asymmetries depend on abdominal muscles strength ß = −0.29, $p = 0.0027$. An increase in the sit-and-reach test score by 1 cm is associated with reducing asymmetries by 0.04. An increase in the sit-ups test by one rep reduces FMS asymmetries number by 0.05.

Table 4. Multiple regression results for FMS asymmetries number.

Dependent Variable	Independent Variables	ß	ß SE	B	b SE	t	p
FMS asymmetries	Hand grip (N/kg)	0.04	0.09	0.01	0.01	0.42	0.6739
	Long jump (cm)	0.01	0.09	0.00	0.00	0.06	0.9553
	Sit-ups (reps/30 s)	−0.29	0.09	−0.05	0.02	−3.08	0.0027
	Sit and reach (cm)	−0.30	0.09	−0.04	0.01	−3.29	0.0014

4. Discussion

The quality of movement patterns and the level of physical performance affect the risk of injury, which raises further questions about their relationship [1,2]. There have been attempts in the literature to answer this type of ambiguity. However, some differences in observation do not allow clear conclusions on this matter, especially considering women due to the low number of studies among females.

Our results showed that flexibility and abdominal muscle strength have an influence on movement patterns quality among young women. The strength of abdominal muscles is crucial in trunk stability, whereas a good level of flexibility aids the optimal range of motion in joints [27,28]. Both mentioned physical performance components allow movement without restrictions in joints with simultaneous stabilization in various body positions, thus avoiding compensations that disturb the movement patterns. [29]. Our results confirm this approach that is supported by the literature which provides related observations [20–22].

Most researchers agree that sex is not a factor that differentiates the overall score of the FMS test within one research group. Schneiders et al. [24] and Miller and Susa [25] did not show a statistically significant difference in the mean FMS score between physically active men and women. On the other hand, diversity can be seen in comparisons between groups from different research studies. The type of physical activity may explain the differences in FMS scores between groups from other studies. This can be seen when comparing the FMS scores results among various sports groups (e.g., footballers [30], volleyball players [31], or runners [8]). The quality of movement patterns can be shaped by appropriate training [32,33].

In the case of assessments of the FMS single motor tasks, sex differences are observed. It was shown that men performed better in a test that required stability and strength (TSPU and RS), whereas women achieved higher scores in a mobility test (SM and ASLR) [24]. A study by Miller and Susa [25] confirms this observation, which indicated that women achieved better results in shoulder mobility (SM) and active straight leg raises (ASLR), while men had higher scores in the trunk stability push-up (TSPU) and in-line lunge (IL-L). Anderson et al. [34] also indicated that women performed a weaker trunk stability push-up (TSPU). Similar observations were made in the study by Chimera et al. [20]. Women achieved better results in tasks requiring flexibility, active straight leg raise (ASLR), and shoulder mobility (SM), whereas men achieved better results than women in trunk stability push-up (TSPU) and rotary stability (RS). These results indicate that, despite averagely comparable results in FMS overall score between sexes, its structure could be differentiated by scores in single tasks. It could be associated with sex differences in physical performance [23]. Therefore, it suggests a need to consider sex differences in targeting the development of physical performance to improve movement quality.

The median value of the FMS overall score of our study sample was 15, indicating high-quality movement patterns associated with low injury risk [26]. Literature shows that high-quality movement patterns characterize young, physically active women. Chimera et al. [6] revealed that female athletes' average FMS overall score was above 14 points. A similar observation was added by Anderson et al. [34], which showed the mean FMS score among females was above 15. Our study sample performed better in the standing long jump than nonathletes females [35]. In the case of the sit-and-reach test, our study sample achieved comparable results to the female athletes from the study by Lopez-Minaro et al. [36]. In the handgrip test and 30 s sit-ups test, our study sample achieved better results than average populations [37,38].

Analyzing the relationship between the quality of movement patterns and physical performance components indicates a high, statically significant correlation between the sit-and-reach test score (flexibility), the FMS overall, and the FMS asymmetries number. The association in single tasks score was observed as an active straight leg raise (ASLR), shoulder mobility (SM), and asymmetries in these tests. A better result in the sit-and-reach test score was also associated with a better hurdle step (HS) score. Additionally, a higher level of flexibility related to a lower number of asymmetries was also observed in better results in the sit-ups test, suggesting that strong abdominal muscles are essential in maintaining functional symmetry. Other physical performance tests showed low and statistically insignificant correlations, suggesting no linear correlation between physical performance tests, such as handgrip or long jump, and the FMS scores. Similar observations were noted in other studies, especially regarding the relationship between flexibility and the quality of movement patterns. However, literature has limited observations considering the association between movement quality and FMS scores with physical performance components such as flexibility or strength. Therefore, it is hard to refer our results to only female groups. Some references must be made to mixed and male groups. Grygorowicz et al. [39] observed that female soccer players have better quality of movement patterns with a higher level of flexibility, which confirms our observations. Glass et al. [40] showed associations between the higher level of strength, balance, and flexibility with the quality of the movement patterns. In mixed groups, Jenkins et al. [41] observed that a better range of hip joint motion was associated with higher quality of movement patterns. Similarly, Yildiz et al. [42] indicated improved FMS scores and flexibility among children during tennis training after using a training intervention. Song et al. [43] noted that flexibility development was associated with improved FMS scores in males. In a study of male baseball players, Liang et al. [44] showed associations of FMS scores with the flexibility of the rectus femoris and speed abilities. Chimera et al. [20] showed that worse ranges of motion in the hip and knee joints negatively affect the movement patterns quality in a mixed study sample. The same authors [18] also observed that stronger trunk muscles positively influenced the FMS scores. Surprisingly, in our research, a higher score in trunk stability push-up (TSPU) was not directly associated with a better result of the sit-ups, whereas the study by Silva et al. [20,21] found links between the trunk stability push-up (TSPU) and the physical fitness of the study group. However, handgrip strength and the FMS scores do not seem to have clear connections [20]. Sannicandro et al. [19] indicated that footballers presented better quality movement patterns that generated greater lower limb power. Willigenburg and Hewett [45] observed correlations between the length of the long jump and the overall FMS score among American football players. In our study, a correlation between the long jump test score and the FMS overall and the deep squat (DS) score was not observed in women. The conclusions drawn from the above observations indicate a clear relationship between the quality of movement patterns and physical performance components. The single motor tasks of the FMS test are specifically related to the level of selected physical performance components. In this type of analysis, there is a need to consider the possible differences between sexes. However, our study shows that flexibility has the most decisive impact on the FMS overall score among female students.

Our analysis also showed that the number of asymmetries observed during the FMS test is related to flexibility and abdominal muscle strength, indicating these factors' significant role in shaping symmetrical movement patterns. However, the literature so far does not pay much attention to the number of FMS asymmetries concerning the level of physical fitness. Athletes with a higher number of asymmetries are 1.8 times more likely to be injured [46]. Similar observations are made by Mokha et al. [9], which also indicated a significant risk of injury due to asymmetries. Considering the relationship between flexibility and muscle strength and the risk of injury [47,48], the importance of these abilities as a key to developing high-quality movement patterns is growing.

5. Conclusions

In young, healthy women, flexibility and abdominal muscles strength are significantly associated with the quality of movement patterns, expressed as an FMS overall score and FMS asymmetries. Furthermore, flexibility is a component of physical performance with the most decisive impact on movement patterns quality in FMS overall score and asymmetries number, whereas abdominal muscle strength only influences on asymmetries in FMS. Our results indicate the importance of flexibility and abdominal muscle strength for movement patterns quality among young women. The appropriate range of motion in joints with abdominal muscle strength that provides trunk stability helps to avoid compensation in movement. It potentially suggests that FMS scores can be shaped throughout the development of flexibility and abdominal muscle strength. However, further studies need to verify if developing these abilities improves movement patterns quality in young women.

We are aware that our study has some limitations. The analysis could be augmented with more physical performance tests measuring other abilities, such as speed and endurance. It is also worth analyzing how the type of physical activity undertaken affects the relationship between the quality of movement patterns and physical performance. These aspects should be considered in further studies.

Author Contributions: Conceptualization, D.K.; methodology, D.K., J.D.; software, J.D.; validation, D.K., J.D.; formal analysis, J.D.; investigation, D.K.; resources, D.K., J.D.; data curation, J.D.; writing—original draft preparation, D.K., J.D.; writing—review and editing, D.K., J.D.; visualization, D.K.; supervision, J.D.; project administration, D.K.; funding acquisition, D.K. All authors have read and agreed to the published version of the manuscript.

Funding: This research received no external funding.

Institutional Review Board Statement: The study was conducted according to the guidelines of the Declaration of Helsinki and approved by the Senate Research Ethics Committee at the University School of Physical Education in Wrocław (ECUPE No. 16/2018; approved on 1 March 2018).

Informed Consent Statement: Informed consent was obtained from all subjects involved in the study.

Data Availability Statement: The datasets used and analyzed during the current study are available from the corresponding author on reasonable request.

Conflicts of Interest: The authors declare no conflict of interest.

References

1. Lisman, P.; O'Connor, F.G.; Deuster, P.A.; Knapik, J.J. Functional movement screen and aerobic fitness predict injuries in military training. *Med. Sci. Sports Exerc.* **2013**, *45*, 636–643. [CrossRef]
2. Koźlenia, D.; Domaradzki, J. Effects of Combination Movement Patterns Quality and Physical Performance on Injuries in Young Athletes. *Int. J. Environ. Res. Public Health* **2021**, *18*, 5536. [CrossRef]
3. van Lummel, R.C.; Walgaard, S.; Pijnappels, M.; Elders, P.J.M.; Garcia-Aymerich, J.; van Dieën, J.H.; Beek, P.J. Physical Performance and Physical Activity in Older Adults: Associated but Separate Domains of Physical Function in Old Age. *PLoS ONE* **2015**, *10*, e0144048. [CrossRef] [PubMed]
4. Beaudart, C.; Rolland, Y.; Cruz-Jentoft, A.J.; Bauer, J.M.; Sieber, C.; Cooper, C.; Al-Daghri, N.; Araujo de Carvalho, I.; Bautmans, I.; Bernabei, R.; et al. Assessment of Muscle Function and Physical Performance in Daily Clinical Practice: A Position Paper Endorsed by the European Society for Clinical and Economic Aspects of Osteoporosis, Osteoarthritis and Musculoskeletal Diseases (ESCEO). *Calcif. Tissue Int.* **2019**, *105*, 1–14. [CrossRef] [PubMed]

5. Cook, G.; Burton, L.; Kiesel, K.; Rose, G.; Brynt, M.F. *Movement: Functional Movement Systems: Screening, Assessment, Corrective Strategies*; On Target Publications; Aptos: Santa Cruz, CA, USA, 2010.
6. Chorba, R.S.; Chorba, D.J.; Bouillon, L.E.; Overmyer, C.A.; Landis, J.A. Use of a Functional Movement Screening Tool to Determine Injury Risk in Female Collegiate Athletes. *N. Am. J. Sports Phys. Ther.* **2010**, *5*, 47–54. [PubMed]
7. Chimera, N.J.; Craig, A.; Smith, C.A.; Warren, M. Injury History, Sex, and Performance on the Functional Movement Screen and Y Balance Test. *J. Athl. Train.* **2015**, *50*, 475–485. [CrossRef] [PubMed]
8. Hotta, T.; Nishiguchi, S.; Fukutani, N.; Tashiro, Y.; Adachi, D.; Morino, S.; Shirooka, H.; Nozaki, Y.; Hirata, H.; Yamaguchi, M.; et al. Functional Movement Screen for Predicting Running Injuries in 18- to 24-Year-Old Competitive Male Runners. *J. Strength Cond. Res.* **2015**, *29*, 2808–2815. [CrossRef] [PubMed]
9. Mokha, M.; Sprague, P.A.; Gatens, D.R. Predicting Musculoskeletal Injury in National Collegiate Athletic Association Division II Athletes From Asymmetries and Individual-Test Versus Composite Functional Movement Screen Scores. *J. Athl. Train.* **2016**, *51*, 276–282. [CrossRef]
10. Kozlenia, D.; Domaradzki, J. Prediction and Injury Risk Based on Movement Patterns and Flexibility in a 6-Month Prospective Study among Physically Active Adults. *PeerJ* **2021**, *9*, e11399. [CrossRef]
11. Chalmers, S.; Fuller, J.T.; Debenedictis, T.A.; Townsley, S.; Lynagh, M.; Gleeson, C.; Zacharia, A.; Thomson, S.; Magarey, M. Asymmetry during Preseason Functional Movement Screen Testing Is Associated with Injury during a Junior Australian Football Season. *J. Sci. Med. Sport* **2017**, *20*, 653–657. [CrossRef]
12. Chalmers, S.; Debenedictis, T.A.; Zacharia, A.; Townsley, S.; Gleeson, C.; Lynagh, M.; Townsley, A.; Fuller, J.T. Asymmetry during Functional Movement Screening and Injury Risk in Junior Football Players: A Replication Study. *Scand. J. Med. Sci. Sports* **2018**, *28*, 1281–1287. [CrossRef]
13. Parsonage, J.R.; Williams, R.S.; Rainer, P.; McKeown, I.; Williams, M.D. Assessment of Conditioning-Specific Movement Tasks and Physical Fitness Measures in Talent Identified under 16-Year-Old Rugby Union Players. *J. Strength Cond. Res.* **2014**, *28*, 1497–1506. [CrossRef]
14. Parchmann, C.J.; McBride, J.M. Relationship between Functional Movement Screen and Athletic Performance. *J. Strength Cond. Res.* **2011**, *25*, 3378–3384. [CrossRef] [PubMed]
15. Lockie, R.; Schultz, A.; Callaghan, S.; Jordan, C.; Luczo, T.; Jeffriess, M. A Preliminary Investigation into the Relationship between Functional Movement Screen Scores and Athletic Physical Performance in Female Team Sport Athletes. *Biol. Sport* **2015**, *32*, 41–51. [CrossRef]
16. Koźlenia, D.; Domaradzki, J.; Trojanowska, I.; Czermak, P. Association between speed and agility abilities with movement patterns quality in team sports players. *Med. Dello Sport* **2020**, *73*, 176–186.
17. Campa, F.; Semprini, G.; Júdice, P.B.; Messina, G.; Toselli, S. Anthropometry, Physical and Movement Features, and Repeatedsprint Ability in Soccer Players. *Int. J. Sports Med.* **2019**, *40*, 100–109. [CrossRef] [PubMed]
18. Chang, W.-D.; Chou, L.-W.; Chang, N.-J.; Chen, S. Comparison of Functional Movement Screen, Star Excursion Balance Test, and Physical Fitness in Junior Athletes with Different Sports Injury Risk. *Biomed. Res. Int.* **2020**, *2020*, 8690540. [CrossRef] [PubMed]
19. Sannicandro, I.; Cofano, G.; Rosa, A.R.; Traficante, P.; Piccinno, A. Functional movement screen and lower limb strength asymmetry in professional soccer players. *Br. J. Sports Med.* **2017**, *51*, 381. [CrossRef]
20. Chimera, N.J.; Knoeller, S.; Cooper, R.; Nicholas, K.; Smith, C.; Warren, M. Prediction of functional movement screen™ performance from lower extremity range of motion and core tests. *Int. J. Sports Phys. Ther.* **2017**, *12*, 173–181.
21. Silva, B.; Clemente, F.M.; Martins, F.M. Associations between Functional Movement Screen Scores and Performance Variables in Surf Athletes. *J. Sports Med. Phys. Fit.* **2018**, *58*, 583–590. [CrossRef]
22. Silva, B.; Rodrigues, L.P.; Clemente, F.M.; Cancela, J.M.; Bezerra, P. Association between motor competence and Functional Movement Screen scores. *PeerJ* **2019**, *7*, e7270. [CrossRef] [PubMed]
23. Kibler, W.B.; Chandler, T.J.; Uhl, T.; Maddux, R.E. A Musculoskeletal Approach to the Preparticipation Physical Examination. Preventing Injury and Improving Performance. *Am. J. Sports Med.* **1989**, *17*, 525–531. [CrossRef] [PubMed]
24. Schneiders, A.G.; Davidsson, A.; Hörman, E.; Sullivan, S.J. Functional Movement Screen Normative Values in a Young, Active Population. *Int. J. Sports Phys. Ther.* **2011**, *6*, 75–82.
25. Miller, J.M.; Susa, K.J. Functional Movement Screen Scores in a Group of Division IA Athletes. *J. Sports Med. Phys. Fit.* **2019**, *59*, 779–783. [CrossRef]
26. Kiesel, K.; Plisky, P.J.; Voight, M.L. Can Serious Injury in Professional Football Be Predicted by a Preseason Functional Movement Screen? *N. Am. J. Sports Phys. Ther.* **2007**, *2*, 147–158.
27. Childs, J.D.; Teyhen, D.S.; Casey, P.R.; McCoy-Singh, K.A.; Feldtmann, A.W.; Wright, A.C.; Dugan, J.L.; Wu, S.S.; George, S.Z. Effects of Traditional Sit-up Training versus Core Stabilization Exercises on Short-Term Musculoskeletal Injuries in US Army Soldiers: A Cluster Randomized Trial. *Phys. Ther.* **2010**, *90*, 1404–1412. [CrossRef]
28. Witvrouw, E.; Danneels, L.; Asselman, P.; D'Have, T.; Cambier, D. Muscle Flexibility as a Risk Factor for Developing Muscle Injuries in Male Professional Soccer Players. A Prospective Study. *Am. J. Sports Med.* **2003**, *31*, 41–46. [CrossRef] [PubMed]
29. Sahrmann, S. *Diagnosis and Treatment of Movement Impairment Syndromes*; Elsevier Mosby: Saint Louis, MO, USA, 2001.
30. Marques, V.B.; Medeiros, T.M.; de Souza Stigger, F.; Nakamura, F.Y.; Baroni, B.M. The functional movement screen (FMS™) in elite young soccer players between 14 and 20 years: Composite score, individual-test scores and asymmetries. *Int. J. Sports Phys. Ther.* **2017**, *12*, 977–985. [CrossRef]

31. Linek, P.; Saulicz, E.; Myśliwiec, A.; Wójtowicz, M.; Wolny, T. The Effect of Specific Sling Exercises on the Functional Movement Screen Score in Adolescent Volleyball Players: A Preliminary Study. *J. Hum. Kinet.* **2016**, *54*, 83–90. [CrossRef]
32. Kiesel, K.; Plisky, P.; Butler, R. Functional Movement Test Scores Improve Following a Standardized Off-Season Intervention Program in Professional Football Players. *Scand. J. Med. Sci. Sports* **2011**, *21*, 287–292. [CrossRef]
33. Bodden, J.G.; Needham, R.A.; Chockalingam, N. The Effect of an Intervention Program on Functional Movement Screen Test Scores in Mixed Martial Arts Athletes. *J. Strength Cond. Res.* **2015**, *29*, 219–225. [CrossRef] [PubMed]
34. Anderson, B.E.; Neumann, M.L.; Huxel Bliven, K.C. Functional Movement Screen Differences between Male and Female Secondary School Athletes. *J. Strength Cond. Res.* **2015**, *29*, 1098–1106. [CrossRef] [PubMed]
35. Koch, A.J.; O'Bryant, H.S.; Stone, M.E.; Sanborn, K.; Proulx, C.; Hruby, J.; Shannonhouse, E.; Boros, R.; Stone, M.H. Effect of Warm-up on the Standing Broad Jump in Trained and Untrained Men and Women. *J. Strength Cond. Res.* **2003**, *17*, 710–714. [CrossRef] [PubMed]
36. López-Miñarro, P.A.; Andújar, P.S.d.B.; Rodrňguez-Garcña, P.L. A Comparison of the Sit-and-Reach Test and the Back-Saver Sit-and-Reach Test in University Students. *J. Sports Sci. Med.* **2009**, *8*, 116–122.
37. Massy-Westropp, N.M.; Gill, T.K.; Taylor, A.W.; Bohannon, R.W.; Hill, C.L. Hand Grip Strength: Age and Gender Stratified Normative Data in a Population-Based Study. *BMC Res. Notes* **2011**, *4*, 127. [CrossRef]
38. Kordi, M.; Fallahi, A.; Sangari, M. Health-Related Physical Fitness and Normative Data in Healthy Women, Tehran, Iran. *Iran J. Public Health* **2010**, *39*, 87–101.
39. Grygorowicz, M.; Piontek, T.; Dudzinski, W. Evaluation of Functional Limitations in Female Soccer Players and Their Relationship with Sports Level–a Cross Sectional Study. *PLoS ONE* **2013**, *8*, e66871. [CrossRef]
40. Glass, S.M.; Schmitz, R.J.; Rhea, C.K.; Ross, S.E. Potential Mediators of Load-Related Decreases in Movement Quality in Young, Healthy Adults. *J. Athl. Train.* **2019**, *54*, 81–89. [CrossRef]
41. Jenkins, M.T.; Gustitus, R.; Iosia, M.; Kicklighter, T.; Sasaki, Y. Correlation between the Functional Movement Screen and Hip Mobility in NCAA Division II Athletes. *Int. J. Exerc. Sci.* **2017**, *10*, 541–549.
42. Yildiz, S.; Pinar, S.; Gelen, E. Effects of 8-Week Functional vs. Traditional Training on Athletic Performance and Functional Movement on Prepubertal Tennis Players. *J. Strength Cond. Res.* **2019**, *33*, 651–661. [CrossRef]
43. Song, H.-S.; Woo, S.-S.; So, W.-Y.; Kim, K.-J.; Lee, J.; Kim, J.-Y. Effects of 16-Week Functional Movement Screen Training Program on Strength and Flexibility of Elite High School Baseball Players. *J. Exerc. Rehabil.* **2014**, *10*, 124–130. [CrossRef]
44. Liang, Y.-P.; Kuo, Y.-L.; Hsu, H.-C.; Hsia, Y.-Y.; Hsu, Y.-W.; Tsai, Y.-J. Collegiate Baseball Players with More Optimal Functional Movement Patterns Demonstrate Better Athletic Performance in Speed and Agility. *J. Sports Sci.* **2019**, *37*, 544–552. [CrossRef] [PubMed]
45. Willigenburg, N.; Hewett, T.E. Performance on the Functional Movement Screen Is Related to Hop Performance But Not to Hip and Knee Strength in Collegiate Football Players. *Clin. J. Sport Med.* **2017**, *27*, 119–126. [CrossRef] [PubMed]
46. Kiesel, K.B.; Butler, R.J.; Plisky, P.J. Prediction of Injury by Limited and Asymmetrical Fundamental Movement Patterns in American Football Players. *J. Sport Rehabil.* **2014**, *23*, 88–94. [CrossRef]
47. de la Motte, S.J.; Gribbin, T.C.; Lisman, P.; Murphy, K.; Deuster, P.A. Systematic Review of the Association Between Physical Fitness and Musculoskeletal Injury Risk: Part 2-Muscular Endurance and Muscular Strength. *J. Strength Cond. Res.* **2017**, *31*, 3218–3234. [CrossRef]
48. de la Motte, S.J.; Lisman, P.; Gribbin, T.C.; Murphy, K.; Deuster, P.A. Systematic Review of the Association Between Physical Fitness and Musculoskeletal Injury Risk: Part 3-Flexibility, Power, Speed, Balance, and Agility. *J. Strength Cond. Res.* **2019**, *33*, 1723–1735. [CrossRef] [PubMed]

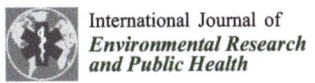

Article

Impact of Rowing Training on Quality of Life and Physical Activity Levels in Female Breast Cancer Survivors

Juan Gavala-González [1,2], Amanda Torres-Pérez [2,3,*] and José Carlos Fernández-García [2,3]

1. Department of Physical Education and Sports, University of Seville, 41013 Seville, Spain; jgavala@us.es
2. Researching in Sport Science: Research Group (CTS-563) of the Andalusian Research Plan, 29010 Malaga, Spain; jcfg@uma.es
3. Department of Didactics of Languages, Arts and Sport, University of Malaga, Andalucía-Tech, IBIMA, 29010 Malaga, Spain
* Correspondence: amandatorres@uma.es

Abstract: The aim of this longitudinal study was to determine whether a rowing training program improved the quality of life and the physical activity levels in female breast cancer survivors ($n = 28$) (stage 1–4.54%; stage 2–36.36%; stage 3–54.54%; and stage 4–4.54%), diagnosed 4.68 ± 3.00 years previously, who had undergone a subsequent intervention (preservation 56.53% and total mastectomy 43.47%) and had a current mean age of 52.30 ± 3.78 years. The participants ($n = 28$) engaged in a 12-week training program, each week comprising three sessions and each session lasting 60–90 min. The short form of the International Physical Activity Questionnaire (IPAQ-SF) and the Short Form 36 Health Survey (SF-36) were also administered. The results showed statistically significant improvements in levels of physical activity and in the dimensions of quality of life. We can conclude that a 12-week rowing training program tailored to women who have had breast cancer increases physical activity levels, leading to improved health status and quality of life.

Keywords: breast cancer; rowing; exercise; quality of life; perceived health; IPAQ-SF; SF-36

1. Introduction

Cancer is the second leading cause of death worldwide, representing about 9.6 million deaths in 2018, which means that one in six deaths globally is due to this disease [1,2]. In women, breast cancer is the most common cancer, affecting around 2.1 million women in 2018, i.e., one in four cancers diagnosed is breast cancer [2–4].

The rise in the number of cancer cases diagnosed in recent years has been associated with population growth, closely linked to increased life expectancy, and therefore with aging, considering age as a fundamental risk factor for developing cancer. It has also been related to the increase in early detection as well as improvements in primary care and in early diagnosis programs, which, although they lead to higher numbers of cases, are in turn related to a decrease in mortality [4–6].

One-third of diagnosed cancer cases could be prevented if exposures to various lifestyle-related risk factors were eliminated or reduced, such as smoking; consumption of harmful substances such as alcohol; an unhealthy, high-calorie diet with a high intake of saturated animal fats and sugars; and/or a sedentary lifestyle [1,4,5,7]. A large body of scientific evidence shows that physical activity has positive effects on the general population, improving health status, mood, body composition, quality of life [7–11], and preventing the onset of numerous diseases, including various types of cancer, such as breast cancer [12–14].

Physical activity has been associated with a lower risk of developing breast cancer [12,13,15], with a decrease in the probability of relapse and with a higher survival rate [13–15]. In individuals with cancer, physical activity has benefits for their health:

reduced fatigue, improved strength levels, and improved quality of life and physical function [15–19].

However, despite the evidence supporting physical activity, two out of three cancer patients do not perform the minimum levels of exercise recommended by the American College of Sports Medicine (ACSM), which considers it essential to perform 150 min of moderate aerobic activity or 75 min of vigorous aerobic activity per week and at least 2 days of resistance training [13,17,20].

The relationship between physical activity and breast cancer has been demonstrated in several studies that analyzed and compared the effects of different exercise programs in breast cancer survivors, finding significant improvements in quality of life [21,22], physical function, and muscle strength [21,23]. More specifically, the study by Wiskemann et al. (2016) based on a 12-week resistance training program showed gains in muscle strength [24]. In several studies where the training programs combined endurance with aerobic exercise for 12 weeks, the improvements were significant in muscle strength, level of physical activity, and quality of life [21,25–29]. In addition, studies on mixed programs combining aerobic and strength exercises [30,31] showed important improvements in aerobic capacity, maximum oxygen consumption, muscle strength, reduction in the percentage of fat mass, and, above all, improved quality of life. Improvements were also found in physical, psychological, social, and quality of life parameters from training programs based on dragon boat rowing in women with breast cancer [18,32–34].

Women breast cancer survivors have found rowing to be an activity that improves the sequelae of the disease [35], such as reducing pain, increasing the range of movement in the upper limbs, improving muscle activation, and increasing strength and muscle function [36,37].

In this sense, rowing is considered one of the most complete water sports, involving the work of the musculature of both the upper and lower limbs [38] and almost all the body's musculature [39]. It is a sport in which symmetrical movements are performed that do not require forced position and that combine the work of strength and aerobic endurance [18]. Several studies have shown that this type of activity improves the quality of life of cancer patients, including psychological, physical, social, and emotional aspects, favoring their rehabilitation, self-esteem, and normalizing their daily life [37,40,41].

In addition, the practice of rowing has psychosocial benefits for cancer survivors [37,42] because it is a team sport that promotes the development of social relationships, and they find the support they need in other women who have gone through or are going through the same situation. Additionally, rowing is an outdoor activity, which provides them with extra motivation to adhere to physical activity and improves their quality of life [41,43,44].

Finally, in studies using the short form of the International Physical Activity Questionnaire (IPAQ-SF) to examine changes in physical activity [28,29] and the Short Form 36 Health Survey (SF-36) for changes in quality of life [27,30] following physical activity interventions in breast cancer patients, it was found that activity levels increased, and the different domains of quality of life improved after completion of the training programs.

The purpose of the present longitudinal study is to determine the influence of a 12-week rowing training program on quality of life and physical activity levels in women who have survived breast cancer.

2. Materials and Methods

2.1. Design and Participants

The study, according to Hernández, Fernández, and Baptista (2014), is a non-experimental longitudinal panel design, given that the same participants have been measured or observed at all times or points in time [45].

Participants (n = 28) aged 52.3 ± 3.8 years were recruited under the condition of having overcome breast cancer. The women were diagnosed 4.7 ± 3.0 years earlier, had different stages of disease, and had undergone surgery, as shown in Table 1.

Breast cancer survivor (BCS) is the name given to women who have been diagnosed with breast cancer and have had to undergo surgery and chemotherapy and/or radiotherapy treatments.

To take part in this research, we searched various breast cancer associations in Malaga for women who wanted to do sports (rowing) and who met the following characteristics: having overcome breast cancer, having completed chemotherapy and radiotherapy treatments, and having the oncologist's approval to do physical activity. No more than 10 years had passed since the cancer diagnosis. All of them were still taking tamoxifen.

The sample was selected based on compliance with these inclusion criteria.

Table 1. Characteristics of the breast cancer survivor sample.

Age (Years)		52.30 ± 3.78
Years from Diagnosis		4.68 ± 3.00
Stage (%)	1	4.54
	2	36.36
	3	54.54
	4	4.54
Surgery (%)	Preservation	56.53
	Total Mastectomy	43.47

The study was carried out at the RC Mediterráneo in Málaga involving women from the Sport Association Málaga D.B. Forty-eight participants were invited to take part: 10 initially withdrew due to compatibility/work/family and transport problems, and 10 were excluded because they did not attend 90% of the sessions.

After the initial selection, the nature of the study was explained to the participants, indicating that their anonymity would be maintained at all times, following the ethical considerations of the Sport and Exercise Science Research [46], as well as the principles included in the Declaration of Helsinki [47], which define the ethical guidelines for research in human subjects. The University of Malaga assigned the identification number 65-2020-H, which is registered with the Ethics Committee. The participants provided written informed consent, and throughout the intervention and afterwards, we acted under the provisions of the Organic Law 3/2018, of December 5, on the Protection of Personal Data and Guarantee of Digital Rights, regarding the protection of personal data under Spanish legislation. After signing the informed consent, the physical activity (IPAQ-SF) and the health-related quality of life (SF-36) questionnaires were administered.

The intervention lasted 12 uninterrupted weeks in which the women carried out two weekly sessions as described above. Both at the beginning and at the end of the program the participants were asked to complete the questionnaires.

2.2. Instruments

The participants also completed the short version of the International Physical Activity (IPAQ-SF) questionnaire to assess physical activity levels over the last 7 days. This questionnaire consists of seven questions that have acceptable measurement properties to monitor physical activity levels for adults aged 18 to 65 years in various settings, and it also reports the number of metabolic equivalents (METS) over the last 7 days [48]. Several studies have demonstrated the reliability of the IPAQ-SF for measuring the level of physical activity or the number of METS achieved during the last 7 days, obtaining similar results to other types of tests such as accelerometry or podometry [49–51].

The SF-36 Health Survey was used to assess health-related quality of life. This questionnaire consists of 36 items that report both positive and negative health status covering eight dimensions: physical function, social function, physical role, emotional role, mental health, vitality, bodily pain, and general health.

2.3. Intervention

Before starting the training program, participants were asked to complete the IPAQ-SF and SF-36 Health Survey questionnaires; in addition, they filled in the informed consent document to participate in the study.

The 12-week rowing training program was carried out at the RC Mediterráneo in Málaga, and it was divided into three parts of 4 weeks each. These stages progressively increased in intensity and were regulated through the participants' subjective perception of effort using the Börg scale [52].

- Initial phase: mobility, proprioceptive, and postural control exercises. Main phase with rowing training. Final phase with stretching. Börg scale 5–6.
- Intermediate phase: mobility, proprioceptive, and postural control exercises. Main phase with rowing training. Final phase with stretching. Börg scale 6–7.
- Final phase: mobility, proprioceptive, and postural control exercises. Main phase with rowing training. Final phase with stretching. Börg scale 7–8.

Throughout the program, a weekly schedule was established consisting of three training days lasting 60–90 min per session. These sessions were supervised by a trainer who ensured attendance, correct execution of the tasks, and intensity of the sessions, in addition to excluding from the study those subjects who did not comply with at least 90% participation. All the exercises in these sessions were performed in a group. Exercises were generic and adjusted for people who have never rowed before. Each of the training sessions had the same structure:

1. Initial phase—performed with warm-up, mobility, proprioceptive, and postural control exercises; all exercises carried out in a multipurpose room (10–15 min).
2. Intermediate phase—performed in the Mediterranean Sea near the port of Malaga (Cruise Terminal/Malagueta Beach) using fixed-bench boats, typical of the Spanish Mediterranean, called Llauts, which are propelled by eight rowers and a coxswain or skipper [53], with each rower holding a single oar (40–60 min).
3. Final phase—flexibility exercises to relax the musculature and bring the body back to its initial state after exercise (10–15 min).

Both at the beginning and at the end of the program sessions were held to discuss issues, and the participants were asked to complete the questionnaires.

2.4. Data Analysis

All analyses were performed with IBM SPSS, version 25 (IBM Corp, Armonk, NY, USA). The significance level was defined as $p < 0.05$. The fit of the different variables to the normal distribution was assessed using graphic procedures and the Shapiro–Wilk test.

To examine the differences resulting from the rowing training performed by the participants, the medians of each variable pre- and post-intervention were analyzed using the Wilcoxon test for related samples (paired data). In addition, graphic analysis of the different variables was carried out using box-and-whisker plots. In addition, the effect size for the Wilcoxon test (r) was calculated by the Z-score [54]. In the Cohen's guidelines for r, a large effect is defined as 0.5, a medium effect as 0.3, and a small effect as 0.1.

3. Results

Descriptive analyses of the different study variables (Table 2), level of physical activity, and quality of life are shown below, differentiating between pre-intervention and post-intervention values.

Table 2. Descriptive analysis of the variables pretest and posttest.

Variables	Mean		Percentiles						Minimum		Maximum	
			25		50 (Mdn)		75					
	Pre	Post	Pre	Post	Pre	Post	Pre	Post	Pre	Post	Pre	Post
IPAQ Walking (METS)	587.8 ± 432.1	1522.1 ± 1353.1	305.3	693.0	495.0	1287.0	693.0	1683.0	0	231	1485	6930
IPAQ Moderate (METS)	185.0 ± 260.0	1250.0 ± 1664.2	0.0	480.0	0.0	720.0	240.0	1140.0	0	240	960	8400
IPAQ Vigorous (METS)	416.7 ± 513.1	1620.0 ± 1608.0	0.0	780.0	80.0	1440.0	960.0	1920.0	0	0	1440	7680
IPAQ Total (METS)	1189.5 ± 835.0	4392.1 ± 3341.7	495.0	2388.0	1075.5	3483.0	1611.0	5442.7	0	1413	3108	16290
IPAQ Sitting (METS)	267.8 ± 155.4	197.8 ± 135.2	120.0	104.3	240.0	150.0	435.0	285.0	30	0	540	520
Physical Function (Points)	75.4 ± 18.8	85.2 ± 13.3	70.0	77.5	82.5	90.0	90.0	93.8	30	50	95	100
Physical Role (Points)	62.5 ± 26.2	76.6 ± 25.4	37.5	62.5	71.9	84.4	85.9	100.0	6.3	12.5	100	100
Bodily Pain (Points)	49.7 ± 18.6	59.3 ± 22.2	41.0	43.5	51.5	61.0	62.0	72.0	10	22	84	100
General Health (Points)	60.1 ± 17.6	67.1 ± 19.9	46.3	50.5	61.0	72.0	72.0	85.8	20	30	92	97
Vitality (Points)	50.0 ± 12.9	59.8 ± 13.4	45.0	50.0	50.0	60.0	60.0	70.0	20	25	70	80
Social Function (Points)	72.4 ± 22.7	87.5 ± 18.4	62.5	75.0	75.0	100.0	87.5	100.0	12.5	37.5	100	100
Emotional Role (Points)	76.0 ± 15.8	89.9 ± 14.7	62.5	77.1	75.0	100.0	89.6	100.0	50	50	100	100
Mental Health (Points)	58.8 ± 13.9	67.0 ± 11.9	48.0	56.0	58.0	68.0	71.0	76.0	32	36	84	84

Pre = pretest; Post = posttest; Mdn = median IPAQ = International Physical Activity Questionnaire; METS = metabolic equivalents; 1 MET = $3.5 \text{ mL } O_2 \times kg^{-1} \times min^{-1}$.

For the variables associated with engaging in physical activity obtained from the IPAQ-SF and the quality of life through the SF-36 questionnaire, the Wilcoxon test was carried out to determine whether significant differences exist between the pretest and posttest data.

Figure 1 depicts all physical activity variables, showing improvements after the intervention in levels of walking (Dif Mdn = 495 < 1287, z = −4.201, p = 0.000, r = 0.79), moderate (Dif Mdn = 0.00 < 720.00, z = −4.314, p = 0.000, r = 0.81), vigorous (Dif Mdn = 80.00 < 1440.00, z = −4.043, p = 0.000, r = 0.76), and total physical activity (Dif Mdn = 1075.50 < 3483.00, z = −4.286, p = 0.000, r = 0.81), all of which were significant. The lower value obtained for the IPAQ sitting variable (Dif Mdn = 240.00 > 150.00, z = −3.075, p = 0.002, r = 0.58) after the intervention compared to before the intervention indicates the participants were more active and spent less time sitting throughout the week. Regarding the effect size, the differences had a large effect and were statistically significant, as they presented values greater than 0.5.

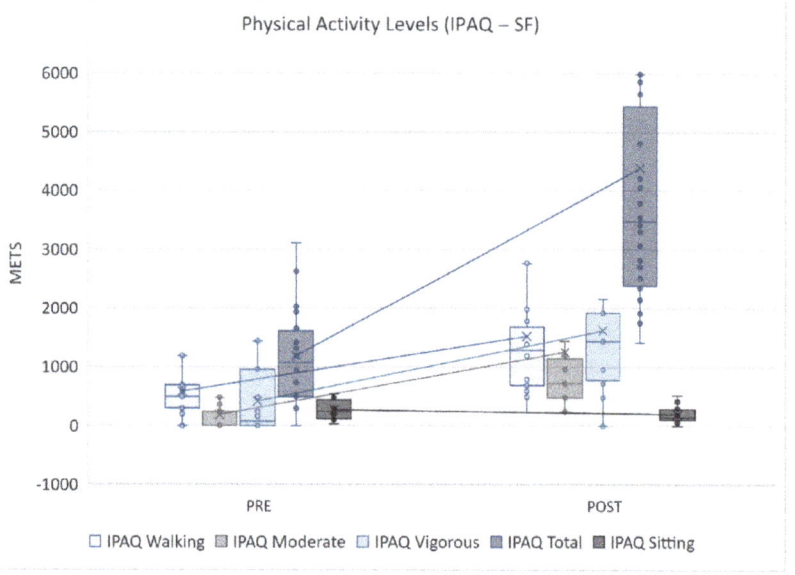

Figure 1. Physical activity levels (IPAQ-SF); PRE = pretest; POST = posttest; METS = metabolic equivalents.

Regarding the variables associated with quality of life, Figure 2 displays the results for the mental dimensions, showing improvements after the intervention in vitality (Dif Mdn = 50.00 < 60.00, z = −2.879, p = 0.004, r = 0.54), social function (Dif Mdn = 75.00 < 100.00, z = −3.247, p = 0.001, r = 0.61), emotional role (Dif Mdn = 75.00 < 100.00, z = −3.268, p = 0.001, r = 0.61), and mental health (Dif Mdn = 58.00 < 68.00, z = −2.836, p = 0.005, r = 0.54), all of which were significant. As for the effect size, its values were relevant as they were above 0.5.

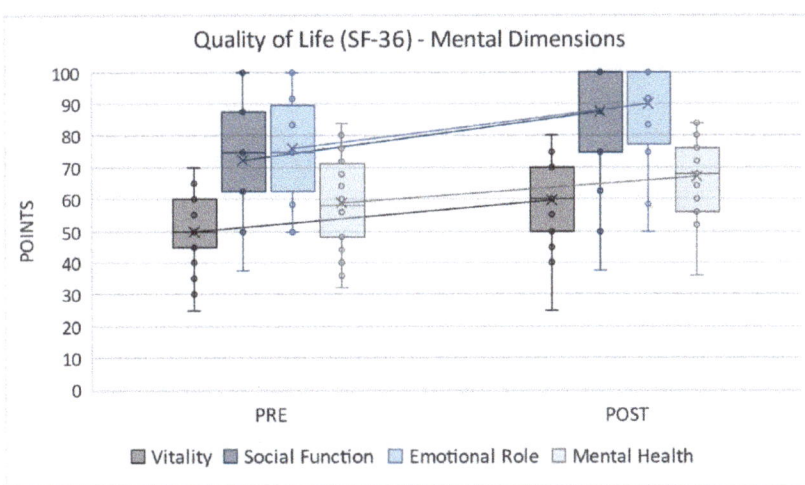

Figure 2. Quality of Life (SF-36)—Mental Dimensions; PRE = pretest; POST = posttest.

Focusing on the physical dimensions, Figure 3 shows that all variables improved significantly after the intervention, including general health (Dif Mdn = 61.00 < 72.00, z = −2.006, p = 0.045, r = 0.37). In the case of the variation in bodily pain (Dif Mdn = 51.50 < 61.00, z = −2.472, p = 0.013, r = 0.47), this may indicate that the participants reported less pain overall after the intervention. In other words, engaging in rowing decreases bodily pain in women who are breast cancer survivors or increases the pain threshold in the women studied. In addition, improvements after the intervention in physical role (Dif Mdn = 71.88 < 84.38, z = −3.866, p = 0.000, r = 0.73) and physical function (Dif Mdn = 82.50 < 90.00, z = −3.256, p = 0.001, r = 0.62) were shown, which indicates that the participants had fewer limitations when performing any physical activity compared to prior to the intervention. In terms of effect size, the data show that the differences were relevant, as they presented values between 0.3 and 0.5. This suggests that a 12-week rowing training program, adapted to women who have had breast cancer, helps to improve the perceived ability to perform other activities.

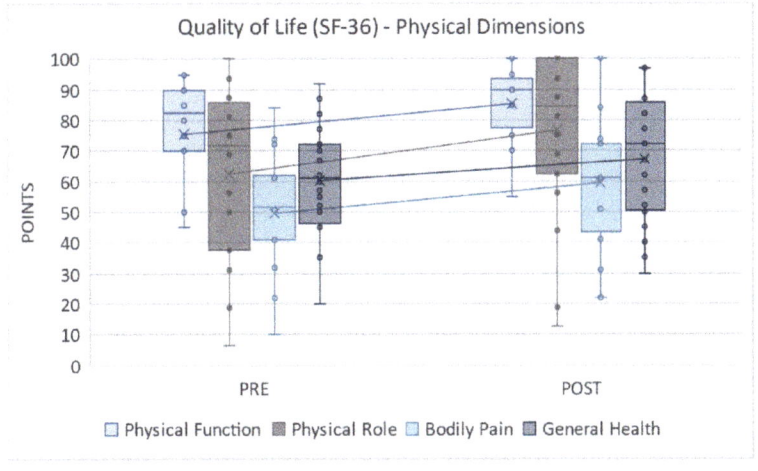

Figure 3. Quality of Life (SF-36)—Physical Dimensions; PRE = pretest; POST = posttest.

Finally, in terms of overall perceived health of the participants, a significant improvement was detected after the physical activity intervention (Figure 4). After completing the rowing program, a tendency towards an improved perception of health emerged: the number of women who reported having poor or fair health decreased, and those who claimed having "very good health" increased, with 75% of the participants reporting their health status to be good or very good.

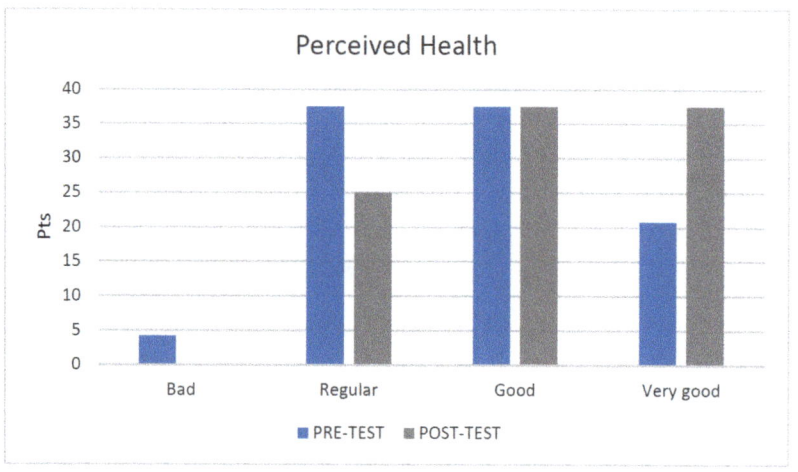

Figure 4. Variation in perceived health; Pts = points.

In summary, after an intervention based on a 12-week rowing training program tailored to women who have had breast cancer, all variables showed significant improvements, including those concerning level of physical activity and quality of life. That is, the participants were more physically active and less sedentary throughout the week. In addition, their perceived physical, emotional, and mental health status improved, which indicates fewer limitations in terms of physical activity, social life, and vitality.

4. Discussion

To date, studies relating rowing to improvements in quality of life or in the level of physical activity in breast cancer survivors are practically non-existent. In this sense, some research can be found in which other types of sports, such as dragon boating [32,33], yoga, Pilates [55,56], or endurance, strength, or aerobic exercise training programs [22,24,31], report improvements at physical, psychological, and social levels in women breast cancer survivors.

More specifically, upon examining studies that used different types of physical activity programs, the 12-week resistance training program proposed by Wiskemann et al. (2016) reported improvements only in muscle strength [24]. Other programs that combined aerobic and strength exercises for 24 weeks led to improvements in muscle strength, aerobic capacity, and only some quality of life dimensions [31], while those that combined resistance and aerobic exercises for 16 weeks showed improvements in the quality of life and physical fitness of the participants [26]. Harris (2012) and McDonough et al. (2018) reported that dragon boat rowing [32,33] led to physical, psychological, and social improvements in women breast cancer survivors.

In our study, based on a rowing training program lasting only 12 weeks, improvements were observed in all levels of physical activity, as measured by the IPAQ-SF, including increased levels of walking, moderate and vigorous physical activity, and total physical activity as well as decreased sedentary activity of the participants; improvements were shown in all dimensions of quality of life. The results obtained in the present research are superior to those reported in previous studies; in addition, a shorter intervention time was required.

These results may be due to the fact that rowing is a sport that involves the muscles of both the lower and upper limbs and almost every muscle in the body [38]. In addition, rowing is a cyclic and symmetrical sport that combines overall strength with aerobic endurance [18]; it is based on cyclic and alternating movements of flexion/extension of the limbs and stabilization of the trunk and back muscles [57]. In this sense, the involvement of the whole body in physical activity, such as rowing, leads to improvements in quality of life and physical function as well as reduction in body fat in women breast cancer survivors [44,58,59].

In the study by Park et al. (2019), through a training program combining aerobic and resistance exercises, physical activity levels increased after the 12-week intervention, rising in 63,4% of the participants. At baseline, 33% of participants were inactive, 49.6% minimally active, and 17.4% health-enhancing physical activity (HEPA) active; after intervention the percentages improved, being 15.3%, 50.4%, and 34.2%, respectively [28]. It is of interest to compare these results with those of our study, which used an intervention of the same duration. In our study, overall physical activity levels increased in all participants after the rowing program with respect to the initial measurement. It should also be noted that prior to the intervention, about 50% of the participants reported no moderate or vigorous physical activity, whereas afterwards, all the participants reported engaging in moderate physical activity, and less than 10% reported no vigorous activity.

Regarding quality of life parameters, the study by Mascherini et al. (2020) shows improvements in physical function, social function, general health, and mental health after 6 months of training [60]. Di Blasio et al. (2017) after 12 weeks of intervention only found improvements in physical function, physical role, bodily pain, and general health [23]. Dolan et al. (2018) also showed that after a 22-week training program all SF-36 quality of life dimensions improved, with the exception of bodily pain [61].

Some of the limitations of this study reside in the scarcity of the sample. Although homogeneity was presented for the variables evaluated in this article, it would be interesting to know what the effects of this rowing program are from different times since the cancer was diagnosed or whether mastectomy is present or not.

The results of the present study demonstrate that rowing training has a greater influence on quality of life in breast cancer survivors than previously reported, as significant improvements were found in all quality of life parameters after an intervention of shorter duration. This implies that perceived physical, emotional, and mental health status and the perceived ability to perform other activities improved to a greater extent after our rowing-based training program. Indeed, 75% of the participants reported their health status as good or very good after the intervention, with a considerable increase compared to the initial data.

5. Conclusions

Previous studies have reported improved quality of life and reduced physical inactivity in female breast cancer survivors through training programs such as aerobic, strength, resistance, and dragon boat exercises. In the present study, we have shown that an intervention of just twelve weeks in length using rowing training tailored to women who have had breast cancer produced improvements in all levels of physical activity and reduced physical inactivity, with respect to the initial measurement. In addition, after the intervention, the physical, emotional, and mental health status of the participants improved, leading to fewer limitations in their daily routines, physical activity, social life, and vitality. Our rowing program showed greater benefits in health and quality of life than other studies of various durations. We can therefore conclude that rowing training contributes to increasing daily physical activity as well as improving health status and the different dimensions of quality of life in women who have survived breast cancer.

Author Contributions: Conceptualization J.G.-G. and A.T.-P.; methodology J.C.F.-G. and J.G.-G.; software, A.T.-P.; validation, J.C.F.-G. and J.G.-G.; formal analysis, J.C.F.-G. and A.T.-P.; investigation J.C.F.-G. and J.G.-G.; resources, J.C.F.-G. and J.G.-G.; data curation, A.T.-P.; writing—original draft preparation, J.G.-G. and A.T.-P.; writing—review and editing, J.G.-G.; J.G.-G. and J.C.F.-G.; visualization, J.G.-G.; A.T.-P. and J.C.F.-G.; supervision, J.C.F.-G.; project administration, J.C.F.-G. and J.G.-G.; funding acquisition, J.C.F.-G. All authors have read and agreed to the published version of the manuscript.

Funding: This research was funded by the "Researching in Sport Sciences" research group (CTS-563) of the Andalusian Research Plan.

Institutional Review Board Statement: The study was conducted according to the guidelines of the Declaration of Helsinki and approved by Ethics Committee of University of Málaga (protocol code 65-2020-H and date of approval 30 September 2020).

Informed Consent Statement: Informed consent was obtained from all subjects involved in the study.

Data Availability Statement: Data consent was obtained from all subjects involved in the study.

Acknowledgments: We would like to thank the Real Club Mediterráneo of Malaga, its rowing captain Juan Carlos Marfil Rodríguez, and the team of the Malaga Dragon Boat BCS for opening their doors to us, letting us use their facilities, and for giving us the most important thing: their time and inspiring us with their impetus and energy, thanks to which we can present the first results of this study. To Maria Repice, for her help with the English version of this manuscript. All authors have read and agreed to the published version of the manuscript.

Conflicts of Interest: The authors declare no conflict of interest.

References

1. World Health Organization Fact Sheets: Cancer. Available online: https://www.who.int/news-room/fact-sheets/detail/cancer (accessed on 10 August 2020).
2. International Agency for Research on Cancer (IARC) Cancer Today. Available online: https://gco.iarc.fr/today/home (accessed on 10 August 2020).
3. World Health Organization Breast Cancer: Prevention and Control. Available online: https://www.who.int/cancer/detection/breastcancer/en/ (accessed on 12 August 2020).
4. Bray, F.; Ferlay, J.; Soerjomataram, I.; Siegel, R.L.; Torre, L.A.; Jemal, A. Global cancer statistics 2018: GLOBOCAN estimates of incidence and mortality worldwide for 36 cancers in 185 countries. *CA. Cancer J. Clin.* **2018**, *68*, 394–424. [CrossRef]
5. Sociedad Española de Oncología Médica Las Cifras del Cáncer en España 2020. Available online: https://seom.org/dmcancer/cifras-del-cancer/ (accessed on 10 August 2020).
6. World Health Organization Early Cancer Diagnosis Saves Lives Cuts Treatments Costs. Available online: https://www.who.int/es/news/item/03-02-2017-early-cancer-diagnosis-saves-lives-cuts-treatment-costs (accessed on 5 December 2020).
7. Loria Calderon, T.M.; Carmona Gómez, C.D. Efecto agudo del baile como ejercicio aeróbico sobre el balance estático en personas mayores de 50 años. *Rev. Iberoam. Ciencias Act. Física Deport.* **2020**, *9*, 61–74. [CrossRef]
8. Gómez-Cabello, A.; Pardos-Mainer, E.; González-Gálvez, N.; Sagarra-Romero, L. Actividad Física y Calidad de Vida en las Personas Mayores: Estudio Piloto PQS. *Rev. Iberoam. Ciencias Act. Fis. Deport.* **2018**, *8*, 96–109. [CrossRef]
9. Warburton, D.E.R.; Bredin, S.S.D. Health benefits of physical activity: A systematic review of current systematic reviews. *Curr. Opin. Cardiol.* **2017**, *32*, 541–556. [CrossRef] [PubMed]
10. Gálvez Fernández, I. Pérdida de Peso y Masa Grasa con Auto-Cargas en Mujeres. *Rev. Iberoam. Ciencias Act. Física Deport.* **2017**, *6*, 30–37. [CrossRef]
11. Díaz, J.; Muñoz, D.; Cordero, J.C.; Robles, M.C.; Courel-Ibañez, J.; Sánchez-Alcaraz, B.J. Estado de Ánimo y Calidad de Vida en Mujeres Adultas practicantes de Pádel. *Rev. Iberoam. Ciencias Act. Fis. Deport.* **2018**, *8*, 34–43. [CrossRef]
12. World Cancer Research Fund (WCRF); American Institute for Cancer Research (AICR). *Diet, Nutrition, Physical Activity and Cancer: A Global Perspective*; World Cancer Research Fund International: London, UK, 2018; ISBN 9781912259465.
13. Pollán, M.; Casla-Barrio, S.; Alfaro, J.; Esteban, C.; Segui-Palmer, M.A.; Lucia, A.; Martín, M. Exercise and cancer: A position statement from the Spanish Society of Medical Oncology. *Clin. Transl. Oncol.* **2020**, *22*, 1710–1729. [CrossRef]
14. Schmidt, M.E.; Chang-Claude, J.; Vrieling, A.; Seibold, P.; Heinz, J.; Obi, N.; Flesch-Janys, D.; Steindorf, K. Association of pre-diagnosis physical activity with recurrence and mortality among women with breast cancer. *Int. J. Cancer* **2013**, *133*, 1431–1440. [CrossRef]
15. Johnsson, A.; Broberg, P.; Krüger, U.; Johnsson, A.; Tornberg, Å.B.; Olsson, H. Physical activity and survival following breast cancer. *Eur. J. Cancer Care* **2019**, *28*, 1–8. [CrossRef]
16. Pennington, K.P.; McTiernan, A. The role of physical activity in breast and gynecologic cancer survivorship. *Gynecol. Oncol.* **2018**, *149*, 198–204. [CrossRef]

17. Mascherini, G.; Tosi, B.; Giannelli, C.; Grifoni, E.; Degl'Innocenti, S.; Galanti, G. Breast cancer: Effectiveness of a one-year unsupervised exercise program. *J. Sports Med. Phys. Fitness* **2018**, *59*, 283–289. [CrossRef]
18. Gavala-González, J.; Gálvez-Fernández, I.; Mercadé-Melé, P.; Fernández-García, J.C. Rowing training in breast cancer survivors: A longitudinal study of physical fitness. *Int. J. Environ. Res. Public Health* **2020**, *17*, 4938. [CrossRef] [PubMed]
19. Furmaniak, A.; Menig, M.; Markes, M. Exercise for women receiving adjuvant therapy for breast cancer. *Cochrane Database Syst. Rev.* **2016**. [CrossRef]
20. De Boer, M.C.; Wörner, E.A.; Verlaan, D.; van Leeuwen, P.A.M. The Mechanisms and Effects of Physical Activity on Breast Cancer. *Clin. Breast Cancer* **2017**, *17*, 272–278. [CrossRef] [PubMed]
21. Courneya, K.S.; McKenzie, D.C.; Mackey, J.R.; Gelmon, K.; Friedenreich, C.M.; Yasui, Y.; Reid, R.D.; Cook, D.; Jespersen, D.; Proulx, C.; et al. Effects of Exercise Dose and Type During Breast Cancer Chemotherapy: Multicenter Randomized Trial. *J. Natl. Cancer Inst.* **2013**, *105*, 1821–1832. [CrossRef]
22. Mishra, S.I.; Scherer, R.W.; Snyder, C.; Geigle, P.; Gotay, C. Are Exercise Programs Effective for Improving Health-Related Quality of Life Among Cancer Survivors? A Systematic Review and Meta-Analysis. *Oncol. Nurs. Forum* **2014**, *41*, E326–E342. [CrossRef] [PubMed]
23. Di Blasio, A.; Morano, T.; Cianchetti, E.; Gallina, S.; Bucci, I.; Di Santo, S.; Tinari, C.; Di Donato, F.; Izzicupo, P.; Di Baldassarre, A.; et al. Psychophysical health status of breast cancer survivors and effects of 12 weeks of aerobic training. *Complement. Ther. Clin. Pract.* **2017**, *27*, 19–26. [CrossRef]
24. Wiskemann, J.; Schmidt, M.E.; Klassen, O.; Debus, J.; Ulrich, C.M.; Potthoff, K.; Steindorf, K. Effects of 12-week resistance training during radiotherapy in breast cancer patients. *Scand. J. Med. Sci. Sport.* **2016**, *27*, 1500–1510. [CrossRef] [PubMed]
25. Soriano-Maldonado, A.; Carrera-Ruiz, Á.; Díez-Fernández, D.M.; Esteban-Simón, A.; Maldonado-Quesada, M.; Moreno-Poza, N.; García-Martínez, M.D.M.; Alcaraz-García, C.; Vázquez-Sousa, R.; Moreno-Martos, H.; et al. Effects of a 12-week resistance and aerobic exercise program on muscular strength and quality of life in breast cancer survivors: Study protocol for the EFICAN randomized controlled trial. *Medicine* **2019**, *98*, 1–9. [CrossRef]
26. Dieli-Conwright, C.M.; Courneya, K.S.; Demark-Wahnefried, W.; Sami, N.; Lee, K.; Sweeney, F.C.; Stewart, C.; Buchanan, T.A.; Spicer, D.; Tripathy, D.; et al. Aerobic and resistance exercise improves physical fitness, bone health, and quality of life in overweight and obese breast cancer survivors: A randomized controlled trial. *Breast Cancer Res.* **2018**, *20*, 1–10. [CrossRef]
27. Thomas, G.A.; Cartmel, B.; Harrigan, M.; Fiellin, M.; Capozza, S.; Zhou, Y.; Ercolano, E.; Gross, C.P.; Hershman, D.; Ligibel, J.; et al. The effect of exercise on body composition and bone mineral density in breast cancer survivors taking aromatase inhibitors. *Obesity* **2017**, *25*, 346–351. [CrossRef] [PubMed]
28. Park, S.W.; Lee, I.; Kim, J.I.; Park, H.; Lee, J.D.; Uhm, K.E.; Hwang, J.H.; Lee, E.S.; Jung, S.Y.; Park, Y.H.; et al. Factors associated with physical activity of breast cancer patients participating in exercise intervention. *Support. Care Cancer* **2019**, *27*, 1747–1754. [CrossRef] [PubMed]
29. Uhm, K.E.; Yoo, J.S.; Chung, S.H.; Lee, J.D.; Lee, I.; Kim, J.I.; Lee, S.K.; Nam, S.J.; Park, Y.H.; Lee, J.Y.; et al. Effects of exercise intervention in breast cancer patients: Is mobile health (mHealth) with pedometer more effective than conventional program using brochure? *Breast Cancer Res. Treat.* **2017**, *161*, 443–452. [CrossRef] [PubMed]
30. Smith, T.M.; Broomhall, C.N.; Crecelius, A.R. Physical and Psychological Effects of a 12-Session Cancer Rehabilitation Exercise Program. *Clin. J. Oncol. Nurs.* **2016**, *20*, 653–659. [CrossRef] [PubMed]
31. De Luca, V.; Minganti, C.; Borrione, P.; Grazioli, E.; Cerulli, C.; Guerra, E.; Bonifacino, A.; Parisi, A. Effects of concurrent aerobic and strength training on breast cancer survivors: A pilot study. *Public Health* **2016**, *136*, 126–132. [CrossRef] [PubMed]
32. Harris, S.R. Were all in the same boat: A review of the benefits of dragon boat racing for women living with breast cancer. *Evidence Based Complement. Altern. Med.* **2012**, *2012*, 1–8. [CrossRef]
33. McDonough, M.H.; Patterson, M.C.; Weisenbach, B.B.; Ullrich-French, S.; Sabiston, C.M. The difference is more than floating: Factors affecting breast cancer survivors' decisions to join and maintain participation in dragon boat teams and support groups. *Disabil. Rehabil.* **2018**, *41*, 1788–1796. [CrossRef] [PubMed]
34. Fong, A.J.; Saxton, H.R.; Kauffeldt, K.D.; Sabiston, C.M.; Tomasone, J.R. "We're all in the same boat together": Exploring quality participation strategies in dragon boat teams for breast cancer survivors. *Disabil. Rehabil.* **2020**, 1–12. [CrossRef]
35. McKenzie, D.C. Abreast in a boat—A race against breast cancer. *CMAJ* **1998**, *159*, 376–378.
36. Asensio-García, M.d.R.; Tomás-Rodríguez, M.I.; Palazón-Bru, A.; Hernández-Sánchez, S.; Nouni-García, R.; Romero-Aledo, A.L.; Gil-Guillén, V.F. Effect of rowing on mobility, functionality, and quality of life in women with and without breast cancer: A 4-month intervention. *Support. Care Cancer* **2020**. [CrossRef]
37. Iacorossi, L.; Gambalunga, F.; Molinaro, S.; De Domenico, R.; Giannarelli, D.; Fabi, A. The effectiveness of the sport "dragon boat racing" in reducing the risk of lymphedema incidence: An observational study. *Cancer Nurs.* **2019**, *42*, 323–331. [CrossRef] [PubMed]
38. Das, A.; Mandal, M.; Syamal, A.K.; Majumdar, P. Monitoring Changes of Cardio-Respiratory Parameters During 2000m Rowing Performance. *Int. J. Exerc. Sci.* **2019**, *12*, 483–490. [PubMed]
39. Yoshiga, C.C.; Higuchi, M. Rowing performance of female and male rowers. *Scand. J. Med. Sci. Sports* **2003**, *13*, 317–321. [CrossRef] [PubMed]
40. McNeely, M.L.; Campbell, K.L.; Courneya, K.S.; Mackey, J.R. Effect of acute exercise on upper-limb volume in breast cancer survivors: A pilot study. *Physiother. Canada* **2009**. [CrossRef]

41. Ray, H.; Jakubec, S.L. Nature-based experiences and health of cancer survivors. *Complement. Ther. Clin. Pract.* **2014**, *20*, 188–192. [CrossRef]
42. Sablston, C.M.; McDonough, M.H.; Crocker, P.R.E. Psychosocial experiences of breast cancer survivors involved in a dragon boat program: Exploring links to positive psychological growth. *J. Sport Exerc. Psychol.* **2007**, *29*, 419–438. [CrossRef]
43. Hadd, V.; Sabiston, C.M.; McDonough, M.H.; Crocker, P.R.E. Sources of stress for breast cancer survivors involved in dragon boating: Examining associations with treatment characteristics and self-esteem. *J. Women's Heal.* **2010**, *19*, 1345–1353. [CrossRef] [PubMed]
44. McDonough, M.H.; Sabiston, C.M.; Ullrich-French, S. The development of social relationships, social support, and posttraumatic growth in a dragon boating team for breast cancer survivors. *J. Sport Exerc. Psychol.* **2011**, *33*, 627–648. [CrossRef] [PubMed]
45. Hernández Sampieri, R.; Fernández Collado, C.; Baptista Lucio, P. *Metodología de la Investigación*, 6th ed.; Editorial McGraw Hill: New York, NY, USA, 2014; ISBN 978-1-4562-2396-0.
46. Harriss, D.; Macsween, A.; Atkinson, G. Standards for Ethics in Sport and Exercise Science Research. *Int. J. Sports Med.* **2017**, *38*, 1126–1131.
47. Ebihara, A. World medical association declaration of Helsinki. *Jpn. Pharmacol. Ther.* **2000**, *28*, 983–986.
48. Barrera, R. Cuestionario Internacional de actividad física (IPAQ). *Rev. Enfermería Trab.* **2017**, *7*, 49–54.
49. Kathleen, Y.; Wolin, D.; Heil, S.; Charles, E.; Gary, G. Validation of the International Physical Activity Questionnaire-Short Among Blacks. *J Phys Act Heal.* **2008**, *5*, 746–760.
50. Cleland, C.; Ferguson, C.; Ellis, C.; Hunter, R. Validity of the International Physical Activity Questionnaire (IPAQ) for assessing moderate-to-vigorous physical activity and sedentary behaviour of older adults in the United Kingdom. *BMC Med Res Methodol.* **2018**, *18*, 176. [CrossRef]
51. Kurtze, N.; Rangul, V.; Hustvedt, B.E. Reliability and validity of the international physical activity questionnaire in the Nord-Trøndelag health study (HUNT) population of men. *BMC Med. Res. Methodol.* **2008**, *8*. [CrossRef]
52. Börg, G. Psychophysical bases of perceived exertion. *Med. Sci. Sports Exerc.* **1982**, *14*, 377–381. [CrossRef]
53. Gavala-González, J. Las Modalidades del Remo: El Remo en Banco Fijo. Available online: http://tv.us.es/las-modalidades-del-remo-el-remo-en-banco-fijo/ (accessed on 12 January 2021).
54. Fritz, C.O.; Morris, P.E.; Richler, J.J. Effect size estimates: Current use, calculations, and interpretation. *J. Exp. Psychol. Gen.* **2012**, *141*, 2–18. [CrossRef]
55. Patsou, E.D.; Alexias, G.D.; Anagnostopoulos, F.G.; Karamouzis, M.V. Effects of physical activity on depressive symptoms during breast cancer survivorship: A meta-analysis of randomised control trials. *ESMO Open* **2017**. [CrossRef] [PubMed]
56. Panchik, D.; Masco, S.; Zinnikas, P.; Hillriegel, B.; Lauder, T.; Suttmann, E.; Chinchilli, V.; McBeth, M.; Hermann, W. Effect of Exercise on Breast Cancer-Related Lymphedema: What the Lymphatic Surgeon Needs to Know. *J. Reconstr. Microsurg.* **2019**. [CrossRef] [PubMed]
57. Aramendi, J.M.G. Remo olímpico y remo tradicional: Aspectos biomecánicos, fisiológicos y nutricionales. Olympic rowing and traditional rowing: Biomechanical, physiological and nutritional aspects. *Arch. Med. Deport.* **2014**, *31*, 51–59.
58. Lane, K.; Jespersen, D.; Mckenzie, D.C. The effect of a whole body exercise programme and dragon boat training on arm volume and arm circumference in women treated for breast cancer. *Eur. J. Cancer Care* **2005**, *14*, 353–358. [CrossRef] [PubMed]
59. Quintana, V.A.; Díaz, K.; Caire, G. Intervenciones para promover estilos de vida saludables y su efecto en las variables psicológicas en sobrevivientes de cáncer de mama: Revisión sistemática. *Nutr. Hosp.* **2018**, *35*, 979–992. [CrossRef] [PubMed]
60. Mascherini, G.; Tosi, B.; Giannelli, C.; Ermini, E.; Osti, L.; Galanti, G. Adjuvant Therapy Reduces Fat Mass Loss during Exercise Prescription in Breast Cancer Survivors. *J. Funct. Morphol. Kinesiol.* **2020**, *5*, 49. [CrossRef] [PubMed]
61. Dolan, L.B.; Barry, D.; Petrella, T.; Davey, L.; Minnes, A.; Yantzi, A.; Marzolini, S.; Oh, P. The Cardiac Rehabilitation Model Improves Fitness, Quality of Life, and Depression in Breast Cancer Survivors. *J. Cardiopulm. Rehabil. Prev.* **2018**, *38*, 246–252. [CrossRef] [PubMed]

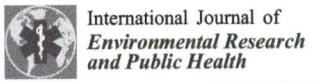

Article

Contribution of Solid Food to Achieve Individual Nutritional Requirement during a Continuous 438 km Mountain Ultramarathon in Female Athlete

Kengo Ishihara [1,*], Naho Inamura [1], Asuka Tani [1], Daisuke Shima [1], Ai Kuramochi [1], Tsutomu Nonaka [2], Hiroshi Oneda [3] and Yasuyuki Nakamura [1,4]

[1] Department of Food Sciences and Human Nutrition, Faculty of Agriculture, Ryukoku University, Shiga 520-2194, Japan; n170316@mail.ryukoku.ac.jp (N.I.); tani@agr.ryukoku.ac.jp (A.T.); n20m005@mail.ryukoku.ac.jp (D.S.); n19m002@mail.ryukoku.ac.jp (A.K.); nakamura@belle.shiga-med.ac.jp (Y.N.)
[2] Tail Ender's Trail Running Life, Tokyo 176-0004, Japan; lacanmood2001@yahoo.co.jp
[3] Nagatasangyo Co., Ltd., Shiso 671-2544, Japan; oneda@nagatasangyo.co.jp
[4] Department of Public Health, Shiga University of Medical Science, Shiga 520-2192, Japan
* Correspondence: kengo@agr.ryukoku.ac.jp; Tel.: +81-77-599-5601 (ext. 2011)

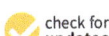

Citation: Ishihara, K.; Inamura, N.; Tani, A.; Shima, D.; Kuramochi, A.; Nonaka, T.; Oneda, H.; Nakamura, Y. Contribution of Solid Food to Achieve Individual Nutritional Requirement during a Continuous 438 km Mountain Ultramarathon in Female Athlete. *Int. J. Environ. Res. Public Health* **2021**, *18*, 5153. https://doi.org/10.3390/ijerph 18105153

Academic Editor: Filipe Manuel Clemente

Received: 21 March 2021
Accepted: 10 May 2021
Published: 13 May 2021

Publisher's Note: MDPI stays neutral with regard to jurisdictional claims in published maps and institutional affiliations.

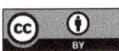

Copyright: © 2021 by the authors. Licensee MDPI, Basel, Switzerland. This article is an open access article distributed under the terms and conditions of the Creative Commons Attribution (CC BY) license (https:// creativecommons.org/licenses/by/ 4.0/).

Abstract: Background: Races and competitions over 100 miles have recently increased. Limited information exists about the effect of multiday continuous endurance exercise on blood glucose control and appropriate intake of food and drink in a female athlete. The present study aimed to examine the variation of blood glucose control and its relationship with nutritional intake and running performance in a professional female athlete during a 155.7 h ultramarathon race with little sleep. Methods: We divided the mountain course of 438 km into 33 segments by timing gates and continuously monitored the participant's glucose profile throughout the ultramarathon. The running speed in each segment was standardized to the scheduled required time-based on three trial runs. Concurrently, the accompanying runners recorded the participant's food and drink intake. Nutrient, energy, and water intake were then calculated. Results: Throughout the ultramarathon of 155.7 h, including 16.0 h of rest and sleep, diurnal variation had almost disappeared with the overall increase in blood glucose levels (25–30 mg/dL) compared with that during resting ($p < 0.0001$). Plasma total protein and triglyceride levels were decreased after the ultramarathon. The intake of protein and fat directly or indirectly contributed to maintaining blood glucose levels and running speed as substrates for gluconeogenesis or as alternative sources of energy when the carbohydrate intake was at a lower recommended limit. The higher amounts of nutrient intakes from solid foods correlated with a higher running pace compared with those from liquids and gels to supply carbohydrates, protein, and fat. Conclusion: Carbohydrate, protein, and fat intake from solid foods contributed to maintaining a fast pace with a steady, mild rise in blood glucose levels compared with liquids and gels when female runner completed a multiday continuous ultramarathon with little sleep.

Keywords: sports nutrition; continuous glucose monitoring; carbohydrate; protein; hydration; trail running; Freestyle Libre

1. Introduction

Ultramarathon is a longer-distance marathon that has increasingly gained popularity in recent years [1]. The total energy expenditure of a 100-mile (160 km) ultramarathon reaches approximately 13,000 kcal in a 180 cm, 75 kg, middle-aged experienced male runner. The carbohydrate-derived energy in 140 min of the mountain marathon was reported to be 68%, which was lower than in 20 to 30 min of track (98%) or mountain running (86%). The percentage of lipid utilization would increase further as time and distance increased [2]. Thus, nutritional strategies are essential for ultramarathon runners wanting to improve their race results and also for those focusing primarily on finishing the event.

For endurance sports, the recommended carbohydrate intake is 30–60 g/h; however, for exercises lasting more than 3 h, the advocated recommendation is higher (i.e., ≤90 g/h and glucose:fructose ratio of 2:1) [3,4]. For a single-stage ultramarathon that generally lasts for more than 3 h, a carbohydrate level of 30–50 g/h is recommended because of numerous barriers to achieve 90 g/h consumption of a multiple-transportable carbohydrate blend [5]. Some of these barriers were described as follows. First, observational studies demonstrated that the actual carbohydrate intake during ultramarathons was less than 60 g/h in most runners [2,6,7], including slower runners consuming 37 g/h [8], and very few reached more than 60 g/h [9,10]. Second, the absolute exercise intensity of an ultramarathon was not as high as some other endurance activities because of its extremely long duration (6, 13, 24, 48, 72, or 10 days) [11]. Third, intestinal absorption might be affected by undertaking highly intensive and long-duration exercises because of the changes in the splanchnic blood flow. In addition, heat, endotoxin, or vertical shaking of their digestive system during rough terrain races could lose the appetite of ultramarathon runners [11,12]. Fourth, ultramarathon runners have to carry their food and fluids in their backpacks during long hours of racing; considering the additional weight being carried, the exercise intensity was increased [8]. Fifth, runners might find food intake difficult while maintaining their balance with both hands when running down steep mountains or climbing steep slopes.

In recent years, races and competitions of over 100 miles have increased, but the specific nutritional and hydration requirements during a continuous multiday ultra-endurance running are still insufficiently known. Reports on races longer than 100 miles [13–18] and especially on the nutritional intake are also limited [19–21].

A review on nutritional supplementation during ultramarathons mainly covers running events of 100–160 km, with a maximum of 217 km [2]. Likewise, a recently published position statement of the International Society of Sports Nutrition [5] and practical recommendations for ultramarathon events [8,14,22] are mainly based on 100–160 km studies.

Since energy intake in an ultramarathon usually exceeds the energy expenditure [5], the effects of energy deficiency would be apparent when the competition time becomes longer than several days and close to a week. The energy deficit could lead to hypoglycemia, degradation of organs, reduction of energy substrates in the blood, and decline in running performance. Firstly, hypoglycemia could reduce the running speed [23]. Hence, the minimum required amount of carbohydrates in each athlete must be identified to maintain their blood glucose levels using a continuous glucose monitoring system. Continuous blood glucose monitoring has widely been used in patients with diabetes and healthy people during exercise [24,25].

Secondly, degradation of tissues could become apparent [8,26,27]. Degradation of tissues could be attenuated by carbohydrate supplementation of 120 g/h, which is far above the recommended amount. However, it cannot enhance running performance and can even increase the incidence of gastrointestinal problems [28,29].

Third, the effects of sleep deprivation on metabolism and athletic performance might be more pronounced. The effects of sleep loss on physiological responses and exercise remain equivocal. An exhaustive review reported that sleep deprivation decreased exercise time to exhaustion, mean power, and increased heart rate [30]. In healthy non-athletes, sleep restriction induced both weight gain and diabetes risk by altering the glucose metabolism, upregulation of appetite, and decreased energy expenditure [31]. However, there are no reports on sleep deprivation and glucose control during ultra-distance events.

Optimal nutrition leads to a decreased risk of energy depletion, better performance [32], the prevention of acute cognitive decline, and improved athlete safety on ultramarathon courses with technical terrain or those requiring navigation [5]. However, the execution of the precise nutrition plan might be difficult for the runner [33] because the nutrient requirements for ultramarathon racing vary greatly, depending on the individual [5], such as age, sex, body mass, or exercise intensity.

A continuous glucose monitoring system encodes individual fluctuations of blood glucose levels in all life situations, including extreme endurance sports [24,25,34–36]. For endurance athletes, wearable devices enable them to compete while maintaining social distance and race across time and space by keeping the records in the cloud [37]. A combination of these devices could potentially improve our understanding of the complex interplay between nutrition and exercise performance.

Through analyzing the relationship between blood glucose fluctuation, running speed, and nutrient intake, one's optimal nutritional requirement could be determined. This approach might help acquire one's appropriate energy and nutrient intake, especially during long-distance events [24,34–36].

This study aimed to examine the variation of blood glucose control and its relationship with the nutritional intake and running performance in a professional female athlete during the 155.7 h of 438 km ultramarathon race with little sleep.

2. Materials and Methods

2.1. Study Design

This case study was designed to define the normal range of blood glucose during a continuous multiday ultramarathon with little sleep and observe the relationships among nutrient intakes, running performance, and blood glucose level. The Ryukoku University Human Research Ethics Review Board (No. 2019-35) approved all our procedures, which complied with the code of ethics of the World Medical Association (Declaration of Helsinki). Written informed consent was obtained from the participant before the study commenced.

2.2. Study Population

A professional female trail runner (age, 44 years; height, 1.52 m; body mass, 42 kg; body mass index, 18.2 kg/m^2, body fat percentage 18%) voluntarily participated in the study. Her annual mileage, elevation gain, and training time were 4440 km, 212,000 m, and 720 h, respectively. She had completed various ultramarathon races, including 330 km certified by the International Trail Running Association, in the last 3 years. In the 35 international races she has competed in, she finished 29 times in the top 10, 16 times in the top 3, and won 4 times. Hence, she is well experienced in ultramarathons.

2.3. Mountain Ultramarathon Course

This study was conducted during a mountain ultramarathon challenge for the fastest-known time in Shiga Round Trail/Shigaichi (https://fastestknowntime.com/route/shiga-round-trail-shiga-ichi-japan, accessed on 12 May 2021) held around the Lake Biwa, the largest lake in Japan (ambient temperature range: 18.3 °C–30.5 °C, relative humidity range: 42–75%), during the first week of June 2020. The distance of the course covered 438 km, and the total elevation gain was 28,300 m. Over 90% of its length unfolded along the unpaved forestry trail. The course was divided into 32 segments by 33 timing gates where investigators recorded each runner's passing time. The distances between each timing gate were 13.69 ± 5.3 SD km (range: 5.9–26.8 km). The running time and speed between each timing gate were obtained by investigators, and the global positioning system (GPS) was recorded by a wristwatch (SUUNTO 9, Suunto, Finland). Furthermore, the location and running speed of the runner were broadcasted live on the internet via a GPS-based tracking system (https://ibuki.run/, archived on 12 May 2021, IBUKI live, ONDO Inc., Kyoto, Japan). Specifically, the running time between each timing gate was 4:52 ± 2:16 h (range: 1:10–11:40 h). During the race, the runner carried her backpack containing necessities, such as food and fluid, which could be replenished at each timing gate. The total running time was 155.7 h, including 16.0 h of rest and sleep. The total hours of rest and sleep each day were 0:20, 1:55, 1:40, 4:00, 3:30, 2:45, 1:50 h:min plus 2 h of fragments of sleep during running.

2.4. Running Pace Data Collection and Standardization

The running performance during the ultramarathon was calculated using the following arbitrary formula:

$$\text{Pace (min/km)} = (E - A)/(\text{Distance of the segment (km)})$$

where

E: the estimated running time of the segment (min);
A: the actual running time of the segment (min).

The pace value was positive when the runner ran faster than the estimated running time but negative when the runner ran slower. Before the ultramarathon, the runner ran 3 1/2 trial laps of this course to determine the estimated running time of the segment.

2.5. Glucose Data Collection and Standardization

All of the blood glucose profile was monitored by flash glucose monitoring (FGM), a minimally invasive method described in previous reports [38–42]. Briefly, the FGM system (FreeStyle Libre; Abbott Diabetes Care, Alameda, CA, USA) mechanically reads and continuously measures the glucose concentration in the interstitial fluid collected right below the skin and subsequently reveals the corresponding ambulatory glucose profile. From one day before the race to three days after the race, the FGM sensor was applied at the back of the runner's upper arm, and glucose concentrations were obtained every 15 min [39]. The highest and lowest glucose concentration levels in each segment and their difference were used as representative values in every segment.

The samples for the plasma clinical parameters were collected after an overnight fast one month before and one week of an off-training period after the ultramarathon and analyzed. The ultramarathon was planned to take place a month earlier, but due to the COVID-19 infection situation and the soft lockdown by the Japanese government, the start of the ultramarathon was delayed by a month. Blood was collected in a clotted vial, and the serum obtained was analyzed by clinical laboratory testing (Falco Biosystems, Inc., Kyoto, Japan). Aspartate aminotransferase (AST), alanine aminotransferase (ALT), and creatine kinase (CK) were estimated by the JSCC standard method. Alkaline phosphatase (ALP) and lactate dehydrogenase (LDH) were estimated by the IFCC standard method. Triglyceride and LDL-cholesterol were estimated by the enzyme colorimetric method. Sodium, potassium, and chloride were estimated by the ion-selective electrode method. Calcium was estimated by the arcenazo III colorimetric test.

2.6. Diet Supply Data Collection

Investigators followed the runner and recorded the entire food and drink intake in relays throughout the ultramarathon. They reported the timing and volume of consumed food and fluid products based on pictures taken during the race. In detail, one or two of the investigators always ran with the runner, taking turns in each segment. They checked the current location, based on GPS, when the runner consumed the refueling meal and recorded the consumption point on a map. Food and fluid products consumed more than 60 min before the start of the ultramarathon were excluded in the nutrient intake calculation with reference to previous studies [23,43]. The nutrition information indicated on the cover of the food and fluid products was our basis when calculating the energy and nutrient intake. If data were unavailable, the intake was calculated according to the standard tables of food composition in Japan 2015 (7th revised edition) [44]. The energy and nutrient intake was expressed relative to the pre-race body weight (kg) per running time (h). In reference to previous research [23,44], all foods were categorized as follows: sports drinks (isotonic and hypertonic formulas), cola, gels, milk product, tea, soup, other liquids (all other drinks consumed), fruits, sweets, bars, noodles, bread, rice products, wheat products, powder, and other solids (all other products consumed).

As shown in Table 1, the runner consumed energy and nutrients from liquids, gels, fruits, sweets, and other solids. The hourly intake of energy, protein, fat, carbohydrate, water, and salt was 170.8 kcal, 5.9 g, 3.1 g, 29.7 g, 263.0 g, and 1.1 g, respectively. The protein:fat:carbohydrate ratio of the ingested nutrients was 13.7:16.5:69.5. The runner consumed 30.1% and 58.3% of their energy from liquids and gels, and solids, respectively. Identically, the intake of carbohydrates from solids (44.4%) was similar to that from liquids or gels (41.4%). Meanwhile, proteins (89.5%) and fats (84.3%) were mostly consumed from solids. Other solids included smoked chicken, potatoes, risotto, lasagna, and protein powder. Other liquids included smoothies and coffee.

Table 1. Total energy and nutrients consumed during the ultramarathon.

	Energy, kcal	Protein, g	Fat, g	Carbohydrate, g	Water, g	Salt, g
Liquids and gels	**7999**	**56**	**17**	**1911**	**35,018**	**84**
Sports drink	1467	5	0	377	6617	13
Cola	87	0	0	21	103	0
Gel	1255	9	0	306	208	44
Milk product	3324	32	6	772	11,889	8
Tea	1120	0	0	284	14,216	14
Soup	331	8	11	48	683	5
Other liquids	415	2	0	103	1302	0
Fruits and sweets	**3075**	**37**	**59**	**657**	**2329**	**1**
Fruit	1122	14	3	291	1601	0
Sweet	1953	23	56	366	728	1
Solids	**15,516**	**815**	**409**	**2047**	**3579**	**77**
Bar	3120	260	91	312	78	8
Noodle	1678	53	29	287	1069	17
Rice product	5334	125	91	965	1050	32
Wheat product	2164	74	88	250	463	7
Powder	651	119	7	22	12	2
Other solids	2569	184	103	211	907	11
Total	**26,590**	**908**	**485**	**4615**	**40,926**	**162**
Average per hour	**171**	**5.9**	**3.1**	**29.7**	**263**	**1.1**

The subtotal of each category is shown in bold.

2.7. Statistics

Herein, numerical data are presented as means and standard deviations unless otherwise specified. Data from a female ultrarunner were processed and analyzed in GraphPad Prism for Mac (version 9.0.1, GraphPad Inc., San Diego, CA, USA). The associations between the running performance, glucose level, and nutrient intake were investigated using Spearman's rank correlation coefficients. The differences among each situation of the blood glucose level were compared by a Mann–Whitney test by ANOVA followed by Dunn's multiple comparison test for the comparison among more than three groups. Results were considered significant when $p < 0.05$. Limitations of the single-subject research design are the generalizability of the study conclusions and were described in the discussion section.

3. Results

3.1. General Results of Blood Glucose Fluctuation during the Ultramarathon

During the 7-day ultramarathon, the regular circadian rhythms, including breakfast, lunch, and dinner, almost disappeared, as detected in the blood glucose levels (Figure 1A). Additionally, the mean blood glucose levels (25–30 mg/dL) were higher than those during the preliminary and post-ultramarathon periods ($p < 0.0001$, Figure 1B). The mean daytime and nighttime blood glucose levels during the ultramarathon were 130.0 ± 16.2 and 124.7 ± 17.3 mg/dL, respectively, with a slight difference ($p < 0.001$, Figure 1C). Moreover, the blood glucose levels during the ultramarathon were controlled within a narrower range than during the preliminary period (Figure 1D).

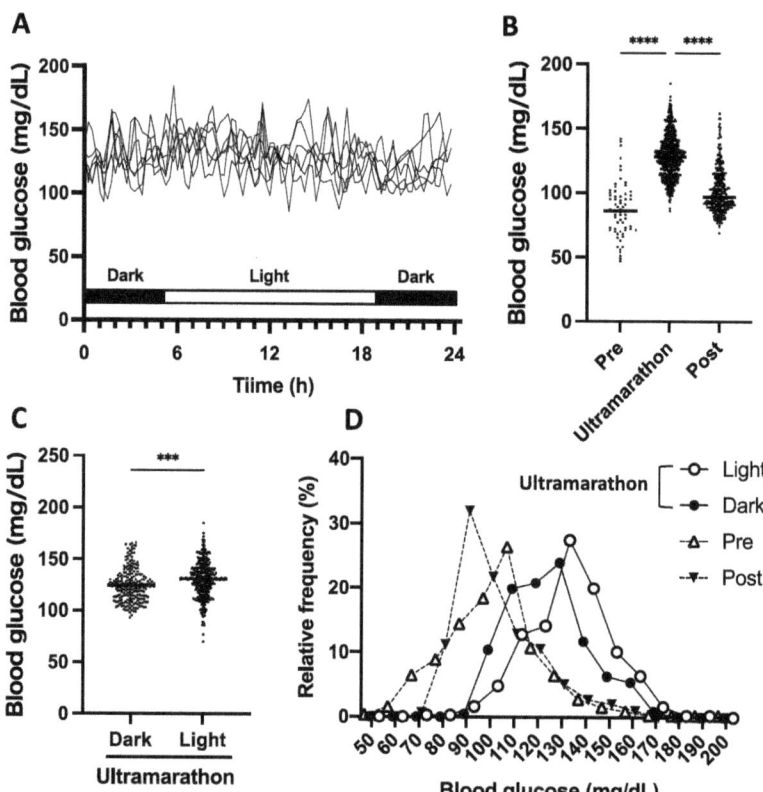

Figure 1. Blood glucose fluctuation during the 7-day ultramarathon. Each solid line represents the daily glucose variation (**A**). Scatter plot of blood glucose during a preliminary, ultramarathon, and post-ultramarathon periods, respectively (**B**). Scatter plot of blood glucose levels during night (dark) and day (light) throughout the ultramarathon (**C**). Histogram of blood glucose fluctuation during preliminary, ultramarathon (night and day), and post-ultramarathon periods (**D**). *** $p < 0.001$, **** $p < 0.0001$ The differences between dark and light were compared by the Mann–Whitney test, and those among pre, ultramarathon post were compared by the Kruskal–Wallis nonparametric ANOVA, followed by Dunn's multiple comparison test.

3.2. Relationship between the Amount of Nutrient Intake and Maintenance of Glucose Level during the Ultramarathon

Significant correlations between the runner's blood glucose levels and nutrient intake were not observed. The lowest glucose level between the segments tended to correlate with protein intake ($p = 0.06$). The highest blood glucose level in the segment was not significantly related to nutrient intake. The difference between the two lines was 50 mg/dL approximately, which was the difference between the highest and lowest blood glucose levels in each segment. Among all nutrients, the difference did not vary significantly from about 50 mg/dL, regardless of the amount consumed (Figure 2).

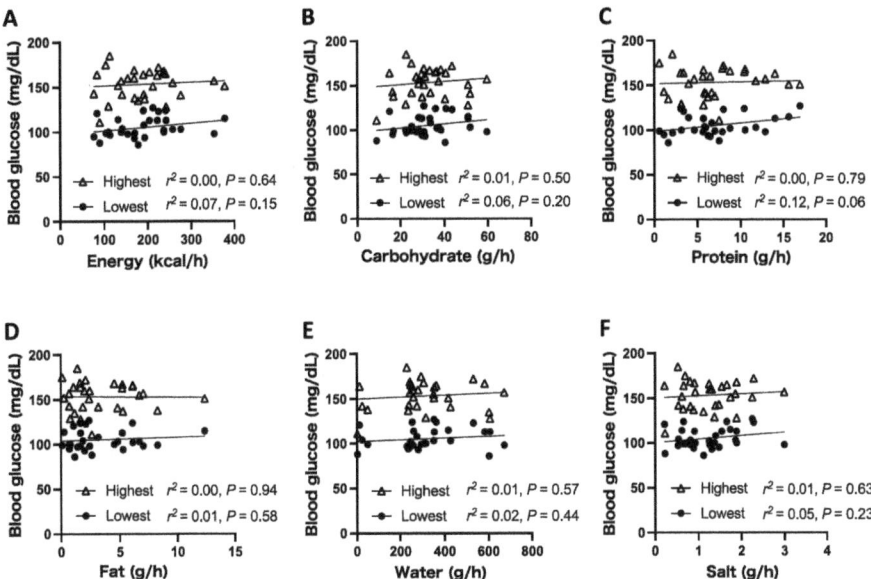

Figure 2. Scatter plots showing the relationships between nutrient intake and blood glucose level. The intake of energy (**A**), carbohydrate (**B**), protein (**C**), fat (**D**), water (**E**), and salt (**F**) was calculated according to the consumed food and fluid products. Each plot indicates one segment.

3.3. Relationship between Glucose Level and Running Pace

During exercise, the runner was within the expected normoglycemic range (86–185 mg/dL), with no extreme hyperglycemia or hypoglycemia (Figure 1). Therefore, the running pace had no significant correlation with the highest blood glucose level ($p = 0.79$), lowest blood glucose level ($p = 0.32$), and delta (difference between the highest and lowest blood glucose levels, $p = 0.36$) between segments (Figure 3).

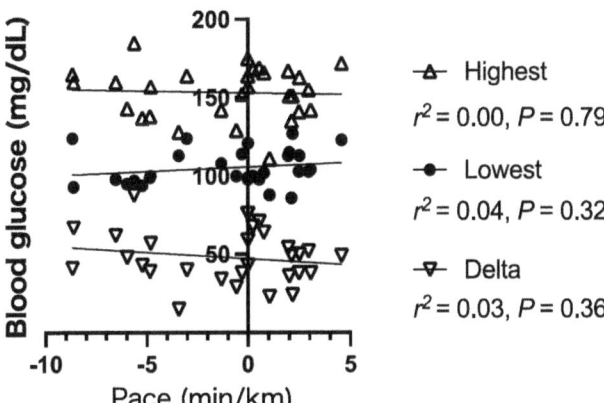

Figure 3. Relationship between the running pace and the highest blood glucose level, lowest blood glucose level, and delta (difference between the highest and lowest blood glucose levels) between segments. The pace was calculated from the difference between the estimated running time and actual running time of the segment, as described in the Methods section. Briefly, the pace value was positive when the runner ran faster than the estimated running time and negative when the runner ran slower.

3.4. Relationship between the Amount of Nutrient Intake and Running Pace during the Ultramarathon

The running pace significantly correlated with energy ($p = 0.02$) and carbohydrates ($p = 0.01$). The running pace tended to correlate with protein ($p = 0.10$) and water intake ($p = 0.06$). Other nutrient intake data did not show the correlation with the running pace (Figure 4).

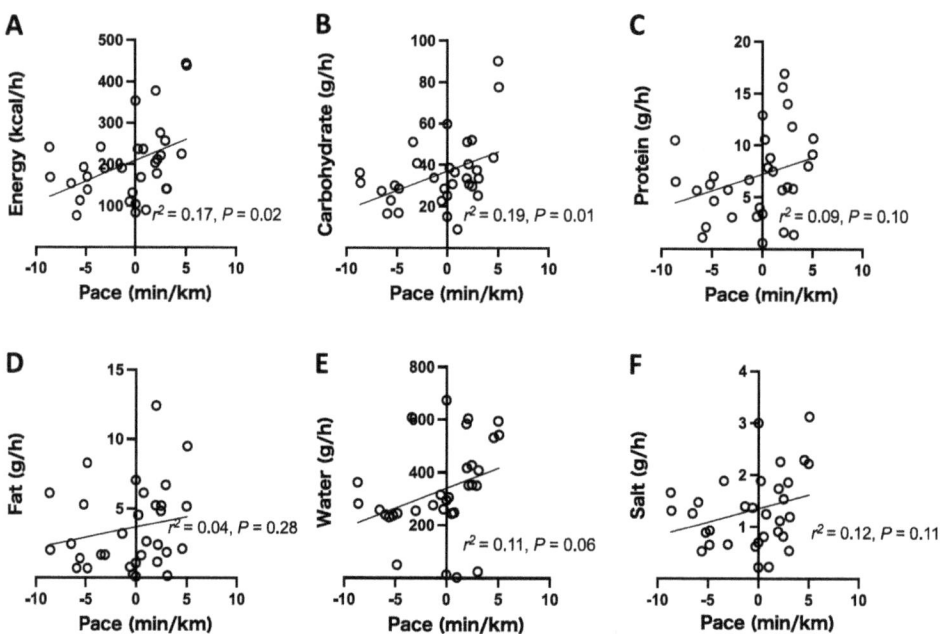

Figure 4. Scatter plots showing the relationships between nutrient intake and running pace. The intake of energy (**A**), carbohydrate (**B**), protein (**C**), fat (**D**), water (**E**), and salt (**F**) was calculated according to the nutrition information of the consumed food and fluid products. Each plot indicates one segment.

3.5. Comparison of Nutrient Intake between Fast and Slow Running Paces

The energy and nutrient intake in the positive running pace (faster than planned) were compared with that in the negative running pace (slower than planned). The energy ($p < 0.01$), carbohydrate ($p < 0.05$), protein ($p < 0.01$), fat ($p < 0.05$), water ($p < 0.01$), and salt ($p < 0.05$) intake in the positive running pace was significantly higher than that in the negative running pace. In the positive running pace, the median hourly nutrient intake for carbohydrate, protein, fat, water, and salt was 38.0 g/h, 9.0 g/h, 5.0 g/h, 413.0 mL/h, and 1.6 g/h, respectively, and the median hourly energy intake was 225 kcal/h (Figure 5).

3.6. Comparison of Food Type between Fast and Slow Running Paces

Food product types used for energy and nutrient consumption were compared in terms of the positivity or negativity of the running pace. When the running pace was positive, the energy and nutrient intake from solids was approximately two times higher than that when it was negative ($p < 0.05$). The water intake was mainly derived from liquids or gels and the intake of liquid (Figure 6).

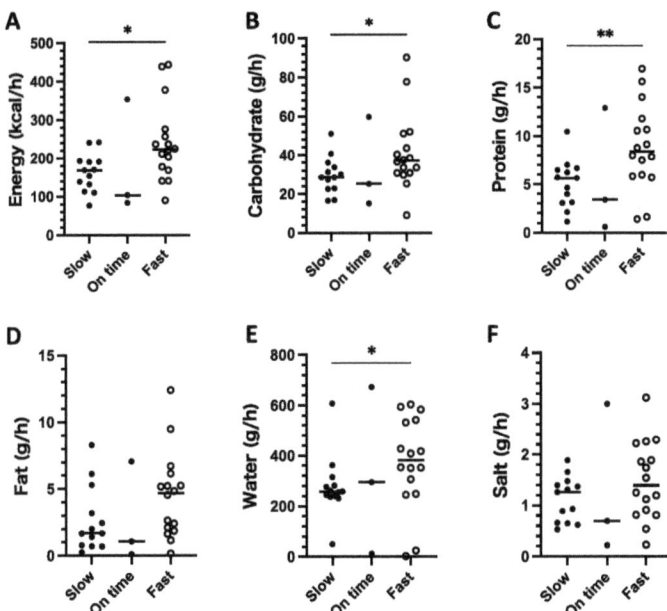

Figure 5. Comparison of energy (**A**), carbohydrate (**B**), protein (**C**), fat (**D**), water (**E**), and salt (**F**) intake among different running paces (fast, when the running pace was faster than planned; on time, when the running pace was the same as planned; slow, when the running pace was slower than planned). * $p < 0.05$ and ** $p < 0.01$ between fast and slow, Mann–Whitney test. The horizontal bar represents the median in each group.

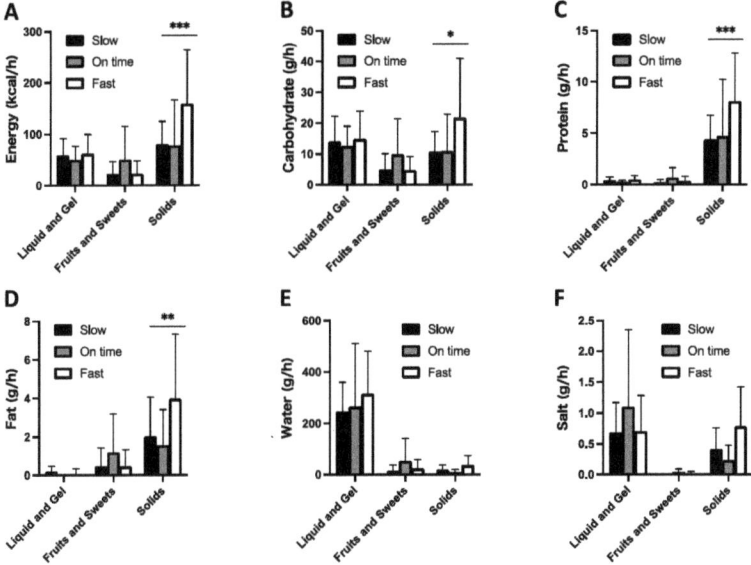

Figure 6. Comparison of product type for energy (**A**), carbohydrate (**B**), protein (**C**), fat (**D**), water (**E**), and salt (**F**) consumption among different running paces (fast, when the running pace was faster than planned; on time, when the running pace was the same as planned; slow, when the running pace was slower than planned). * $p < 0.05$, ** $p < 0.01$, *** $p < 0.001$ between fast and slow, Mann–Whitney test. Values are means ± SEM.

3.7. Change of Serum Parameters Pre- and Post-Ultramarathon

Triglycerides in the blood were greatly reduced, suggesting that lipid utilization contributed significantly to energy production. The total protein in the blood was also slightly decreased. The decrease in ALP could be due to insufficient zinc intake. On the other hand, there was only a slight increase in AST and ALT compared to the marked increase in LDH and CK, suggesting that although there was muscle damage, the damage on the liver function was small (Table 2).

Table 2. Serum parameters pre- and post-ultramarathon compared with the Japanese population.

		Normal Range Mean (95% CI)	Ultramarathon Pre	Ultramarathon Post
Total protein	g/dL	7.4 ± 0.5 (6.5–8.3)	6.9	5.8 [L]
Triglyceride	mg/dL	89.5 ± 30.4 (30.0–149.0)	140	33
LDL-cholesterol	mg/dL	104.5 ± 17.6 (70.0–139.0)	65 [L]	42 [L]
AST	U/L	23.0 ± 7.7 (8.0–38.0)	31	87 [H]
ALT	U/L	23.5 ± 9.9 (4.0–43.0)	35	84 [H]
ALP	U/L	232.0 ± 62.2 (110.0–354.0)	258	70 [L]
LDH	U/L	183.0 ± 31.6 (121.0–245.0)	184	428 [H]
CK	U/L	117.0 ± 40.3 (38.0–196.0)	102	1312 [H]
Na	mEq/L	142.5 ± 3.8 (135.0–150.0)	137	142
Cl	mEq/L	104.0 ± 3.1 (98.0–110.0)	101	106
K	mEq/L	4.4 ± 0.5 (3.5–5.3)	4.7	3.9
Ca	mg/dL	9.3 ± 0.5 (8.4–10.2)	9	8.5

[L], lower than normal range CI; [H], higher than normal range; AST, aspartate aminotransferase; ALT, alanine aminotransferase; ALP, alkaline phosphatase; lactate dehydrogenase; LDH, lactate dehydrogenase; CK, creatine kinase.

4. Discussion

This study aimed to examine the variation of blood glucose control and its relationship with nutritional intake and running performance in a professional female athlete during the continuous over 400 km ultramarathon race with little sleep. Diurnal variation had almost disappeared with the overall average glucose increase of approximately 30 mg/dL compared to resting. A significantly faster running speed correlated with a higher energy and nutrient intake from solid foods than from gels and liquids. Interestingly, the median energy and carbohydrate intake in the fast-running pace were within the recommended energy and carbohydrate intake, mainly covered 100–160 km ultramarathon [5,6].

Protein intake contributed to the maintenance of blood glucose levels as carbohydrate intake was at the lower end of the recommended amount. Sufficient energy and nutrient intake prevented hypoglycemia, thereby maintaining the running speed during the ultramarathon. Consistent with the findings from a 100-mile race [23], the highest blood glucose concentration obtained was not associated with the running speed, indicating that instead of the rapid availability of carbohydrates, nutrient intake from solid foods for controlling glucose homeostasis was the key determinant of performance especially in an ultramarathon of over 400 km.

Recording the amount of energy and nutrient intake during prolonged exercise events had corresponding difficulties. A bicycle equipped with a camera cycled alongside the runner to accurately record the results [45]. In the present study, given that the course mostly covered a single track where bicycles could not pass, the ultramarathon runners were followed by other runners to record the food and drink intake; hence, the energy and nutrient intake recorded was precise and valuable. This ultramarathon gained considerable attention that several runners took turns to accompany the ultramarathon runner for approximately one week to keep track of her meals and drinks.

Gluconeogenesis played an essential role in maintaining blood glucose levels during an ultramarathon, considering that meeting carbohydrate consumption throughout the entire ultramarathon race was not feasible, not even in typical durations of an ultramarathon (6–48 h). Energy deficiency was common in ultramarathons [5–7,32,45–48]. Studies using a doubly labeled water technique or respiratory gas analysis estimated that the energy expenditure during 160 km ultramarathons was approximately 13,000 kcal [2,49,50]. The previously reported rates of gluconeogenesis and hepatic glycogenolysis in a resting state in low-carbohydrate–fed subjects were 0.07 and 0.03 g/kg/h, respectively [51]. The sum of these two values (0.1 g/kg/h), otherwise known as endogenous glucose production, would be the minimum required amount of carbohydrates to maintain blood glucose levels during a resting state. The endogenous glucose production significantly increased to 0.36 g/kg/h during exercise at 55% of peak power output [51] or 0.48 g/kg/h during exercise at the lactate threshold level in fasted, well-trained subjects [52]. In accordance with this calculation, the runner in the present study required 29.7 and 5.9 g/h of carbohydrate and protein intake, respectively, to maintain her blood glucose concentrations during the ultramarathon.

Consuming mostly solid foods alongside other carbohydrate forms can be a practical option for the supplementation of adequate energy and nutrients with fewer gastrointestinal problems, especially for a race that lasts for several days. Previous reports using ^{13}C-labeled isotopes revealed that carbohydrates from solid foods (as well as from liquids) were effectively oxidized during exercise and could suppress gastric emptying compared with the liquid form [43]. Solid foods slightly elevated blood glucose levels and secreted less insulin [53] and glucose-dependent insulinotropic peptide compared with liquid foods [54]. Furthermore, gastric emptying of semisolid food was not affected by exercises at intensities of the 40% VO_2 peak [55]. Solid foods could maintain the same blood glucose levels as gel foods and perform the same intensity of cycle exercise and time trials [56]. According to recent reports, ingestion of a larger volume of carbohydrate solution at less frequent intervals during prolonged submaximal running spared endogenous carbohydrate oxidation rates. It did not cause increased markers of gastrointestinal discomfort compared with the smaller volumes at more frequent intervals [57].

A marked increase in CK, compared with the other biochemical markers, such as ALT, AST, LDH, were reported in previous studies on 130 to 160 km of ultramarathon [26,27]. In a longer-distance ultramarathon, a significant increase in CK was observed [8]. On the other hand, ALP was mildly elevated in this previous study but decreased in the present study. The reduction of ALP might be due to insufficient zinc intake in this study.

In the present study, there was a correlation between nutrient intake and speed, as the intake of energy and nutrients were insufficient compared with the energy expenditure during the ultramarathon. Insufficient intake was speculated by the decrease in blood triglycerides and total protein concentration in the present ultramarathon. Our previous study also revealed that the lowest blood glucose level in each section was the cause of the running speed reduction, though the highest blood glucose level in each section of the run was not related to the running speed [23]. Fatigue is caused by various factors, and excessive intake did not entirely enhance performance. The weak correlation between the blood glucose level and the running speed could be explained by the previously reported gender-specific differences in fuel utilization during exercise. Females showed higher lipid oxidation caused by higher plasma adiponectin levels [58], higher muscle triglyceride utilization [59], low plasma glucose levels [60], and higher fasting hepatic glucose uptake than males [61].

Levels of glucose increased by an average of approximately 20 percent during the early part of nocturnal sleep but returned to baseline levels in the morning because of reduced glucose utilization during sleep [62]. Similarly, glucose tolerance was optimal in the morning and reached its minimum in the middle of the night [63,64]. Another study revealed an association between sleep and glucose regulation during constant glucose infusion, which was a condition that inhibited endogenous glucose production and, therefore, revealed changes in glucose utilization [62].

The intravenous glucose tolerance test during the sleep restriction condition demonstrated that the rate of glucose clearance was approximately 40% lower and the acute insulin response to glucose was 30% lower compared to the sleep extension condition [65].

Interestingly, the diurnal rhythm of blood glucose levels in the present study was almost abolished compared to the resting state, and the difference between daytime and nighttime blood glucose levels was significant but not pronounced. This change was caused by the combined factors of running and sleep deprivation, but the mean and SD of blood glucose levels did not gradually increase along with the accumulation of sleep deprivation during the ultramarathon. These results suggested that running in a sleep-deprived state for at least up to a week did not cause extreme fluctuations in blood glucose levels.

Sleep deprivation of 30 to 72 h did not drastically affect cardiovascular and respiratory responses to exercise of varying intensity or the aerobic and anaerobic performance capability [66]. For example, during prolonged treadmill walking at about 80% of the VO_{2max}, the reduction of work time to exhaustion was only 11% after 30 h of sleep deprivation [67]. Another study reported that the maximal isometric and isokinetic muscular strength and endurance of selected upper and lower body muscle groups, the performance of the Wingate Anaerobic Power Test, simple reaction time, the blood lactate response to cycle exercise at 70% VO_{2max}, and most of the cardiovascular and respiratory responses to treadmill running at 70% and 80% VO_{2max}, were not significantly altered as a result of sleep deprivation of 60 h [68]. Although the sleep deprivation in this study was 155.7 h, the runner was not in complete sleep deprivation, and its relationship to performance needed to be carefully examined.

Meanwhile, the main limitation of this study was the number of subjects. It was not feasible to have sufficient subjects, as few people even attempt to run through the entire route of the 438 km of a mountain ultramarathon for continuous several days. In the present ultramarathon, another runner started simultaneously but retired in the middle of the race. Though this research was a case study, our study athlete set the fastest time; thus, our record could be considered valuable. Our observational study supported the effectiveness of the position statement of the International Society of Sports Nutrition [5] and practical recommendation for ultramarathon participants to prevent hypoglycemia during exercise.

The limitations of the single-subject research design were the generalizability of the study conclusions and the methodological and statistical assumptions that were typically needed for inferential statistical tests. A single-subject design provided limited support for conclusions regarding populations of subjects [69]. Nonetheless, single-subject studies have been conducted in rehabilitation, disability [70,71], or psychological research [72]. These study designs employ a comparison in the AB design. In this design, A represents the baseline, and B represents the treatment. The subject is treated repeatedly as AB or ABA [73,74]. Similarly, ABAB or other extensions of AB designs are stronger designs than the simple phase change of an AB design [71]. In the present study, the statistical data was processed as an extended AB design consisting of segments of faster or slower than the planned pace. In the future, these findings need to be accumulated to reach a general conclusion.

Another methodological limitation was the large fluctuations in running speed during the ultramarathon. The running speed in the mountain ultramarathon usually varied by vast diversities of terrain [75] and physiological changes such as muscle fatigue and energy deficiency. We could not measure the heart rate as the runners did not tolerate the discomfort of wearing the belt for six days. We used a GPS tracking system to monitor this run, but it was difficult to calculate the intensity from the distance and slope because more than 90% of this route was a track in the forest, and the surface was diverse. Therefore, the running speed values of the runner were standardized using the preliminary planned running time, which was obtained by allowing the runner to run 3 1/2 trial laps of this course before the ultramarathon. The precise and objective power meters were already applicable in cycling studies [76].

Continuous glucose monitoring systems were less accurate than the gold standard for intermittent self-measurement of blood glucose [40]. The present research adopted the system, which was pronounced as superior performance during exercise compared with the other GM systems [41]. Although we rarely observed hypoglycemia in this study, caution should be exercised regarding the accuracy of values at low blood glucose levels as the median absolute relative difference between the reference values and those obtained by the sensor across the glycemic range overall was 22 (13.9–29.7)% and was 36.3 (24.2–45.2)% during hypoglycemia, 22.8 (14.6–30.6)% during euglycemia and 15.4 (9–21)% during hyperglycemia [77].

GPS monitoring throughout the entire running and sharing the runner's location was linked to the assured dietary support and safety of the runner in the present study. Sharing the blood glucose level as well was expected to ensure further safety. Accurate physical workload calculation based on GPS monitoring or running power meter would enable a more accurate analysis of the running performance and blood glucose fluctuations.

5. Conclusions

In conclusion, the diurnal variation of the plasma glucose level had almost disappeared with the overall slight glucose increase during a continuous multiday ultramarathon in a female athlete. The intake of protein and fat directly or indirectly contributed to maintaining the blood glucose levels and running speed as gluconeogenesis source or energy source when the intake of carbohydrates was at the lower limit of dietary recommendation. Carbohydrate, protein, and fat intake from solid foods contributed to maintaining a fast pace compared with liquids and gels.

Author Contributions: Conceptualization, K.I.; methodology, K.I., N.I., and A.T.; software, K.I., N.I., and A.T.; validation, K.I. and N.I.; formal analysis, N.I.; investigation, K.I., N.I., D.S., and A.K.; resources, K.I. and H.O.; data curation, K.I., N.I., and T.N.; writing—original draft preparation, K.I.; writing—review and editing, K.I. and Y.N.; visualization, K.I. and N.I.; supervision, K.I., and Y.N.; project administration, K.I.; funding acquisition, K.I. and H.O. All authors have read and agreed to the published version of the manuscript.

Funding: This research was funded by the Ryukoku University and Nagatasangyo.co. (Hyogo, Japan).

Institutional Review Board Statement: The study was conducted according to the guidelines of the Declaration of Helsinki, and approved by the Institutional Review Board of Ryukoku University (Protocol no. 2019-35, Date of approval: 18 Februay 2020).

Informed Consent Statement: Informed consent was obtained from all subjects involved in the study. Written informed consent has been obtained from the patient to publish this paper.

Acknowledgments: We express our gratitude and deep appreciation to Kaori Niwa, Hitomi Matsubara, and Noriyuki Niwa for their kind support. We also thank all the participants for their cooperation in the investigation.

Conflicts of Interest: The authors declare no conflict of interest. The funders had no role in the design of the study; in the collection, analyses, or interpretation of data; in the writing of the manuscript, or in the decision to publish the results.

References

1. Stöhr, A.; Nikolaidi, P.T.; Villiger, E.; Sousa, C.V.; Scheer, V.; Hill, L.; Knechtle, B. An analysis of participation and performance of 2067 100-km ultra-marathons worldwide. *Int. J. Environ. Res. Public Health* **2021**, *18*, 362. [CrossRef]
2. Arribalzaga, M.; Ruano, G.; Saiz, S. Review of the Food Guidelines in Continuous Ultramarathon. *J. Nutr. Food Sci.* **2017**, *7*. [CrossRef]
3. Wilson, G.; Drust, B.; Morton, J.P.; Close, G.L. Weight-making Strategies in Professional Jockeys: Implications for Physical and Mental Health and Well-being. *Sport. Med.* **2014**, *44*, 785–796. [CrossRef]
4. Rodriguez, N.N.R.; Di Marco, N.; Langley, S.; DiMarco, N.M. American College of Sports Medicine, American Dietetic Association, and Dietitians of Canada Joint Position Statement: Nutrition and Athletic Performance. *Med. Sci. Sports Exerc.* **2009**, *41*, 709–731. [CrossRef] [PubMed]
5. Tiller, N.B.; Roberts, J.D.; Beasley, L.; Chapman, S.; Pinto, J.M.; Smith, L.; Wiffin, M.; Russell, M.; Sparks, S.A.; Duckworth, L.; et al. International Society of Sports Nutrition Position Stand: Nutritional Considerations for Single-stage Ultra-marathon Training and Racing. *J. Int. Soc. Sports Nutr.* **2019**, *16*, 1–23. [CrossRef]

6. Costa, R.J.S.; Gill, S.K.; Hankey, J.; Wright, A.; Marczak, S. Perturbed Energy Balance and Hydration Status in Ultra-endurance Runners During a 24 h Ultra-marathon. *Br. J. Nutr.* **2014**, *112*, 428–437. [CrossRef] [PubMed]
7. Clark, H.R.; Barker, M.E.; Corfe, B.M. Nutritional Strategies of Mountain Marathon Competitors-An Observational Study. *Int. J. Sport Nutr. Exerc. Metab.* **2005**, *15*, 160–172. [CrossRef]
8. Costa, R.J.S.; Knechtle, B.; Tarnopolsky, M.; Hoffman, M.D. Nutrition for Ultramarathon Running: Trail, Track, and Road. *Int. J. Sport Nutr. Exerc. Metab.* **2019**, *29*, 130–140. [CrossRef] [PubMed]
9. Hoffman, M.D.; Stuempfle, K.J. Hydration Strategies, Weight Change and Performance in a 161 km Ultramarathon. *Res. Sport. Med.* **2014**, *22*, 213–225. [CrossRef]
10. Zalcman, I.; Guarita, H.V.; Juzwiak, C.R.; Crispim, C.A.; Antunes, H.K.M.; Edwards, B.; Tufik, S.; de Mello, M.T. Nutritional Status of Adventure Racers. *Nutrition* **2007**, *23*, 404–411. [CrossRef] [PubMed]
11. Knechtle, B.; Nikolaidis, P.T. Physiology and Pathophysiology in Ultra-marathon Running. *Front. Physiol.* **2018**, *9*, 634. [CrossRef] [PubMed]
12. Stuempfle, K.J.; Valentino, T.; Hew-Butler, T.; Hecht, F.M.; Hoffman, M.D. Nausea is associated with Endotoxemia during a 161-km Ultramarathon. *J. Sports Sci.* **2016**, *34*, 1662–1668. [CrossRef]
13. Alcock, R.; McCubbin, A.; Camões-Costa, V.; Costa, R.J.S. Case Study: Providing Nutritional Support to an Ultraendurance Runner in Preparation for a Self-Sufficient Multistage Ultramarathon: Rationed Versus Full Energy Provisions. *Wilderness Environ. Med.* **2018**, *29*, 508–520. [CrossRef] [PubMed]
14. Kerschan-Schindl, K.; Thalmann, M.M.; Weiss, E.; Tsironi, M.; Föger-Samwald, U.; Meinhart, J.; Skenderi, K.; Pietschmann, P. Changes in Serum Levels of Myokines and Wnt-Antagonists After an Ultramarathon Race. *PLoS ONE* **2015**, *10*, e0132478. [CrossRef]
15. Edwards, K.H.; Elliott, B.T.; Kitic, C.M. Carbohydrate Intake and Ketosis in Self-sufficient Multi-stage Ultramarathon Runners. *J. Sports Sci.* **2019**. [CrossRef] [PubMed]
16. Seal, A.D.; Anastasiou, C.A.; Skenderi, K.P.; Echegaray, M.; Yiannakouris, N.; Tsekouras, Y.E.; Matalas, A.L.; Yannakoulia, M.; Pechlivani, F.; Kavouras, S.A. Incidence of Hyponatremia During a Continuous 246-km Ultramarathon Running Race. *Front. Nutr.* **2019**, *6*, 161. [CrossRef]
17. David Cotter, J.; Gatterer, H.; Vernillo, G.; Savoldelli, A.; Skafidas, S.; Zignoli, A.; La Torre, A.; Pellegrini, B.; Giardini, G.; Trabucchi, P.; et al. An Extreme Mountain Ultra-Marathon Decreases the Cost of Uphill Walking and Running. *Front. Physiol.* **2016**, *7*, 530. [CrossRef]
18. Fallon, K.E.; Sivyer, G.; Sivyer, K.; Dare, A. The Biochemistry of Runners in a 1600 km Ultramarathon. *Br. J. Sport. Med.* **1999**, *33*, 264–269. [CrossRef]
19. Abernethy, P.J.; Eden, B. Changes in Blood Glucose Levels during a 1005-km Running Race: A Case Study. *Br. J. Sports Med.* **1992**, *26*, 66–68. [CrossRef]
20. Dempster, S.; Britton, R.; Murray, A.; Costa, R.J.S. Case Study: Nutrition and Hydration Status during 4,254 km of Running Over 78 Consecutive Days. *Int. J. Sport Nutr. Exerc. Metab.* **2013**, *23*, 533–541. [CrossRef]
21. Rontoyannis, G.P.; Skoulis, T.; Pavlou, K.N. Energy Balance in Ultramarathon Running. *Am. J. Clin. Nutr.* **1989**, *49*, 976–979. [CrossRef]
22. Costa, R.J.S.; Hoffman, M.D.; Stellingwerff, T. Considerations for Ultra-endurance Activities: Part 1- Nutrition. *Res. Sport. Med.* **2019**. [CrossRef] [PubMed]
23. Ishihara, K.; Uchiyama, N.; Kizaki, S.; Mori, E.; Nonaka, T.; Oneda, H. Application of Continuous Glucose Monitoring for Assessment of Individual Carbohydrate Requirement During Ultramarathon Race. *Nutrients* **2020**, *12*, 1121. [CrossRef] [PubMed]
24. Nikolaidis, P.T.; Knechtle, B. Ultramarathon with Type 1 Diabetes. *Praxis* **2018**, *107*, 777–781. [CrossRef]
25. Sengoku, Y.; Nakamura, K.; Ogata, H.; Nabekura, Y.; Nagasaka, S.; Tokuyama, K. Continuous Glucose Monitoring During a 100-km Race: A Case Study in an Elite Ultramarathon Runner. *Int. J. Sports Physiol. Perform.* **2015**, *10*, 124–127. [CrossRef]
26. Arakawa, K.; Hosono, A.; Shibata, K.; Ghadimi, R.; Fuku, M.; Goto, C.; Imaeda, N.; Tokudome, Y.; Hoshino, H.; Marumoto, M.; et al. Changes in blood biochemical markers before, during, and after a 2-day ultramarathon. *Open Access J. Sport Med.* **2016**, *7*, 43–50. [CrossRef] [PubMed]
27. Hoffman, M.D.; Ingwerson, J.L.; Rogers, I.R.; Hew-Butler, T.; Stuempfle, K.J. Increasing creatine kinase concentrations at the 161-km western states endurance run. *Wilderness Environ. Med.* **2012**, *23*, 56–60. [CrossRef] [PubMed]
28. Viribay, A.; Arribalzaga, S.; Mielgo-Ayuso, J.; Castañeda-Babarro, A.; Seco-Calvo, J.; Urdampilleta, A. Effects of 120 g/h of Carbohydrates Intake During a Mountain Marathon on Exercise-induced Muscle Damage in Elite Runners. *Nutrients* **2020**, *12*, 1367. [CrossRef]
29. Urdampilleta, A.; Arribalzaga, S.; Viribay, A.; Castañeda-Babarro, A.; Seco-Calvo, J.; Mielgo-Ayuso, J. Effects of 120 vs. 60 and 90 g/h Carbohydrate Intake During a Trail Marathon on Neuromuscular Function and High Intensity Run Capacity Recovery. *Nutrients* **2020**, *12*, 2094. [CrossRef]
30. Watson, A.M. Sleep and Athletic Performance. *Curr. Sports Med. Rep.* **2017**, *16*, 413–418. [CrossRef]
31. Knutson, K.L.; Spiegel, K.; Penev, P.; Van Cauter, E. The metabolic consequences of sleep deprivation. *Sleep Med. Rev.* **2007**, *11*, 163–178. [CrossRef]
32. Williamson, E. Nutritional Implications for Ultra-endurance Walking and Running Events. *Extrem. Physiol. Med.* **2016**, *5*, 1–18. [CrossRef]

33. Pruitt, K.A.; Hill, J.M. Optimal Pacing and Carbohydrate Intake Strategies for Ultramarathons. *Eur. J. Appl. Physiol.* **2017**, *117*, 2527–2545. [CrossRef] [PubMed]
34. Gawrecki, A.; Zozulinska-Ziolkiewicz, D.; Matejko, B.; Hohendorff, J.; Malecki, M.T.; Klupa, T. Safe Completion of a Trail Running Ultramarathon by Four Men with Type 1 Diabetes. *Diabetes Technol. Ther.* **2018**, *20*, 147–152. [CrossRef] [PubMed]
35. Kordonouri, O.; Vazeou, A.; Scharf, M.; Würsig, M.; Battelino, T. Striving for Control: Lessons Learned from a Successful International Type 1 Diabetes Youth Challenge. *Acta Diabetol.* **2017**, *54*, 403–409. [CrossRef] [PubMed]
36. Belli, T.; de Macedo, D.V.; Scariot, P.P.M.; de Araújo, G.G.; dos Reis, I.G.M.; Lazarim, F.L.; Nunes, L.A.S.; Brenzikofer, R.; Gobatto, C.A. Glycemic Control and Muscle Damage in 3 Athletes with Type 1 Diabetes During a Successful Performance in a Relay Ultramarathon: A Case Report. *Wilderness Environ. Med.* **2017**, *28*, 239–245. [CrossRef]
37. Emig, T.; Peltonen, J. Human Running Performance from Real-world Big Data. *Nat. Commun.* **2020**, *11*, 1–9. [CrossRef]
38. Al Hayek, A.A.; Robert, A.A.; Al Dawish, M.A. Evaluation of FreeStyle Libre Flash Glucose Monitoring System on Glycemic Control, Health-Related Quality of Life, and Fear of Hypoglycemia in Patients with Type 1 Diabetes. *Clin. Med. Insights Endocrinol. Diabetes* **2017**, *10*. [CrossRef]
39. Fokkert, M.J.; Van Dijk, P.R.; Edens, M.A.; Abbes, S.; De Jong, D.; Slingerland, R.J.; Bilo, H.J.G. Performance of the Freestyle Libre Flash Glucose Monitoring System in Patients with Type 1 and 2 Diabetes Mellitus. *BMJ Open Diabetes Res. Care* **2017**, *5*. [CrossRef]
40. Fokkert, M.J.; Damman, A.; Van Dijk, P.R.; Edens, M.A.; Abbes, S.; Braakman, J.; Slingerland, R.J.; Dikkeschei, L.D.; Dille, J.; Bilo, H.J.G. Use of FreeStyle Libre Flash Monitor Register in the Netherlands (FLARE-NL1): Patient Experiences, Satisfaction, and Cost Analysis. *Int. J. Endocrinol.* **2019**, *2019*. [CrossRef]
41. Aberer, F.; Hajnsek, M.; Rumpler, M.; Zenz, S.; Baumann, P.M.; Elsayed, H.; Puffing, A.; Treiber, G.; Pieber, T.R.; Sourij, H.; et al. Evaluation of subcutaneous glucose monitoring systems under routine environmental conditions in patients with type 1 diabetes. *Diabetes. Obes. Metab.* **2017**, *19*, 1051–1055. [CrossRef] [PubMed]
42. Moser, O.; Mader, J.K.; Tschakert, G.; Mueller, A.; Groeschl, W.; Pieber, T.R.; Koehler, G.; Messerschmidt, J.; Hofmann, P. Accuracy of continuous glucose monitoring (CGM) during continuous and high-intensity interval exercise in patients with type 1 diabetes mellitus. *Nutrients* **2016**, *8*, 489. [CrossRef]
43. Pfeiffer, B.; Stellingwerff, T.; Zaltas, E.; Jeukendrup, A.E.; Pfeeffer, B.; Stellingwerff, T.; Zaltas, E.; Jeukendrup, A.E.; Pfeiffer, A.B.; Stellingwertf, T.; et al. Oxidation of Solid Versus Liquid CHO Sources During Exercise. *Med. Sci. Sports Exerc.* **2010**, *42*, 2030–2037. [CrossRef] [PubMed]
44. Office for Resources, P.D.S.T. P.B. *Standard Tables of Food Composition in Japan-2015-(Seventh Revised Version)*; Ministry of Education, Culture, Sports, Science and Technology: Tokyo, Japan, 2015.
45. Arnaoutis, G.; Leveritt, M.; Wardenaar, F.C.; Hoogervorst, D.; Versteegen, J.J.; Van Der Burg, N.; Lambrechtse, K.J.; Bongers, C.C.W.G. Real-Time Observations of Food and Fluid Timing During a 120 km Ultramarathon. *Front. Nutr.* **2018**, *5*, 32. [CrossRef]
46. Wardenaar, F.C.; Dijkhuizen, R.; Ceelen, I.J.M.; Jonk, E.; de Vries, J.H.M.; Witkamp, R.F.; Mensink, M. Nutrient Intake by Ultramarathon Runners: Can They Meet Recommendations? *Int. J. Sport Nutr. Exerc. Metab.* **2015**, *25*, 375–386. [CrossRef] [PubMed]
47. Stuempfle, K.J.; Hoffman, M.D.; Weschler, L.B.; Rogers, I.R.; Hew-Butler, T. Race Diet of Finishers and Non-finishers in a 100 Mile (161 km) Mountain Footrace. *J. Am. Coll. Nutr.* **2011**, *30*, 529–535. [CrossRef]
48. Martinez, S.; Aguilo, A.; Rodas, L.; Lozano, L.; Moreno, C.; Tauler, P. Energy, Macronutrient and Water Intake During a Mountain Ultramarathon Event: The Influence of Distance. *J. Sports Sci.* **2018**, *36*, 333–339. [CrossRef]
49. Hill, R.J.; Davies, P.S. Energy Expenditure during 2 wk of an Ultra-endurance Run around Australia. *Med. Sci. Sports Exerc.* **2001**, *33*, 148–151. [CrossRef]
50. Dumke, C.L.; Shooter, L.; Lind, R.H.; Nieman, D.C. Indirect Calorimetry during Ultradistance Running: A Case Report. *J. Sports Sci. Med.* **2006**, *5*, 692–698.
51. Webster, C.C.; Noakes, T.D.; Chacko, S.K.; Swart, J.; Kohn, T.A.; Smith, J.A.H. Gluconeogenesis During Endurance Exercise in Cyclists Habituated to a Long-term Low Carbohydrate High-fat Diet. Authors. *J. Physiol. C* **2016**, *594*, 4389–4405. [CrossRef]
52. Emhoff, C.A.W.; Messonnier, L.A.; Horning, M.A.; Fattor, J.A.; Carlson, T.J.; Brooks, G.A. Gluconeogenesis and Hepatic Glycogenolysis During Exercise at the Lactate Threshold. *J. Appl. Physiol.* **2013**, *114*, 297–306. [CrossRef] [PubMed]
53. Roberts, R.A.; Mcminn, S.B.; Mermier, C.; Hi, G.L.; Ruby, B.; Quinn, C. Blood Glucose and Glucoregulatory Hormone Responses to Solid and Liquid Carbohydrate Ingestion during Exercise. *Int. J. Of Sport Nutr.* **1998**, *8*, 70–83. [CrossRef]
54. Peracchi, M.; Santangelo, A.; Conte, D.; Fraquelli, M.; Tagliabue, R.; Gebbia, C.; Porrini, M. The Physical State of a Meal Affects Hormone Release and Postprandial Thermogenesis. *Br. J. Nutr.* **2000**, *83*, 623–628. [CrossRef]
55. Mattin, L.R.; Yau, A.M.W.; McIver, V.; James, L.J.; Evans, G.H. The Effect of Exercise Intensity on Gastric Emptying Rate, Appetite and Gut Derived Hormone Responses After Consuming a Standardised Semi-Solid Meal in Healthy Males. *Nutrients* **2018**, *10*, 787. [CrossRef] [PubMed]
56. Ishihara, K.; Taniguchi, H.; Akiyama, N.; Asami, Y. Easy to Swallow Rice Cake as a Carbohydrate Source During Endurance Exercise Suppressed Feelings of Thirst and Hunger Without Changing Exercise Performance. *Nutr. Sci. Vitaminol.* **2020**, *66*, 128–135. [CrossRef] [PubMed]
57. Mears, S.A.; Boxer, B.; Sheldon, D.; Wardley, H.; Tarnowski, C.A.; James, L.J.; Hulston, C.J. Sports Drink Intake Pattern Affects Exogenous Carbohydrate Oxidation During Running. *Med. Sci. Sports Exerc.* **2020**, *52*, 1976–1982. [CrossRef]

58. Geer, E.B.; Shen, W. Gender Differences in Insulin Resistance, Body Composition, and Energy Balance. *Gend. Med.* **2009**, *6*, 60–75. [CrossRef]
59. Wismann, J.; Willoughby, D. Gender Differences in Carbohydrate Metabolism and Carbohydrate Loading. *J. Int. Soc. Sports Nutr.* **2006**, *3*, 28–32. [CrossRef]
60. Soeters, M.R.; Sauerwein, H.P.; Groener, J.E.; Aerts, J.M.; Ackermans, M.T.; Glatz, J.F.C.; Fliers, E.; Serlie, M.J. Gender-related Differences in the Metabolic Response to Fasting. *J. Clin. Endocrinol. Metab.* **2007**, *92*, 3646–3652. [CrossRef]
61. Keramida, G.; Peters, A.M. Fasting Hepatic Glucose Uptake is Higher in Men than Women. *Physiol. Rep.* **2017**, *5*. [CrossRef]
62. Scheen, A.J.; Byrne, M.M.; Plat, L.; Leproult, R.; Van Cauter, E. Relationships between sleep quality and glucose regulation in normal humans. *Am. J. Physiol. Endocrinol. Metab.* **1996**, *271*. [CrossRef]
63. Shapiro, E.T.; Polonsky, K.S.; Copinschi, G.; Bosson, D.; Tillil, H.; Blackman, J.; Lewis, G.; Van Cauter, E. Nocturnal elevation of glucose levels during fasting in noninsulin-dependent diabetes. *J. Clin. Endocrinol. Metab.* **1991**, *72*, 444–454. [CrossRef]
64. Cauter, E.; Van Désir, D.; Decoster, C.; Féry, F.; Balasse, E.O. Nocturnal Decrease in Glucose Tolerance During Constant Glucose Infusion. *J. Clin. Endocrinol. Metab.* **1989**, *69*, 604–611. [CrossRef]
65. Spiegel, K.; Leproult, R.; Van Cauter, E. Impact of sleep debt on metabolic and endocrine function. *Lancet* **1999**, *354*, 1435–1439. [CrossRef]
66. Van Helder, T.; Radoki, M.W. Sleep Deprivation and the Effect on Exercise Performance. *Sports Med.* **1989**, *7*, 235–247. [CrossRef]
67. Martin, B.J. Effect of sleep deprivation on tolerance of prolonged exercise. *Eur. J. Appl. Physiol. Occup. Physiol.* **1981**, *47*, 345–354. [CrossRef]
68. Symons, J.D.; Vanhelder, T.; Myles, W.S. Physical performance and physiological responses following 60 hours of sleep deprivation. *Med. Sci. Sports Exerc.* **1988**, *20*, 374–380. [CrossRef]
69. Janosky, J.E. Use of the single subject design for practice based primary care research. *Postgrad. Med. J.* **2005**, *81*, 549–551. [CrossRef]
70. Bobrovitz, C.D.; Ottenbacher, K.J. Comparison of visual inspection and statistical analysis of single- subject data in rehabilitation research. *Am. J. Phys. Med. Rehabil.* **1998**, *77*, 94–102. [CrossRef] [PubMed]
71. Zhan, S.; Ottenbacher, K.J. Single subject research designs for disability research. *Disabil. Rehabil.* **2001**, *23*, 1–8. [CrossRef] [PubMed]
72. Guyatt, G.H. N of 1 Randomized Trials for Investigating New Drugs. In *Drug Epidemiology and Post-Marketing Surveillance*; Springer: Boston, MA, USA, 1992; pp. 125–134. [CrossRef]
73. McReynolds, L.V.; Thompson, C.K. Flexibility of single-subject experimental designs. Part I: Review of the basics of single-subject designs. *J. Speech Hear. Disord.* **1986**, *51*, 194–203. [CrossRef] [PubMed]
74. McLaughlin, T.F. An Examination and Evaluation of Single Subject Designs Used in Behavior Analysis Research in School Settings. *Educ. Res. Q.* **1983**, *7*, 35–42.
75. Brown, J.S.; Connolly, D.A. Selected Human Physiological Responses during Extreme Heat: The Badwater Ultramarathon. *J. Strength Cond. Res.* **2015**, *29*, 1729–1736. [CrossRef]
76. Paton, C.D.; Hopkins, W.G. Tests of Cycling Performance. *Sport. Med.* **2001**, *31*, 489–496. [CrossRef] [PubMed]
77. Moser, O.; Eckstein, M.L.; Mueller, A.; Birnbaumer, P.; Aberer, F.; Koehler, G.; Sourij, C.; Kojzar, H.; Holler, P.; Simi, H.; et al. Impact of physical exercise on sensor performance of the FreeStyle Libre intermittently viewed continuous glucose monitoring system in people with Type 1 diabetes: A randomized crossover trial. *Diabet. Med.* **2019**, *36*, 606–611. [CrossRef] [PubMed]

Article

Effects of the Menstrual Cycle on Jumping, Sprinting and Force-Velocity Profiling in Resistance-Trained Women: A Preliminary Study

Felipe García-Pinillos [1,2], Pascual Bujalance-Moreno [3,*], Carlos Lago-Fuentes [4,5,†], Santiago A. Ruiz-Alias [1], Irma Domínguez-Azpíroz [5,6], Marcos Mecías-Calvo [4] and Rodrigo Ramirez-Campillo [7,8]

[1] Department of Physical Education and Sports, Universidad de Granada, 18010 Granada, Spain; fegarpi@gmail.com (F.G.-P.); santiagoalejoruizalias@hotmail.com (S.A.R.-A.)
[2] Department of Physical Education, Sports and Recreation, Universidad de La Frontera, Temuco 4811230, Chile
[3] Department of Corporal Expression, University of Jaen, 23071 Jaen, Spain
[4] Faculty of Education and Sports Sciences, University of Vigo, 36310 Pontevedra, Spain; carloslagofuentes@hotmail.com (C.L.-F.); marcos.mecias@uneatlantico.es (M.M.-C.)
[5] Faculty of Health Sciences, European University of Atlantic, 39011 Santander, Spain; irma.dominguez@uneatlantico.es
[6] Department of Education, Universidad Internacional Iberoamericana, Campeche 24560, Mexico
[7] Human Performance Laboratory, Quality of Life and Wellness Research Group, Deparment of Physical Activity Sciences, Universidad de Los Lagos, Osorno 5200000, Chile; r.ramirez@ulagos.cl
[8] Centro de Investigación en Fisiología del Ejercicio, Facultad de Ciencias, Universidad Mayor, Santiago 7500000, Chile
* Correspondence: pascualbujalancemoreno@gmail.com; Tel.: +34-695537155
† Current Address: Department of Education, Universidad Internacional Iberoamericana, Campeche 24560, Mexico.

Abstract: The aim of this study was to examine the effects of the menstrual cycle on vertical jumping, sprint performance and force-velocity profiling in resistance-trained women. A group of resistance-trained eumenorrheic women (n = 9) were tested in three phases over the menstrual cycle: bleeding phase, follicular phase, and luteal phase (i.e., days 1–3, 7–10, and 19–21 of the cycle, respectively). Each testing phase consisted of a battery of jumping tests (i.e., squat jump [SJ], countermovement jump [CMJ], drop jump from a 30 cm box [DJ30], and the reactive strength index) and 30 m sprint running test. Two different applications for smartphone (My Jump 2 and My Sprint) were used to record the jumping and sprinting trials, respectively, at high speed (240 fps). The repeated measures ANOVA reported no significant differences ($p \geq 0.05$, ES < 0.25) in CMJ, DJ30, reactive strength index and sprint times between the different phases of the menstrual cycle. A greater SJ height performance was observed during the follicular phase compared to the bleeding phase ($p = 0.033$, ES = −0.22). No differences ($p \geq 0.05$, ES < 0.45) were found in the CMJ and sprint force-velocity profile over the different phases of the menstrual cycle. Vertical jump, sprint performance and the force-velocity profiling remain constant in trained women, regardless of the phase of the menstrual cycle.

Keywords: female athletes; ovarian cycle; plyometric exercises; testing; velocity

1. Introduction

Lower-limb ballistic movements, or stretch-shortening cycle (SSC) muscle actions, have been identified as key determinants of physical performance in women [1], and jumping and sprinting tests are widely used to assess the mechanical capabilities of the lower-limbs and the efficiency of the SSC [1,2]. The individual force-velocity (F-v) relationship has been proposed as a valid marker of the athlete's mechanical profile [3], providing more useful information for training prescription and monitoring training adaptations than isolated jumping or sprinting tests [4]. Moreover, with the constant advances in technology, more practical and easy-to-access alternatives have emerged in the past years, with different applications for jumping and sprinting assessment [5,6].

Traditionally, the adaptations to training and responses to exercise have been assumed as equal for both men and women [7]. However, a growing body of evidence [8,9] points to cyclical variations in steroids hormones (i.e., estrogen and progesterone) during an ovulatory menstrual cycle (MC). Despite the theoretical implications for physical performance, the available evidence about the influence of hormone variations related to MC on physical performance is controversial [7,9–11]. Some previous works have found cyclical variations in muscular performance parameters over an MC, such as handgrip, standing long jump and consecutive drop jumps [12,13], whereas other studies did not report differences in variables such as bench press or Smith machine squat, counter movement jump (CMJ), repeated sprint, or other no-muscular performance test [14–17]. Since an ovulatory MC implies alterations in the estrogen levels, and given that tendon and ligaments stiffness, and thereby SSC efficiency, has been shown to be impaired in the presence of high levels of estrogen [9], the use of single-joint isokinetic measurements, which minimize the SSC requirements, might overlook the influence of the MC and the hormone alterations.

Lastly, Thompson et al. [18] reviewed the effects of the MC on resistance training, suggesting that strength stimulus during the follicular phase (FP) will increase performance on this capacity. However, this study only registered 10 researches of acute responses, and most of them were focused only on biochemical parameters. Additionally, a recent review of this topic observed only a few studies that have analyzed performance associated to SSC requirements, due to most of them including single-joint isokinetic movements to test muscle strength and performance, or related to aerobic power [19–21]. Taking this into account, the lack of a consensus in the current scientific literature highlights the need to conduct further studies that analyze the relationship among the different phases of the MC and actions with SSC requirements.

Taken altogether, the purpose of this study is to examine the effect of the MC on vertical jump, sprint performance and F-v profiling in resistance-trained women. We hypothesized changes in vertical jump, sprint performance and some alterations in the F-v profile according to the phases of the MC with a better performance during the follicular phase.

2. Methods

In order to test our hypothesis, resistance-trained women completed a battery of loaded and unloaded vertical jump and linear sprint tests on three different days, according to their MC phases, including the early follicular phase, the late-follicular phase, and the mid-luteal phase.

2.1. Participants

A group of nine healthy eumenorrheic and trained women (age: 28.7 ± 3.6 years; height: 1.63 ± 0.05 m; body mass: 61.1 ± 5.6 kg) voluntarily participated in this study. The inclusion criteria were: (I) not to take any hormonal contraceptive; (II) to have a regular MC (i.e., 26 to 32 days of duration) for the last six months confirmed by the athletes through bleeding phase verification using the phone application "Clue"; (III) to train regularly (i.e., at least three times per week (over 200 min per week) for the last six months); (IV) to include resistance and endurance training in their training plan for the last six months. The sample size was selected by convenience and a post hoc analysis of the achieved power for this sample size was conducted (G*Power software vs. 3.1), given $\alpha = 0.05$, $(1 - \beta) = 0.8$, effect size = 0.5, statistical test = mean difference between matched pairs. This analysis revealed a low to moderate power (0.4). After receiving detailed information on the objectives and procedures of the study, each participant signed an informed consent form in order to participate, which complied with the ethical standards of the World Medical Association's Declaration of Helsinki, Finland (2013). The study was approved by the Institutional Review Board.

2.2. Procedures

Participants performed a total of four testing sessions, held between 17:00 and 20:00 h to avoid the influence of the circadian rhythms during the months of June and July. The day before a testing protocol, participants were instructed to perform a low-intensity workout. During the training period, participants were encouraged to maintain their dietary routine. This procedure is based on a similar previous study [14].

A preliminary session (i.e., session 1) was used to ensure that all participants were able to perform the vertical jumping and linear sprinting tests with a proper technique, despite all participants being experienced in loaded and unloaded plyometric jump and sprint exercises. The following testing sessions (i.e., sessions 2–4) were conducted in three different phases across the MC: (I) phase 1—bleeding or early follicular phase (i.e., testing between days 1–3); (II) phase 2—follicular or late-follicular phase (i.e., testing between days 7–10) and; (III) phase 3—luteal or mid-luteal phase (i.e., testing between days 19–21) (Figure 1). The selection of these phases were based on previous studies [11,14,19,22] and it has been suggested that those phases represent the main events during an MC, including menses, pre-ovulation and post-ovulation, respectively [11,15]. Phases of the MC were defined based on the first day of menses.

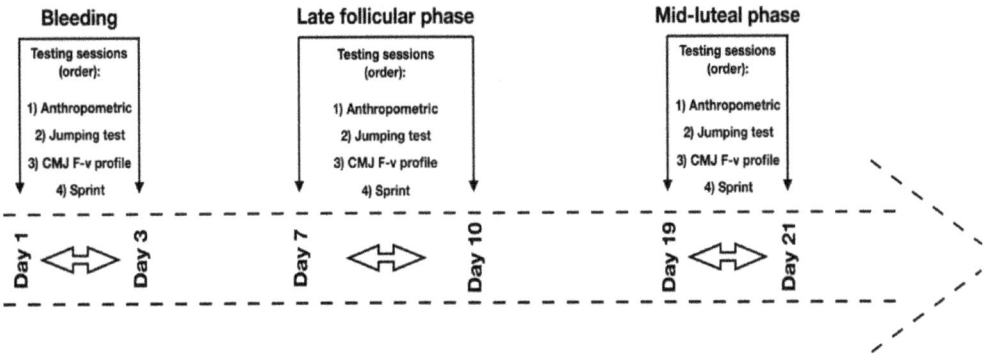

Figure 1. Visual representation of the timeline of the testing procedure.

Identical testing protocols were performed in sessions 2–4. First, the anthropometric characteristics of the participants were measured, including standing height, body mass and measurements needed to determine the push-off distance (leg length and initial height) [3,23]. Then, after a standardized 10-min warm-up protocol based on dynamic stretching and preparatory exercises, including jumping and sprinting exercises, the participants performed a battery of vertical jumping tests, and an incremental vertical loaded-jump protocol, and two 30 m linear sprints (see below for further details). Every testing session was conducted on one specific day, including anthropometric measurements, jumping and sprinting test—in that order. The testing protocols were performed indoors, and weather conditions were registered for the subsequent analysis. Participants were encouraged to achieve maximum performance during each test, and the personal best attempt for each test was selected for the subsequent analysis.

Anthropometric measurements. A stadiometer (Seca 202, Seca Ltd., Hamburg, Germany), a weighing scale (Seca 803, Seca Ltd., Hamburg, Germany) and a non-stretchable tape (Seca 201, Seca Ltd., Hamburg, Germany) were used to measure height, body mass and push-off distance.

Jumping tests. The participants performed a battery of vertical jumping tests including two maximal attempts for the squat jump (SJ), countermovement jump (CMJ) and drop jump from a 30 cm box (DJ30). Jumping tests were performed in that order. The resting period lasted 15 s between repetitions and 4 min between tests. As described by a previous study [24], during SJ, participants were instructed to adopt a flexed knee position (approximately 90 degrees) for 3 s before jumping, while during the CMJ no restriction was imposed over the knee angle achieved before jumping. Jumping tests were executed with arms akimbo. Takeoff and landing were standardized to full knee and ankle extension on the same spot. During the DJ30, participants were instructed to maximize jump height and to minimize ground contact time after dropping down [25]. Jump heights (m) were registered for each test. Additionally, the reactive strength index (RSI) was obtained from DJ30 (i.e., RSI = flight time [ms]/contact time [ms]).

All these assessments were performed through the My Jump 2 app (v.5.0.5). This is based on high-speed video analysis (i.e., 240 fps) and it has been shown as valid and reliable to determine jump height during CMJ, SJ and DJ tests [5], as well as to determine related parameters such as temporal variables and RSI [26]. The instructions provided by the developer were followed for collecting data [5]. A researcher, laying prone on the ground, held the smartphone (iPhone; Apple, Inc., Cupertino, CA, USA) and recorded each jump from a frontal plane, at approximately 1.5 m.

CMJ F-v profiling. Thereafter, the participants were assessed for the F-v profiling, performing two maximal CMJs under an unloaded and loaded condition, including at least three loads from 10 to 45 kg [23]. Loads were increased until the jump height was shorter than 10 cm [27]. The resting period lasted 15 s between repetitions and 4 min between sets. The same equipment and protocol previously described (i.e., My Jump 2 app, v.5.0.5) was used for these measurements.

This method has been shown as valid and reliable for computing mechanical parameters, and thereby F-v profiles, from the CMJ [23]. As previously recommended [4], the variables extracted from the F-v protocol included the theoretical maximal force at null velocity (F_0), the theoretical maximal velocity of lower-limbs extension under zero load (v_0), maximal power output against different loads (P_{max}), and the slope of the linear F-v relationship (S_{fv}).

30 m sprint test. The participants performed two maximal-effort 30 m linear sprints, with 5 min rest in between, on a synthetic indoor track. An application for smartphone (i.e., My Sprint app) was used to record and analyze (i.e., split times: 5, 10, 15, 20, 25 and 30 m) the trials. The system is based on high-speed video analysis (i.e., 240 fps) and it has been shown as valid and reliable to evaluate linear sprint performance in relation to two different reference systems such as timing photocells and radar gun [6]. The testing protocol was based on the procedures described by the developer in a previous paper [6]. The recording was conducted through an iPhone 7, which was mounted to a tripod and located 10 m perpendicular to the sprint direction, just in front of the 15 m marker.

Sprint F-v profiling. Video analysis provided split times during the linear 30 m sprint test. Following a simple method proposed by Samozino and colleagues [3], those data along with anthropometric characteristics and weather conditions let the researchers obtain power, force and velocity properties as well as mechanical effectiveness during linear sprint running. This method has been examined and it has been shown as valid to determine mechanical parameters during linear sprint [3]. As identified by a previous work [4], the variables of interest from this profile are the theoretical maximal horizontal force (HZT-F_0), maximal running velocity (HZT-v_0), associated maximal power output (P_{max}), the slope of the F-v relationship that determined the mechanical profile (Fv_{slope}), the maximum value of ratio of force (RF_{max}) and the rate of decrease in the ratio of force with increasing speed during sprint acceleration as a measure of the index of the effectiveness of ground force orientation (D_{RF}).

2.3. Statistical Analysis

All data are presented as mean and standard deviation (mean ± SD). The normality assumption was confirmed by the Shapiro–Wilk test ($p > 0.05$). One-way repeated measures analysis of variance (ANOVA) with Bonferroni post-hoc tests were conducted to compare the outcome variables at three different phases during the MC (i.e., bleeding, follicular and luteal phases). The F-v relationships were established by means of least squares linear regression models [4,28]. The Hedges g effect size (ES) was also calculated to determine the magnitude of differences, interpreted as follows: trivial (<0.2), small (0.2–0.59), moderate (0.60–1.19), large (1.20–2.0), and extremely large (>2.0) [29]. Statistical significance was set at $\alpha < 0.05$. The SPSS software (version 25.0, SPSS Inc., Chicago, IL, USA) was used.

3. Results

Table 1 shows the vertical jumping and linear sprinting performance of participants at the three different phases of the MC. The repeated measures ANOVA reported no significant differences between phases in CMJ, DJ30, RSI nor sprint performance ($p \geq 0.05$, ES < 0.25). However, differences ($p = 0.033$, ES = -0.22) were found in SJ, with the post-hoc test revealing a greater performance during the follicular phase compared to the bleeding phase.

Table 1. Comparison of the vertical jumping and 30 m sprint performance parameters obtained from three different phases of the menstrual cycle.

Parameter	Phase 1	Phase 2	Phase 3	p-Value	ES Phase 1 vs. Phase 2	ES Phase 1 vs. Phase 3	ES Phase 2 vs. Phase 3
CMJ (cm)	23.46 ± 5.17	24.50 ± 5.60	23.74 ± 5.57	0.322	−0.18	−0.05	0.13
SJ (cm)	21.75 ± 5.36 ^	22.98 ± 5.50 ^	21.70 ± 4.75	0.033 *	−0.22	0.01	0.24
DJ30 (cm)	23.22 ± 5.22	23.80 ± 5.48	23.33 ± 5.93	0.422	−0.10	−0.01	0.08
RSI	1.07 ± 0.28	1.09 ± 0.30	1.10 ± 0.23	0.833	−0.07	−0.11	−0.04
Sprint 5 m (s)	1.65 ± 0.15	1.62 ± 0.15	1.62 ± 0.12	0.562	0.19	0.21	0.01
Sprint 10 m (s)	2.51 ± 0.19	2.48 ± 0.19	2.48 ± 0.16	0.321	0.15	0.16	0.01
Sprint 15 m (s)	3.37 ± 0.27	3.32 ± 0.25	3.32 ± 0.23	0.283	0.18	0.19	0.01
Sprint 20 m (s)	4.19 ± 0.33	4.14 ± 0.32	4.13 ± 0.29	0.233	0.15	0.18	0.03
Sprint 25 m (s)	4.95 ± 0.40	4.88 ± 0.38	4.88 ± 0.34	0.151	0.17	0.18	0.01
Sprint 30 m (s)	5.66 ± 0.46	5.58 ± 0.44	5.57 ± 0.39	0.113	0.17	0.20	0.01

Values as mean (± standard deviation); * denotes significant differences between phases ($p < 0.05$); ^ indicates where the between-phase difference is. ES: g Hedges effect size; phase 1: bleeding phase; phase 2: follicular phase; phase 3: luteal phase; CMJ: countermovement jump; SJ: squat jump; DJ30: drop jump from a 30 cm box; RSI: reactive strength index (flight time [ms]/contact time [ms]).

The CMJ F-v relationship parameters at the three different phases of the MC are indicated in the Table 2. No significant differences ($p \geq 0.327$, ES < 0.45) were found between phases in any parameter (i.e., F_0, v_0, P_{max} and S_{fv}).

Table 2. Comparison of the F-v relationship parameters obtained from three different phases of the menstrual cycle during an incremental loading protocol for the countermovement jump (CMJ) test.

Parameter	Phase 1	Phase 2	Phase 3	p-Value	ES (g) Phase 1 vs. Phase 2	ES (g) Phase 1 vs. Phase 3	ES (g) Phase 2 vs. Phase 3
F_0 (N)	26.49 ± 2.97	28.02 ± 5.17	25.87 ± 5.04	0.441	−0.35	0.14	0.40
v_0 (m·s^{-1})	2.98 ± 0.81	2.85 ± 0.59	3.45 ± 1.68	0.327	0.17	−0.34	−0.44
P_{max} (W)	20.31 ± 5.74	19.63 ± 3.19	22.13 ± 8.08	0.757	0.14	−0.25	−0.39
S_{fv} (N·s·m^{-1})	−8.71 ± 2.80	−9.69 ± 4.30	−8.61 ± 5.55	0.774	0.26	−0.02	−0.21

Values as mean (± standard deviation); ES (g): g Hedges effect size; phase 1: bleeding phase; phase 2: follicular phase; phase 3: luteal phase; F-v: force-velocity; F_0: the theoretical maximal force at null velocity; v_0: the theoretical maximal velocity of lower-limbs extension under zero load; P_{max}: maximal power output against different loads; S_{fv}: slope of the linear F-v relationship.

Table 3 shows the mechanical parameters associated to the F-v relationship during the 30 m linear sprint test in different phases of the MC. No between-phase significant differences ($p \geq 0.340$, ES < −0.36) were found in any parameter.

Table 3. Power–force–velocity relationship parameters during a 30 m linear sprint test obtained from three different phases of the menstrual cycle.

Parameter	Phase 1	Phase 2	Phase 3	p-Value	ES Phase 1 vs. Phase 2	ES Phase 1 vs. Phase 3	ES Phase 2 vs. Phase 3
HZT-F_0 (N·kg^{-1})	5.72 ± 1.01	5.86 ± 1.20	5.73 ± 0.86	0.710	−0.12	−0.01	0.12
HZT-v_0 (m·s^{-1})	6.96 ± 0.73	7.06 ± 0.64	7.11 ± 0.60	0.340	−0.13	−0.21	−0.08
P_{max} (W·kg^{-1})	10.05 ± 2.71	10.45 ± 3.06	10.26 ± 2.37	0.377	−0.13	−0.08	0.07
Fv_{slope}	−0.82 ± 0.15	−0.83 ± 0.13	−0.79 ± 0.08	0.360	0.07	−0.24	−0.35
RF_{max} (%)	35.33 ± 4.21	36.11 ± 4.40	35.89 ± 3.62	0.386	−0.17	−0.14	0.05
D_{RF} (%)	−7.90 ± 1.15	−7.93 ± 1.09	−7.70 ± 0.70	0.613	0.03	−0.20	−0.24

Values as mean (± standard deviation); ES: g Hedges effect size; phase 1: bleeding phase; phase 2: follicular phase; phase 3: luteal phase; HZT-F_0: theoretical maximal horizontal force; HZT-v_0: maximal running velocity; P_{max}: associated maximal power output; Fv_{slope}: slope of the F-v relationship that determined the mechanical profile; RF_{max}: maximal ratio of force; D_{RF}: rate of decrease in the ratio of force with increasing speed during sprint acceleration.

4. Discussion

This study aimed to examine the effects of three different phases of the MC on vertical jumping, linear sprinting performance and F-v profiling in resistance-trained women. The main finding rejects our initial hypothesis, as athletic performance in these explosive tasks (i.e., jumping and sprinting) and the F-v profiling requiring SSC muscle actions suffer no significant variation in trained women over the course of their ovarian MC.

Although there are theoretical implications for athletic performance, there is no conclusive evidence about cyclical variations during the MC in sportswomen [7,9,10,14]. Focused on the influence of the MC on muscular performance and muscle strength, the lack of consensus is remarkable, with previous studies reporting opposing findings. As mentioned earlier, some previous works have found variations in muscular performance parameters over an MC [12,13], whereas other studies did not find differences [14,20,30,31]. The authors suggest that between-study differences might be attributed to some methodological issues (e.g., exercise testing, timing of measurements or definition of the MC phases). Related to this, the last review about this topic matches with this finding, due to the differences among phases analyzed and level of participants, including non-homogeneous participant groups, among others. However, our study presents a small but homogeneous sample, similar to the mean of previous studies, among 10 to 15 trained women [32]. Nonetheless, more studies should analyze muscular performance with the same methodology to ensure the existence, or not, of differences among the different phases of MC, including the bleeding, late-follicular and mid-luteal phases [32].

In this context, it is noteworthy that some previous studies have used maximal voluntary contraction or maximal voluntary isometric force through isokinetic measurements [19,20] to examine the influence of the MC on muscular performance. Variations in steroid hormones affect tendons and ligaments, with a high level of estrogen decreasing musculotendinous stiffness [9]. Therefore, it is possible that the effect of the MC may be modulated by the type of muscle action being performed, with those requiring high levels of musculotendinous stiffness (i.e., SSC muscle actions) more prone to be affected by the MC. However, the current study provides some insights into the influence of the MC phases on explosive tasks with high SSC requirements (i.e., jumping and sprinting), with both athletic performance and mechanical parameters showing no differences over different phases of the MC. Regarding this, the rise of estrogen during the follicular phase has been signaled as the main influencing factor to affect the muscular performance [32]; meanwhile, during the luteal phase the CK concentrations increases and decreases the strength levels [18]. However, its influence on short–high intensity efforts such as jumps, among others, is not clear. The body composition has also been described as a potential influencing factor on athletic performance. Traditionally, it has been suggested that the fat oxidation increases during the follicular phase because of the anabolic effect of estrogen, meanwhile fluid retentions can influence the lowest performance during the luteal phase. However, a recent study with trained women compared different body composition variables throughout the three main MC phases and found no significant differences in these parameters [33]. So, this factor should be cautiously considered as an influencing parameter to explain plausible differences on athletic performance over the ovarian cycle.

Regarding jumping performance, few studies have analyzed the effect of the MC phases on this physical fitness outcome, and conflicting results have been reported. Whereas Davies et al. (1991) reported an improvement in standing long jump test in the bleeding phase compared to the follicular phase, other previous works did not find differences in performance over the course of an ovarian MC in the CMJ-comparing only the early follicular phase vs. the mid-luteal phase in soccer players [16], SJ [34] nor in the DJ-comparing only the follicular phase vs. the ovulation phase in active women [13]. Nevertheless, the participants of these studies did not report previous experience in resistance training, which might be relevant for this type of efforts. Of note, any of the aforementioned studies provided mechanical parameters related to vertical jumping, which might better describe the differences among different MC phases. Recently, another study performed with a similar sample (i.e., trained athletes with six months of experience in resistance training) registered three different variables to determine each MC phase to test force, velocity and power output in the concentric phase in a Smith machine half squat exercise [15]. This work neither found differences in performance comparing these three phases (bleeding, follicular and luteal phases), which concur with our main findings for similar outcomes. Lastly, our results are also in line with a recent study with high-level team sport players, which did not show differences among MC phases in CMJ performance in eumenorrheic athletes, analyzed with serum hormonal levels by blood sample [35]. Therefore, the current study confirms the lack of MC effect on vertical jumping performance and, as a novelty, provides information about the dynamic of the F-v relationship parameters over the different phases of MC.

Concerning the linear sprint performance, previous studies have considered the effect of the MC in cycling sprints [17,34,36] and linear running sprints [16,30,31], with all those works reporting no effect of the MC in maximal anaerobic performance. With the focus on studies testing linear running sprint, some works [30,31] have used a 30-s non-motorized treadmill sprinting test in different phases of the MC, reporting no differences in performance (i.e., in terms of mean and peak power output and sprint total time) in trained women. Likewise, in an experiment performed outdoors (i.e., on field testing) [16], the authors found no differences in 30 m linear sprint time during the different phases of MC in female soccer players. Another recent study found differences in 20 m linear sprint with high-level team sport players [35]. However, as previously indicated, the authors of these studies only compared the follicular phase with the luteal phase, dismissing the bleeding phase, one of the most important physiological moments of the MC due to the lower concentrations of estrogen and progesterone [8,9]. In fact, a recent systematic review reinforces the need to include this phase in further studies on the relationship between athletic performance and MC [32]. This study observed that performance could be reduced during the bleeding phase compared with the rest of the MC phases. Due to the small number of studies which performed CMJ or sprinting tests including this stage, our findings provide a novel result which suggests that performance does not increase during the first days of the MC. That is, the current study provides support about the lack of effect of MC phases on linear running sprint performance comparing the three main phases, and it builds up the available information on the MC influence on sprint mechanical parameters and F-v profile.

Finally, some limitations must be taken into consideration to properly interpret these findings: first, the verification of the MC phases with no hormone concentration measurements [37]; second, the limited number of participants (n = 9) with low to moderate statistical power for this sample size; third, the performance level of the subjects; fourth, the methods for assessing jump performance parameters based on high-speed video analysis and with no information regarding jump strategy (e.g., time to take-off or CMJ displacement) [38]. Notwithstanding these limitations, the current study provides some insights into the effects of MC on jumping, sprinting and F-v profiling in women by using low-cost and easy-to-access tools and measures.

Practical Applications

The current study confirms the lack of MC effect on vertical jumping performance, but a small difference was found in SJ, with a greater performance during the follicular phase compared to the bleeding phase. Likewise, the linear running sprint performance was not influenced by MC phases, supporting the aforementioned research projects. From a practical standpoint, given the lack of differences in muscular performance (in terms of F-v profile) during different MC phases, the hormone variations over the course of an ovarian cycle do not seem to play a key role for athletic performance in high-intensity muscle activities such as jumping or sprinting for non-competitive eumenorrheic trained women.

Considering the lack of consensus, the authors claim the convenience of further studies to highlight, on the one hand, if the training response (i.e., internal load to an external load) might change over the course of an ovarian MC and, on the other hand, if training programmes based on MC phases are more efficient and safer for eumenorrheic women than traditional plans based on training outcomes.

5. Conclusions

Vertical jumping, linear sprinting performance and the F-v profiling requiring stretch-shortening cycle muscle actions suffer no significant variation in eumenorrheic sportswomen over the course of an ovarian MC.

Author Contributions: F.G.-P. participated in the design of the study, data reduction/analysis and interpretation of results; P.B.-M. participated in the design of the study and contributed to data collection; C.L.-F. contributed to data analysis and interpretation of results; R.R.-C., I.D.-A., S.A.R.-A. and M.M.-C. participated in the design of the study and interpretation of results. All authors contributed to the manuscript writing. All authors have read and agreed to the published version of the manuscript.

Funding: This research was supported by the Pre-competitive Projects for Early Stage Researchers Programme from the University of Granada (ref: PPJIA2020.03)

Institutional Review Board Statement: The study was conducted according to the guidelines of the Declaration of Helsinki, and approved by the Ethics Committee of University of Jaen, Jaen, Spain (protocol code ABR.19/13.PRY and date of approval 29 April 2019).

Informed Consent Statement: Informed consent was obtained from all subjects involved in the study.

Data Availability Statement: Data will be available by request.

Conflicts of Interest: The authors declare that they have no competing interests.

References

1. Hennessy, L.; Kilty, J. Relationship of the Stretch-Shortening Cycle to Sprint Performance in Trained Female Athletes. *J. Strength Cond. Res.* **2001**, *15*, 326–331. [CrossRef]
2. Klavora, P. Vertical-jump Tests: A Critical Review. *Strength Cond. J.* **2000**, *22*, 70–75. [CrossRef]
3. Samozino, P.; Morin, J.-B.; Hintzy, F.; Belli, A. A simple method for measuring force, velocity and power output during squat jump. *J. Biomech.* **2008**, *41*, 2940–2945. [CrossRef] [PubMed]
4. Morin, J.-B.; Samozino, P. Interpreting Power-Force-Velocity Profiles for Individualized and Specific Training. *Int. J. Sports Physiol. Perform.* **2016**, *11*, 267–272. [CrossRef] [PubMed]
5. Balsalobre-Fernández, C.; Glaister, M.; Lockey, R.A. The validity and reliability of an iPhone app for measuring vertical jump performance. *J. Sports Sci.* **2015**, *33*, 1574–1579. [CrossRef] [PubMed]
6. Romero-Franco, N.; Jiménez-Reyes, P.; Castaño-Zambudio, A.; Capelo-Ramírez, F.; Rodríguez-Juan, J.J.; González-Hernández, J.; Toscano-Bendala, F.J.; Cuadrado-Peñafiel, V.; Balsalobre-Fernández, C. Sprint performance and mechanical outputs computed with an iPhone app: Comparison with existing reference methods. *Eur. J. Sport Sci.* **2016**, *17*, 386–392. [CrossRef] [PubMed]
7. Sims, S.T.; Heather, A.K. Myths and Methodologies: Reducing scientific design ambiguity in studies comparing sexes and/or menstrual cycle phases. *Exp. Physiol.* **2018**, *103*, 1309–1317. [CrossRef]

8. Stricker, R.; Eberhart, R.; Chevailler, M.-C.; Quinn, F.A.; Bischof, P.; Stricker, R. Establishment of detailed reference values for luteinizing hormone, follicle stimulating hormone, estradiol, and progesterone during different phases of the menstrual cycle on the Abbott ARCHITECT® analyzer. *Clin. Chem. Lab. Med.* **2006**, *44*, 883–887. [CrossRef] [PubMed]
9. Chidi-Ogbolu, N.; Baar, K. Effect of Estrogen on Musculoskeletal Performance and Injury Risk. *Front. Physiol.* **2019**, *9*, 1834. [CrossRef]
10. Constantini, N.W.; Dubnov, G.; Lebrun, C.M. The Menstrual Cycle and Sport Performance. *Clin. Sports Med.* **2005**, *24*, e51–e82. [CrossRef]
11. De Jonge, X.A.K.J. Effects of the menstrual cycle on exercise performance. *Sports Med.* **2003**, *33*, 833–851. [CrossRef] [PubMed]
12. Davies, B.N.; Elford, J.C.; Jamieson, K.F. Variations in performance in simple muscle tests at different phases of the menstrual cycle. *J. Sports Med. Phys. Fit.* **1991**, *31*, 532–537.
13. Sipavičienė, S.; Daniusevičiūtė, L.; Klizienė, I.; Kamandulis, S.; Skurvydas, A. Effects of Estrogen Fluctuation during the Menstrual Cycle on the Response to Stretch-Shortening Exercise in Females. *BioMed Res. Int.* **2013**, *2013*, 1–6. [CrossRef]
14. García-Pinillos, F.; Lago-Fuentes, C.; Bujalance-Moreno, P.; Pérez-Castilla, A. Effect of the Menstrual Cycle When Estimating 1 Repetition Maximum from the Load-Velocity Relationship During the Bench Press Exercise. *J. Strength Cond. Res.* **2020**. [CrossRef]
15. Romero-Moraleda, B.; Del Coso, J.; Gutiérrez-Hellín, J.; Ruiz-Moreno, C.; Grgic, J.; Lara, B. The Influence of the Menstrual Cycle on Muscle Strength and Power Performance. *J. Hum. Kinet.* **2019**, *68*, 123–133. [CrossRef] [PubMed]
16. Julian, R.; Hecksteden, A.; Fullagar, H.H.K.; Meyer, T. The effects of menstrual cycle phase on physical performance in female soccer players. *PLoS ONE* **2017**, *12*, e0173951. [CrossRef] [PubMed]
17. Wiecek, M.; Szymura, J.; Maciejczyk, M.; Cempla, J.; Szygula, Z.; Information, R. Effect of sex and menstrual cycle in women on starting speed, anaerobic endurance and muscle power. *Acta Physiol. Hung.* **2016**, *103*, 127–132. [CrossRef] [PubMed]
18. Thompson, B.; Almarjawi, A.; Sculley, D.; De Jonge, X.J. The Effect of the Menstrual Cycle and Oral Contraceptives on Acute Responses and Chronic Adaptations to Resistance Training: A Systematic Review of the Literature. *Sports Med.* **2020**, *50*, 171–185. [CrossRef]
19. Gür, H. Concentric and eccentric isokinetic measurements in knee muscles during the menstrual cycle: A special reference to reciprocal moment ratios. *Arch. Phys. Med. Rehabil.* **1997**, *78*, 501–505. [CrossRef]
20. Abt, J.P.; Sell, T.C.; Laudner, K.G.; McCrory, J.L.; Loucks, T.L.; Berga, S.L.; Lephart, S.M. Neuromuscular and biomechanical characteristics do not vary across the menstrual cycle. *Knee Surg. Sports Traumatol. Arthrosc.* **2007**, *15*, 901–907. [CrossRef]
21. Elliott-Sale, K.J.; McNulty, K.L.; Ansdell, P.; Goodall, S.; Hicks, K.M.; Thomas, K.; Swinton, P.A.; Dolan, E. The Effects of Oral Contraceptives on Exercise Performance in Women: A Systematic Review and Meta-analysis. *Sports Med.* **2020**, *50*, 1785–1812. [CrossRef] [PubMed]
22. Pallavi, L.C.; Souza, U.J.D.; Shivaprakash, G. Assessment of Musculoskeletal Strength and Levels of Fatigue during Different Phases of Menstrual Cycle in Young Adults. *J. Clin. Diagn. Res.* **2017**, *11*, CC11–CC13. [CrossRef] [PubMed]
23. Jiménez-Reyes, P.; Samozino, P.; Pareja-Blanco, F.; Conceição, F.; Cuadrado-Peñafiel, V.; González-Badillo, J.J.; Morin, J.-B. Validity of a Simple Method for Measuring Force-Velocity-Power Profile in Countermovement Jump. *Int. J. Sports Physiol. Perform.* **2017**, *12*, 36–43. [CrossRef] [PubMed]
24. Ramírez-Campillo, R.; Andrade, D.C.; Izquierdo, M. Effects of Plyometric Training Volume and Training Surface on Explosive Strength. *J. Strength Cond. Res.* **2013**, *27*, 2714–2722. [CrossRef] [PubMed]
25. Young, W.B.; Pryor, J.F.; Wilson, G.J. Effect of Instructions on characteristics of Countermovement and Drop Jump Performance. *J. Strength Cond. Res.* **1995**, *9*, 232–236. [CrossRef]
26. Haynes, T.; Bishop, C.; Antrobus, M.; Brazier, J. The validity and reliability of the My Jump 2 app for measuring the reactive strength index and drop jump performance. *J. Sports Med. Phys. Fit.* **2019**, *59*, 253–258. [CrossRef] [PubMed]
27. García-Ramos, A.; Pérez-Castilla, A.; Jaric, S. Optimisation of applied loads when using the two-point method for assessing the force-velocity relationship during vertical jumps. *Sports Biomech.* **2021**, *20*, 274–289. [CrossRef]
28. Yamauchi, J.; Ishii, N. Relations Between Force-Velocity Characteristics of the Knee-Hip Extension Movement and Vertical Jump Performance. *J. Strength Cond. Res.* **2007**, *21*, 703–709. [CrossRef]
29. Hopkins, W.G.; Marshall, S.W.; Batterham, A.M.; Hanin, J. Progressive Statistics for Studies in Sports Medicine and Exercise Science. *Med. Sci. Sports Exerc.* **2009**, *41*, 3–13. [CrossRef]
30. Tsampoukos, A.; Peckham, E.A.; James, R.; Nevill, M.E. Effect of menstrual cycle phase on sprinting performance. *Graefes Arch. Clin. Exp. Ophthalmol.* **2010**, *109*, 659–667. [CrossRef]
31. Sunderland, C.; Tunaley, V.; Horner, F.; Harmer, D.; Stokes, K.A. Menstrual cycle and oral contraceptives' effects on growth hormone response to sprinting. *Appl. Physiol. Nutr. Metab.* **2011**, *36*, 495–502. [CrossRef] [PubMed]
32. McNulty, K.L.; Elliott-Sale, K.J.; Dolan, E.; Swinton, P.A.; Ansdell, P.; Goodall, S.; Thomas, K.; Hicks, K.M. The Effects of Menstrual Cycle Phase on Exercise Performance in Eumenorrheic Women: A Systematic Review and Meta-Analysis. *Sports Med.* **2020**, *50*, 1813–1827. [CrossRef]
33. Rael, B.; Romero-Parra, N.; Alfaro-Magallanes, V.M.; Barba-Moreno, L.; Cupeiro, R.; de Jonge, X.J.; Peinado, A.B. Body Composition Over the Menstrual and Oral Contraceptive Cycle in Trained Females. *Int. J. Sports Physiol. Perform.* **2021**, *16*, 375–381. [CrossRef]
34. Giacomoni, M.; Bernard, T.; Gavarry, O.; Altare, S.; Falgairette, G. Influence of the menstrual cycle phase and menstrual symptoms on maximal anaerobic performance. *Med. Sci. Sports Exerc.* **2000**, *32*, 486–492. [CrossRef] [PubMed]

35. Dasa, M.S.; Kristoffersen, M.; Ersvær, E.; Bovim, L.P.; Bjørkhaug, L.; Moe-Nilssen, R.; Sagen, J.V.; Haukenes, I. The Female Menstrual Cycles Effect on Strength and Power Parameters in High-Level Female Team Athletes. *Front. Physiol.* **2021**, *12*, 164. [CrossRef] [PubMed]
36. Botcazou, M.; Gratas-Delamarche, A.; Allain, S.; Jacob, C.; Bentué-Ferrer, D.; Delamarche, P.; Zouhal, H. Influence de la phase du cycle menstruel sur les réponses en catécholamines à l'exercice de sprint chez la femme. *Appl. Physiol. Nutr. Metab.* **2006**, *31*, 604–611. [CrossRef] [PubMed]
37. Janse, D.E.; Jonge, X.; Thompson, B.; Han, A. Methodological Recommendations for Menstrual Cycle Research in Sports and Exercise. *Med. Sci. Sports Exerc.* **2019**, *51*, 2610–2617. [CrossRef]
38. Pérez-Castilla, A.; Fernandes, J.F.T.; Rojas, F.J.; García-Ramos, A. Reliability and Magnitude of Countermovement Jump Performance Variables: Influence of the Take-off Threshold. *Meas. Phys. Educ. Exerc. Sci.* **2021**, 1–9. [CrossRef]

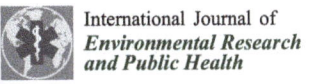

Article

Exploring the Determinants of Repeated-Sprint Ability in Adult Women Soccer Players

Lillian Gonçalves [1,*], Filipe Manuel Clemente [2,3], Joel Ignacio Barrera [4], Hugo Sarmento [4], Francisco Tomás González-Fernández [5], Markel Rico-González [6,7] and José María Cancela Carral [1]

1. Faculty of Educational Sciences and Sports Sciences, University of Vigo, 36005 Pontevedra, Spain; chemacc@uvigo.es
2. Escola Superior Desporto e Lazer, Instituto Politécnico de Viana do Castelo, Rua Escola Industrial e Comercial de Nun'Álvares, 4900-347 Viana do Castelo, Portugal; filipe.clemente5@gmail.com
3. Instituto de Telecomunicações, Delegação da Covilhã, 1049-001 Lisboa, Portugal
4. University of Coimbra, Research Unit for Sport and Physical Activity, Faculty of Sport Sciences and Physical Education, 3004-531 Coimbra, Portugal; jibarrera@outlook.pt (J.I.B.); hg.sarmento@gmail.com (H.S.)
5. Department of Physical Activity and Sport Sciences, Pontifical University of Comillas (Centro de Estudios Superiores Alberta Giménez), 07013 Palma, Spain; francis.gonzalez.fernandez@gmail.com
6. BIOVETMED & SPORTSCI Research Group, University of Murcia, 30720 San Javier, Spain; markeluniv@gmail.com
7. Department of Physical Education and Sport, University of the Basque Country, UPV-EHU, Lasarte 71, 01007 Vitoria-Gasteiz, Spain
* Correspondence: lilliangoncalves@ipvc.pt

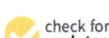

Citation: Gonçalves, L.; Clemente, F.M.; Barrera, J.I.; Sarmento, H.; González-Fernández, F.T.; Rico-González, M.; Carral, J.M.C. Exploring the Determinants of Repeated-Sprint Ability in Adult Women Soccer Players. *Int. J. Environ. Res. Public Health* **2021**, *18*, 4595. https://doi.org/10.3390/ijerph18094595

Academic Editor: Veronique Billat

Received: 25 March 2021
Accepted: 24 April 2021
Published: 26 April 2021

Publisher's Note: MDPI stays neutral with regard to jurisdictional claims in published maps and institutional affiliations.

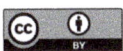

Copyright: © 2021 by the authors. Licensee MDPI, Basel, Switzerland. This article is an open access article distributed under the terms and conditions of the Creative Commons Attribution (CC BY) license (https://creativecommons.org/licenses/by/4.0/).

Abstract: This study aimed to explore the main determinants of repeated-sprint ability (RSA) in women soccer players considering aerobic capacity, sprinting performance, change-of-direction, vertical height jump, and hip adductor/abductor isometric strength. Twenty-two women soccer players from the same team participating in the first Portuguese league were observed. Fitness assessments were performed three times during a 22-week cohort period. The following assessments were made: (i) hip abductor and adductor strength, (ii) squat and countermovement jump (height), (iii) change-of-direction test, (iv) linear sprinting at 10- and 30-m, (v) RSA test, and (vi) Yo-Yo intermittent recovery test level 1. Positive moderate correlations were found between peak minimum RSA and adductor and abductor strength (r = 0.51, $p < 0.02$ and r = 0.54, $p < 0.01$, respectively). Positive moderate correlations were also found between peak maximum RSA and adductor and abductor strength (r = 0.55, $p < 0.02$ and r = 0.46, $p < 0.01$, respectively). Lastly, a moderate negative correlation was found between fatigue index in RSA and YYIR1 test performance (r = −0.62, $p < 0.004$). In conclusion, abductor and adductor isometric strength-based coadjutant training programs, together with a high degree of aerobic endurance, may be suitable for inducing RSA in female soccer players.

Keywords: football; athletic performance; anaerobic; aerobic; sports training

1. Introduction

Soccer is a team sport practiced by many athletes throughout the world, with an estimated 4–26 million female participants [1–4] and approximately 238 million male participants [5]. The number of female soccer players has increased in the last years in approximately 50% considering the last report of FIFA [3,6]. Due to the challenges associated with this rapid increase in the number of participants, it is important to better understand the characteristics of these players, their physiological/physical demands, and their training processes [1,2,7].

As an intermittent exercise, a women's soccer match involves activities with different intensities, such as walking, jogging, moderate running, high-intensity running, and sprinting [8–10]. It is well-known that low-intensity movements are predominant during women's matches [9,11,12], although high-intensity activities are also considered important components of physical performance, and they are often crucial to the outcomes of matches because they are associated with offensive attacks [12,13]. Usually, women soccer players cover between 8.5 and 11 km in a match, of which 1.5–1.8 km are spent performing high-speed running and from 14.9 to 460 m are spent sprinting [4,9,10,14,15].

To support the demands of the match, a proper fitness status should be sustained. As an example, in previous research on women soccer players, a strong correlation was observed between Yo-Yo intermittent recovery test performance and the amount of high-intensity running performed in games [9,16]. Additionally, a strong correlation between sprinting skills and high-intensity performance was found in a previous study [2]. In fact, many decisive phases during a soccer match require players to exercise at a high intensity [17]. Therefore, the ability of a soccer player to recover and to reproduce their performance in subsequent sprints is a vital fitness condition [10]. In the particular case of elite level, the intermittent high-intensity endurance and the ability to repeatedly sprint in short time intervals (RSA) are considered relevant fitness conditions for competitive soccer players [18–22].

As a multifactorial factor, the RSA can be influenced by anaerobic and aerobic metabolism [18,23–25]. From a physiological perspective, RSA is a complex quality that is correlated with motor unit activation and is essential to achieving maximal sprint speed and oxidate capacity for phosphocreatine (PCr) recovery and hydrogen (H+) buffering to provide the ability to repeated sprints [26]. Following the same line of thinking, other authors have shown that better sprinters use more of their accessible PCr stores than weaker sprinters [27]. This idea could be related to the strong relationship between PCr resynthesis and power output recovery following 30-s sprints [27,28].

The RSA test simulates intermittent exercise and identifies a player's capacity to maintain maximal effort and recovery during multiple successive high-speed running or sprinting efforts [20,29–31]. Therefore, RSA is an essential factor for determining success in soccer, alongside other qualities like technical and tactical skills, strength, explosive power, speed, and endurance [26,32]. When RSA is compared with aerobic capacities, it was concluded that players with a higher aerobic capacity and faster oxygen kinetics recover faster after high-intensity exercise [29]. These athletes also exhibited better overall RSA performance and recovery performance during the RSA test [29]. Another study showed that subjects with a higher maximal oxygen consumption (VO_2max) value present smaller sprint decrements, suggesting that VO_2max contributes to maintaining performance during repeated-sprint efforts [27].

Beside the metabolic perspective that supports RSA, physical capacities also play a determinant role in RSA. As example, a well-developed neuromuscular system allows a better activation of motor unit [26], while lower-limb strength and power support the acceleration and the maximal speed in the first repetitions and aerobic capacity sustain the performance over the last sprints [33]. The efficiency of RSA could also depend on the player's agility, as this factor is known to be correlated with linear sprint ability [34–36].

The ability to perform repeated sprints while requiring minimal recovery periods between efforts (RSA) appears to be an important aspect of field-based team sport [37]. However, it is difficult to understand which determinants are related to RSA. Thus, some doubts and non-consensual evidence remain in this regard in women's soccer. For that reason, it is important to identify which physical capacities could explain RSA in women's soccer. Such identification may help coaches define better strategies for improving RSA. Therefore, the purpose of this study was to analyze the determinants of RSA based on aerobic performance, linear sprinting and change-of-direction, vertical height jump, and abductor and adductor isometric strength. We hypothesize that strength and power will be determinants for maximum and minimum peak power RSA, while aerobic performance will be determinant for sustaining the performance (fatigue index) [33].

2. Materials and Methods

2.1. Experimental Approach to the Study

This study followed an observational analytic cohort design. The period of observation was 22 consectutive weeks. Fitness assessment were performed three times during the cohort (Figure 1). Between the first and second assessment occurred 4 weeks (pre-season) and between the second and third assessment 18 weeks (end of the first half of the season). The aim was to explore determinants of RSA based on the measures of aerobic capacity, sprinting performance, change-of-direction, vertical height jump and hip adductor/abductor isometric strength. From the initial twenty-five participants, twenty-two remained. Three were excluded based on the fact that did not participated in all the assessments.

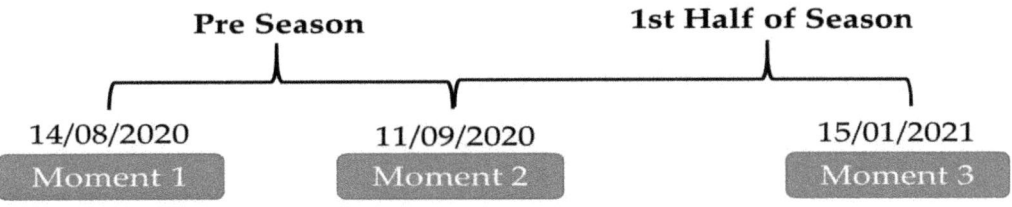

Figure 1. Timeline of the study.

2.2. Participants

Twenty-two women soccer players from the same team participating in the first Portuguese league were observed during the study. In the beginning of the season, the participants presented a mean age of 22.7 ± 5.21 years old, 162.51 ± 7.08 cm of height, 59.1 ± 9.50 kg of body mass. In the second assessment the mean of body mass was 59.01 ± 9.31 kg and in the third evaluation the mean body mass was 61.10 ± 9.94 kg. The eligibility criteria for including in the final sample was: (i) participants were assessed in the three moments of the cohort; (ii) participants participated in, at least, 85% of the total number of training sessions during the cohort; (iii) players had injuries or illness no longer than 4 consecutive weeks; and (iv) players should had a minimum of two years of experience to volunteered for this study. Among the included participants, three were goalkeepers, four were external defenders, four were central defenders, six were midfielders, and five were attackers. The team had three training sessions per week plus an official match in the weekends. Before the cohort begin, all the players were informed about the study design and procedures. After that, each player signed an informed consent. The study was approved by the local university (code: CTC-ESDL-CE001-2021) and followed the ethical standards of Declaration of Helsinki for the study in humans.

2.3. Data Collection

In the three moments of assessment, the tests were made always at the same hour (7:30 p.m.) and days of the week, with a rest period of 48 h (considering the last match/training). Additionally, the assessments two and three were preceded by the same type of microcycle. In each moment of the assessment, the tests were split over three days (interspaced by 24 h). In the first training session of the week players were tested for their anthropometry and hip adductor and abductor strength. In the second training session it was assessed the vertical jump, changes of direction and linear speed. In the third session it were applied the repeated sprint ability test and the Yo-Yo intermittent recovery test. Before the first assessment of each day, a standard warm-up protocol was implemented, by group of players, since they were organized in groups of three to have the same duration between the end of warm-up and beginning of the test. All the players followed the same order. Between tests, there was a minimum of 3 min of rest. The anthropometry, abductor and adductor strength and squat and countermovement jump were performed in a private room, with a stable temperature of 23 °C and relative humidity of 55%. The sprinting tests, RSA test and the Yo-Yo intermittent recovery test were executed in a synthetic turf with a mean temperature of 19.5 ± 3.4 °C and relative humidity of 63 ± 4%. No raining conditions occurred in the assessments.

2.3.1. Anthropometry

There was collected the height and body mass in the three moments of evaluation, at the same hour and at the same day of the week. The evaluation of the height was executed by using the stadiometer (SECA 213, Birmingham, UK), players were asked to remove shoes and other accessories that influence the assessment, they also should be in a vertical and immobile position, with the arms extended along the body and keep a fixed stare, straight ahead and in an upright position. The evaluation of the body mass was executed with a digital balance (SECA 869, Birmingham, UK), it was asked to the players to be barefoot and only in light clothing. For each measure, only one measured was collected.

2.3.2. Hip Adductor and Abductor Isometric Strength

Hip adductor and abductor isometric strength measurement was tested with the dynamometer (Smart Groin Trainer, Neuro excellence, Braga, Portugal). The dynamometer was positioned in the thigh area. Players were asked to lie down in the supine position, with 45° of hip flexion and around 90° of knee flexion [38]. Players were instructed to execute the maximum squeeze in accordance with a previous study [38], although with changes to 20 s for the present protocol. Three trials were made for abductor and adductor, with 10 s of rest between trials. Abductor were tested first (all the trials) and then adductor (all the trials). The highest strength in kilograms were extracted as the main outcome. The best score among trials was obtained for the data treatment.

2.3.3. Squat and Countermovement Jump

The squat and countermovement jumps were performed. The squat jump (SJ) consisted in standing with the knees at 90 degrees, as the position of squat, with no movement, hand in the waist, with no help of the upper limbs the player should jump and extend the legs, falling in the same place. The players waited 3 s in squat position before each jump. The countermovement jump (CMJ) started in standing position with the hands in the waist, being realized with the flexion of the legs and immediately the extension with the jump, the legs will be in extension and they will fall in the same place. For each movement, three trials were executed, with a rest period of 30 s between. The SJ and CMJ were tested with an optical measurement system consisting of a transmitting and receiving bar (Optojump, Microgate, Bolzano, Italy). The Optojump allows a repeatable measurement of flight time as confirmed in a reliability experiment with an intraclass correlation test of 0.95 [39]. The outcome extracted in each trial was the jump height (cm). For each movement, it was considered the highest jump for data treatment.

2.3.4. Change-of-Direction Test

Agility was assess by using the test zig-zag 20 m [40], this test consisted in four sections of 5 m each set out at 100°. The time was recorded using photocells timing gates (Photocells, Brower Timing System, UT, USA), with resolution of 1 thousandth of seconds. Typical error of the Photocells was between 0.04 and 0.06 (s), while the smallest worthwhile change was between 0.11 and 0.17 (s) [41]. This test was performed in the fields, before the training session. Subjects performed three trials of the test, with 3 min of rest between all trials and tests. The outcome extracted was the best time (lowest time in seconds) considering the trials.

2.3.5. Linear Sprinting

Linear Sprint was assessed over 10-m and 30-m using photocell timing gates (Photocells, Brower Timing System, USA), with resolution of 1 thousandth of seconds. The participants started 0.5 m behind the initial timing gate in a two point split stance and were instructed to set off in their own time and run at the maximal speed until the last gate. Each participant performed three trials at maximal effort. The outcome extracted was the time (seconds) for completing the run. The best score in each running distance was considered for the data treatment.

2.3.6. Running Anaerobic Sprint test

The protocol used for testing the RSA consisted in 35 linear meters (no change-of-direction), performed six times and with a recovery time between efforts of 10 s [42]. The participants started their sprint 0.5 m behind the starting timing gate. Photocell timing gate (Photocells, Brower Timing System, UT, USA), with resolution of 1 thousandth of seconds were positioned in the beginning and at the end lines to record the time of each sprint effort. The time (seconds) for each trial was collected. After that, the minimum and maximum peak power was determined by using the equation [43] Power = $\frac{\text{Body mass} \times \text{Distance}^2}{\text{Time}^3}$, as well as the fatigue index used the following equation [43] Fatigue index = $\frac{\text{max}_{power} - \text{min}_{power}}{\text{Sum of 6 sprints (s)}}$.

2.3.7. Yo-Yo Intermittent Recovery Test—Level 1

The Yo-Yo IR1 test consisted of repeated 20-m runs back and forth between two markers with a progressive increase in speed, which was regulated by an audio player. Between each 40-m run, the athlete recovered with 10 s of jogging (shuttle runs of 2 × 5 m). Yo-yo level 1 starts at 10 km/h and level 2 at 13 km/h, with both levels progressively increasing in speed throughout the test. The test was completed when the athlete reached voluntary exhaustion or failed to maintain her running pace in synchrony with the audio recording. The number of completed levels and shuttles and the total distance covered were recorded at the end of the test. The total distance (meters) was extracted as the outcome. The maximal oxygen Uptake (VO_2max in mL/min/kg) was estimated by the next equation [44]: VO_2max = final distance (m) × 0.0084 + 36.4.

2.4. Statistical Analysis

For the treatment of the data, we use adequate statistical methods to calculate percentages and central and dispersion parameters (arithmetic mean and standard deviation). Descriptive statistics were calculated for each variable (See Table 1, for more information). In ADD and ABD two subjects missed the data collection, and they were excluded from the item analysis. Similarly occurred with one participant in YYIRT. Before any parametric statistical analysis was performed, the assumption of normality was tested with the Kolmogorov–Smirnov test on each variable. The changes over the season were determined by a one-way ANOVA with repeated measures. Significant main effects were subsequently analyzed using a Bonferroni post hoc test. Effect size is indicated with partial eta squared for Fs. To interpret the magnitude of the eta squared we adopted the following criteria: $\eta^2 = 0.02$, small; $\eta^2 = 0.06$, medium; and $\eta^2 = 0.14$ large. Pearson correlation coefficient r was used to examine the relationship between RSA (Pmax, Pmin, and Fatigue index) and the remaining variables (ADDs, ABDs, SJ, CMJ, 10 and 30 m sprint, COD and YYIRT1). To interpret the magnitude of these correlations we adopted the following criteria: $r \leq 0.1$, trivial; $0.1 < r \leq 0.3$, small; $0.3 < r \leq 0.5$, moderate; $0.5 < r \leq 0.7$, large; $0.7 < r \leq 0.9$, very large; and $r > 0.9$, almost perfect [45]. Confidence intervals (95% CI) were calculated for each correlation. Multiple regression analysis was used to model the prediction of RSA from remaining variables. In this regression analysis, were examined separately all variables. Data were analyzed using software Statistica (version 10.0; Statsoft, Inc., Tulsa, OK, USA).

Table 1. Anthropometrical and fitness variables in the three moments of assessment (Mean ± SD).

	Women Soccer Players ($n = 22$)						
	Moment 1	Moment 2	Moment 3	CI (95%)	Upper CI (95%)	Lower CI (95%)	Repeated Measures ANOVA (p)
Hip strength							
ADDs (kg)		34.66 ± 7.81	35.06 ± 8.12	3.39	37.93	31.15	$p = 0.97, \eta^2 = 0.001$.
ABDs (kg)		33.48 ± 5.87	34.19 ± 6.23	2.72	36.14	30.69	$p = 0.98, \eta^2 = 0.001$.
Squat and countermovement jump							
SJ (cm)	25.33 ± 2.98	26.24 ± 3.09	24.39 ± 3.95	1.38	26.62	23.84	$p = 0.003 *, \eta^2 = 0.35$.
CMJ (cm)	27.26 ± 2.98	27.40 ± 3.51	24.65 ± 3.93	1.39	27.70	24.90	$p = 0.001 *, \eta^2 = 0.60$.
Linear sprinting							
10 m (s)	1.87 ± 0.08	1.90 ± 0.10	1.88 ± 0.10	0.05	1.94	1.85	$p = 0.26, \eta^2 = 0.09$.
30 m (s)	4.79 ± 0.23	4.78 ± 0.22	4.75 ± 0.23	0.11	4.90	4.68	$p = 0.07, \eta^2 = 0.16$.
Change-of-direction test							
COD (s)	5.73 ± 0.19	5.75 ± 0.18	5.79 ± 0.23	0.09	5.86	5.67	$p = 0.32, \eta^2 = 0.08$.
Repeated sprint ability test (RSA test)							
Pmin (s)	240.44 ± 46.87	267.15 ± 46.29	293.09 ± 36.49	18.29	281.51	244.93	$p = 0.001 *, \eta^2 = 0.48$.
Pmax (s)	380.81 ± 68.38	401.77 ± 74.47	444.38 ± 72.96	31.40	441.72	378.92	$p = 0.001 *, \eta^2 = 0.40$.
FI (%)	4.61 ± 1.85	4.42 ± 1.66	4.96 ± 1.87	0.70	5.53	4.11	$p = 0.38, \eta^2 = 0.07$.
Yo-Yo intermittent recovery test- Level 1							
YYIR1. Distance (m)	677.78 ± 203.72	788.00 ± 219.89	863.33 ± 218.73	89.40	833.84	655.04	$p = 0.001 *, \eta^2 = 0.53$.
VO$_2$max (mL/kg/min)	41.74 ± 5.33	43.02 ± 1.85	43.82 ± 1.82	0.82	43.40	41.75	$p = 0.001 *, \eta^2 = 0.55$.

ADD: adductor isometric strength; ABD: abductor isometric strength; SJ: squat jump; CMJ: countermovement jump; 10 m: 10-m sprint; 30 m: 30-m sprint; COD: change-of-direction; YYIRT1: Yo-Yo intermittent recovery test level 1; Pmin: peak power (minimum); Pmax: peak power (maximum); FI: fatigue index; cm: centimeters; s: seconds. * denotes significance at $p < 0.01$.

3. Results

Descriptive statistics were calculated for each variable (See Table 1, for more information).

Different repeated measures ANOVAs with participants' mean ADDs, ABDs, 10 m, 30 m, COD and FI, did not revealed any effect of moment $F (1.16) = 0.00080, p = 0.97, \eta^2 = 0.001$, $F (1.16) = 0.00063, p = 0.98, \eta^2 = 0.001, F (2.28) = 1.39, p = 0.26, \eta^2 = 0.09, F (2.28) = 2.81, p = 0.07, \eta^2 = 0.16, F (2.26) = 1.18, p = 0.32, \eta^2 = 0.08$, and $F (2.26) = 0.99, p = 0.38, \eta^2 = 0.07$, respectively. Continuing with the same type of repeated measures ANOVA analysis with participant´s mean SJ, CMJ, Pmin, Pmax, YYIR1 and VO$_2$max revealed a significant effect of moment, $F (2.26) = 7.03, p = 0.003, \eta^2 = 0.35, F (2.26) = 20.20, p = 0.001, \eta^2 = 0.60, F (2.26) = 12.41, p = 0.001, \eta^2 = 0.48, F (2.26) = 8.84, p = 0.001, \eta2 = 0.40, F (2.18) = 10.26, p = 0.001, \eta^2 = 0.53$, and $F (2.16) = 9.84, p = 0.001, \eta^2 = 0.55$.

The correlation coefficients between RSA indices (Pmax, Pmin, and Fatigue index) and fitness variables are summarized in Table 2. No significant correlations were found between all RSA indices and SJ, CMJ, 10m, 30m and COD. However, positive moderate correlations were found between Pmin and ADDs and ABDs [$r = 0.51, p < 0.02$ and $r = 0.54, p < 0.01$, respectively (See Figure 2]. In the same line, positive moderate correlations were found between Pmax and ADDs and ABDs ($r = 0.55, p < 0.02$ and $r = 0.46, p < 0.01$, respectively (see Figure 3)). Last, other interest and negative moderate correlation was found between FI and YYIR1 test [$r = -0.62, p < 0.004$ (Figure 4)].

The regression analysis to predict RSA from physical fitness variables was in agreement with the correlation analysis (See Table 3). On the one hand, ADDs and ABDs were predictor variables of Pmin ($r = 0.53$ and $r = 0.55$, respectively). On the other hand, ABDs was predictor variable of Pmax ($r = 0.48$). Finally, YYIR1 test was a predictor variable of IF ($r = -0.53$).

Table 2. Pearson correlation coefficient between RSA indices and fitness variables ($n = 22$).

RSA Indices	ADDs (kg)	ABDs (kg)	SJ (cm)	CMJ (cm)	10m (s)	30m (s)	COD (s)	YYIR1 (m)
Pmin (s)	r = 0.51 p = 0.02 **	r = 0.54 p = 0.01 **	r = 0.13 p = 0.58	r = 0.04 p = 0.84	R = 0.10 p = 0.67	r = 0.09 p = 0.70	r = −0.00 p = 0.99	r = −0.08 p = 0.72
Pmax (s)	r = 0.55 p = 0.01 **	r = 0.46 p = 0.04 *	r = 0.19 p = 0.41	r = 0.05 p = 0.81	r = −0.10 p = 0.65	r = −0.24 p = 0.30	r = −0.12 p = 0.61	r = −0.38 p = 0.10
FI (%)	r = 0.33 p = 0.16	r = 0.18 p = 0.45	r = 0.16 p = 0.50	r = 0.03 p = 0.87	r = −0.24 p = 0.30	r = −0.43 p = 0.06	r = −0.17 p = 0.47	r = −0.62 p = 0.04 *

ADD: adductor isometric strength; ABD: abductor isometric strength; SJ: squat jump; CMJ: countermovement jump; 10 m: 10-m sprint; 30 m: 30-m sprint; COD: change-of-direction; YYIRT1: Yo-Yo intermittent recovery test level 1; Pmin: peak power (minimum); Pmax: peak power (maximum); FI: fatigue index; cm: centimeters; s: seconds. * Denotes significance at $p < 0.05$, and ** denotes significance at $p < 0.01$.

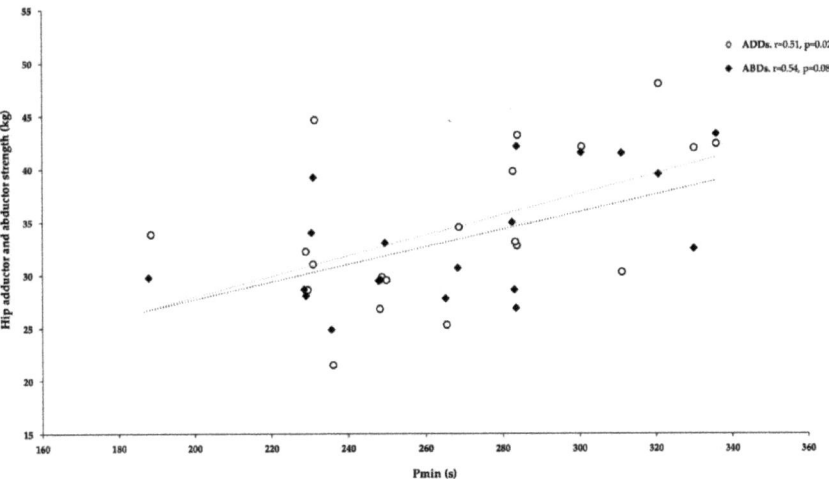

Figure 2. Relationship between hip adductor and abductor isometric strength (ADDs and ABDs) and Pmin of RSA test.

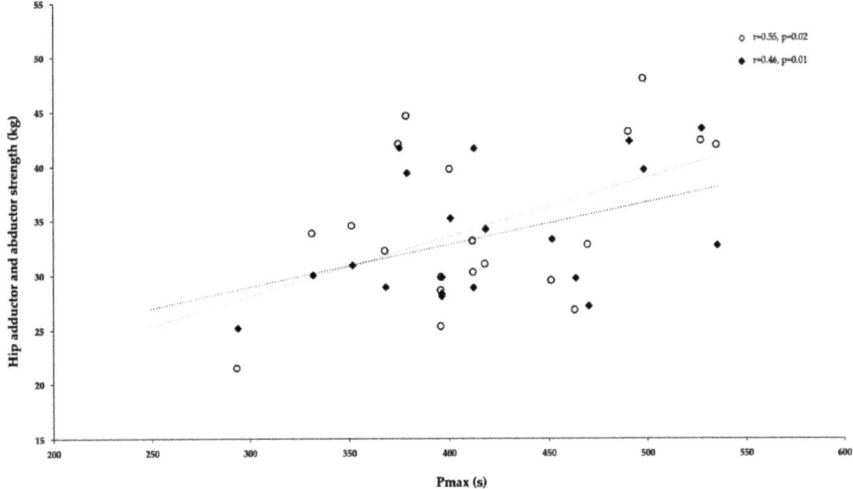

Figure 3. Relationship between hip adductor and abductor isometric strength (ADDs and ABDs) and Pmax of RSA test.

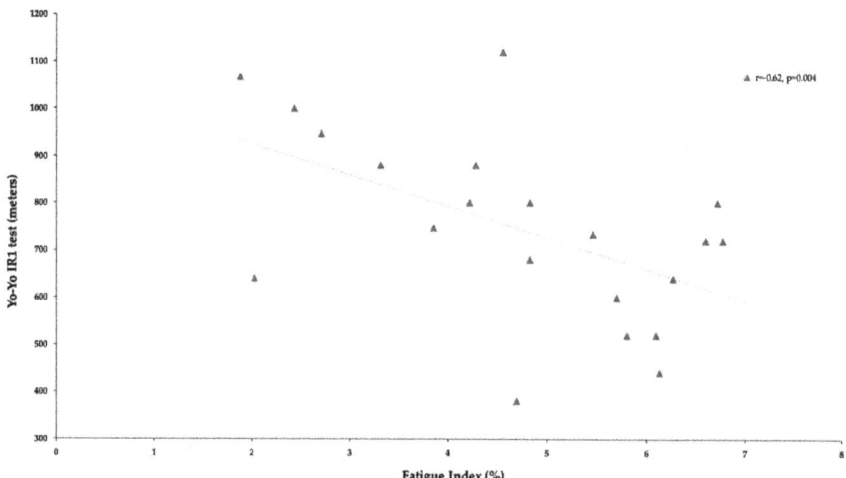

Figure 4. Relationship between Yo-Yo IR1 test and fatigue index (FI) of repeated-sprint ability test.

Table 3. Values of regression analysis explaining, Pmax, Pmin and Fatigue index based on the remaining variables.

RSA Indices		R	R^2	Adjusted R^2	F	P	SE
Pmin (s)	ADDS	0.53	0.27	0.23	6.86	0.01	34.25
	ABDs	0.55	0.30	0.26	8.01	0.01	33.49
Pmax (s)	ADDs	0.48	0.23	0.19	5.52	0.03	57.60
FI (%)	YYIR1	−0.53	0.28	0.24	7.39	0.01	1.35

Pmin: peak power (minimum); Pmax: peak power (maximum); FI: fatigue index; s: seconds.

4. Discussion

The present study aimed to analyze the determinants of RSA based on aerobic performance, linear sprinting and change-of-direction, vertical height jump, and abductor and adductor isometric strength. The main findings were as follows: (i) power in repeated sprints can be improved and predicted through exercises of ABD´s and ADD´s strength, and (ii) RSA can be improved and forecasted through aerobic endurance-based exercises such as the YYIR1 test. Additionally, it was found that RSA, and cardiorespiratory fitness had meaningfully improved over the season, while vertical jump had decreased.

The assessments performed repeatedly over the season revealed a meaningful improvement in RSA and aerobic performance. On the other hand, vertical jump decreased over the season, possibly due to the lack of reactive strength training or oriented training for this physical quality. Usually, both RSA and aerobic performance are key determinants of physical performance in soccer and match running-performance is associated with those capacities [16,46,47], thus it can be expected that over the season the training and match load may explain positive changes in RSA and aerobic performance [48,49].

High-intensity efforts, such as sprints, are essential components explaining soccer players´ behavior [50]. However, in addition to sprints in isolation, players perform repeated high-intensity efforts in short intervals, drawing from their aerobic endurance to do so [10]. In this sense, RSA seems to be a suitable method for inducing optimal improvements in anaerobic and aerobic metabolism [18,23–25], thus giving a team an advantage over the opponent during moments in matches characterized by high-speed efforts.

It seems that RSA can be improved through any soccer-specific training program [51], supporting the improvements found in this study over four- and 18-week female soccer training programs. However, the main determinants of RSA test performance among female soccer players are still unclear. Therefore, the authors of the present study tried to analyze the most relevant variables of RSA by comparing indicators from the RSA test (power and fatigue index) with aerobic endurance (YYIR1 test), linear sprinting with COD, vertical height jump (SJ and CMJ test), and ABDs and ADD strength. The primary moderate correlations were established between power and ABD/ADD isometric strength (Pmin and ADD [r = 0.51], Pmin and ABDs [r = 0.54], Pmax and ADDs [r = 0.55], and Pmax and ABDs [r = 0.46]) and between fatigue and YYIR1 test outcomes [r = −0.62]. No other correlations were found between RSA parameters and other tests.

The relationship between power and ABD/ADD isometric strength may be due to the implication of these muscle groups in sprinting efforts [52]. From an anatomy-based or biomechanic viewpoint, ADD assists hip flexion and neutralizes the abduction and external rotation caused by tensor fascia latae and Sartorius. In addition, during the mid-to-late swing, when the hip is flexed, adductors work as synergists of the gluteus maximus, helping with hip extension and counterbalancing external rotation [52]. On the other hand, the ABDs stabilize the femoral head during high-speed running efforts. They lengthen eccentrically while helping to stabilize the pelvis and control femoral adduction in the transverse plane [53].

Researchers have tried to analyze the implications of hypertrophy of these muscles during sprints. For example, Nuell et al. [52] and Tottori [54] highlighted the implications of and the close relationship between ADD and sprint performance, while Fredericson and Weir [53] highlighted the implications of ABD in gait and sprints. Interestingly, it seems that the implication of ADD correlates with sprinting time [52] and with sprinting distance [54]. These findings encourage physical fitness and conditioning coaches to design coadjutant training programs based on ADD and ABD isometric strength to improve female soccer players' sprint performance. However, no relationship was found between RSA parameters and exercises with significant quadriceps implications (i.e., SJ, CMJ, and COD).

This idea seems consistent among experts in this topic [55,56], who have concluded that the quadriceps are not related to sprint performance. Instead of the quadriceps, it may be anatomically due to the anterior and middle parts of the gluteus medius, which have a stronger vertical pull and help initiate abduction, which is then completed by the tensor fascia lata [53].

Nevertheless, in addition to strength exercises, aerobic endurance remains crucial during female soccer matches. In the present study, the authors found correlations between fatigue and YYIR1 test results ($p < 0.004$; Figure 4). This finding is supported by Gabrys et al. [57], who concluded that the anaerobic glycolytic system is more sensitive to long, repetitive sprints, highlighting that RSA is a suitable strategy for avoiding insufficient aerobic energy systems, which lead to early decreases in performance [57]. All of these results indicate the value of forecasting Pmax from ADD and ABD isometric strength values (r = 0.53 and r = 0.55, respectively), Pmax from ABD values (r = 0.48), and fatigue from YYIR1 (r = −0.53).

This study had some limitations. The force platforms were not used to calculate the rate of force development during vertical jumps, and this could be interesting. Additionally, an isometric mid-thigh pull test would be interesting to associated with RSA. Future studies should consider analyzing the influence of each physical capacity in different number of sprints, and also consider analyzing COD deficit and asymmetries trying to understand if this can be related with RSA ability. Other limitation is associated with small sample and the specificity of being conducted in women, thus not being possible to generalize for other populations. More research should be conducted to test the replication of results in different scenarios (other competitive contexts, age-groups and populations).

As practical applications, the coadjutant training program—mainly based on these determinants (ABD and ADD isometric strength exercises and YYIR1)—may induce improvements in female soccer players' RSA and better outcomes during critical moments of matches. Although it was declared that straight sprinting is the most frequent action taken before goals, both for scoring and assisting players [51], the current trend highlights that sprints during soccer games are curvilinear [58–60]. As such, they may lead to different demands than straight sprints [57]. Therefore, further studies should assess the main determinants of curvilinear sprinting performance during RSA tests.

5. Conclusions

Power and fatigue are notable RSA-related parameters. Power during RSA is mainly determined by ABD and ADD isometric strength, while fatigue is related to YYIR1. Therefore, physical fitness and conditioning coaches are encouraged to improve ABD and ADD isometric strength alongside aerobic endurance. Doing so may lead to improvements in RSA, subsequently giving the player an advantage over the opponent during critical game situations. However, since it seems that most sprint efforts are made in a curvilinear trajectory, future studies should replicate the present study, focusing on these efforts.

Author Contributions: L.G., F.M.C. and J.M.C.C. lead the project, established the protocol and wrote and revised the original manuscript; J.I.B. and H.S. collected the data, wrote and revised the original manuscript; F.T.G.-F. and M.R.-G. wrote and revised the original manuscript. All authors have read and agreed to the published version of the manuscript.

Funding: This research received no external funding.

Institutional Review Board Statement: The study was conducted according to the guidelines of the Declaration of Helsinki and approved by the Institutional Review Board (or Ethics Committee) of Polytechnic Institute of Viana do Castelo, School of Sport and Leisure (code: CTC-ESDL-CE001-2021).

Informed Consent Statement: Informed consent was obtained from all subjects involved in the study.

Acknowledgments: Filipe Manuel Clemente: This work is funded by Fundação para a Ciência e Tecnologia/Ministério da Ciência, Tecnologia e Ensino Superior through national funds and when applicable co-funded EU funds under the project UIDB/50008/2020. Hugo Sarmento gratefully acknowledge the support of a Spanish government subproject Integration ways between qualitative and quantitative data, multiple case development, and synthesis review as main axis for an innovative future in physical activity and sports research [PGC2018-098742-B-C31] (Ministerio de Economía y Competitividad, Programa Estatal de Generación de Conocimiento y Fortalecimiento Científico y Tecnológico del Sistema I+D+i), that is part of the coordinated project 'New approach of research in physical activity and sport from mixed methods perspective (NARPAS_MM) [SPGC201800X098742CV0]'.

Conflicts of Interest: The authors declare no conflict of interest.

References

1. Sedan, S.; Vaeyens, R.; Philippaerts, R.M.; Redondo, J.C.; Cuadrado, G. Anthropometric and anaerobic fitness profile of elite and non-elite female soccer players. *J. Sports Med. Phys. Fit.* **2009**, *49*, 387–394.
2. Haugen, T.A.; Tønnessen, E.; Seiler, S. Speed and countermovement-jump characteristics of elite female soccer players, 1995–2010. *Int. J. Sports Physiol. Perform.* **2012**, *7*, 340–349. [CrossRef]
3. Milanović, Z.; Sporiš, G.; James, N.; Trajković, N.; Ignjatović, A.; Sarmento, H.; Trecroci, A.; Mendes, B. Physiological demands, morphological characteristics, physical abilities and injuries of female soccer players. *J. Hum. Kinet.* **2017**, *60*, 77–83. [CrossRef] [PubMed]
4. Manson, S.; Brughelli, M.; Harris, N. Physiological characteristics of International female soccer players. *J. Strength Cond. Res.* **2014**, *28*, 308–318. [CrossRef] [PubMed]
5. Mufty, S.; Bollars, P.; Vanlommel, L.; Van Crombrugge, K.; Corten, K.; Bellemans, J. Injuries in male versus female soccer players: Epidemiology of a nationwide study. *Acta Orthop. Belg.* **2015**, *81*, 289–295. [PubMed]
6. Reilly, T. Energetics of high-intensity exercise (soccer) with particular reference to fatigue. *J. Sports Sci.* **1997**, *15*, 257–263. [CrossRef] [PubMed]
7. Ramos, G.; Nakamura, F.Y.; Pereira, L.A.; Wilke, C.F. Movement patterns of an U-20 National female soccer team during competitive matches: Influence of playing position and performance in the first half. *Int. J. Sports Med.* **2017**, *38*, 747–754. [PubMed]
8. Ingebrigtsen, J.; Dillern, T.; Shalfawi, S.A.I. Aerobic Capacities and Anthropometric Characteristics of Elite Female Soccer Players. *J. Strength Cond. Res.* **2011**, *25*, 3352–3357. [CrossRef] [PubMed]
9. Mohr, M.; Krustrup, P.; Andersson, H.; Kirkendal, D.; Bangsbo, J. Match Activities of Elite Women Soccer Players at Different Performance Levels. *J. Strength Cond. Res.* **2008**, *22*, 341–349. [CrossRef] [PubMed]

10. McCormack, W.; Stout, J.; Wells, A.; Gonzalez, A.; Mangine, G.; Hoffman, J. Predictors of high-intensity running capacity in collegiate women during a soccer game. *J. Stregth Cond. Res.* **2014**, *28*, 964–970. [CrossRef]
11. Wells, A.; Hoffman, J.; Beyer, K.; Hoffman, M.; Jajtner, A.; Fukuda, D.; Stout, J. Regular and postseason comparisons of playing time and measures of running performance in NCAA Division I women soccer players. *App. Phys. Nut. Metab.* **2015**, *40*, 907–917. [CrossRef] [PubMed]
12. Mohr, M.; Krustrup, P.; Bangsbo, J. Match performance of high-standard soccer players with special reference to development of fatigue. *J. Sports Sci.* **2003**, *21*, 519–528. [CrossRef] [PubMed]
13. Datson, N.; Drust, B.; Weston, M.; Jarman, I.; Lisboa, P.; Gregson, W. Match physical performance of elite female soccer player during international competition. *J. Stregth Cond. Res.* **2017**, *31*, 2379–2387. [CrossRef] [PubMed]
14. Datson, N.; Hulton, A.; Andersson, H.; Lewis, T.; Weston, M.; Drust, B.; Gregson, W. Applied physiology of female soccer: An update. *Sports Med.* **2014**, *44*, 1225–1240. [CrossRef] [PubMed]
15. Davis, J.A.; Brewer, J. Applied physiology of female soccer players. *Sports Med.* **1993**, *16*, 180–189. [CrossRef]
16. Krustrup, P.; Mohr, M.; Ellingsgaard, H.; Bangsbo, J. Physical Demands during an Elite Female Soccer Game: Importance of Training Status. *Med. Sci. Sports Exerc.* **2005**, *37*, 1242–1248. [CrossRef]
17. Bangsbo, J.; Mohr, M.; Krustrup, P. Physical and metabolic demands of training and match-play in the elite football player. *J. Sports Sci.* **2006**, *24*, 665–674. [CrossRef]
18. Chaouachi, A.; Manzi, V.; Wong, D.; Chaalali, A.; Laurencelle, L.; Chamari, K.; Castagna, C. Intermittent endurance and repeated sprint ability in soccer players. *J. Strength Cond. Res.* **2010**, *24*, 2663–2669. [CrossRef]
19. Krustrup, P.; Mohr, M.; Steensberg, A.; Bencke, J.; Klær, M.; Bangsbo, J. Muscle and blood metabolites during a soccer game: Implications for sprint performance. *Med. Sci. Sports Exerc.* **2006**, *38*, 1165–1174. [CrossRef]
20. Rampinini, E.; Coutts, A.J.; Castagna, C.; Sassi, R.; Impellizzeri, F.M. Variation in top level soccer match performance. *Int. J. Sports Med.* **2007**, *28*, 1018–1024. [CrossRef]
21. Gabbett, T.; Wiig, H.; Spencer, M. Repeated high-intensity running and sprinting in elite women's soccer competition. *Int. J. Sports Physiol. Perform.* **2013**, *8*, 130–138. [CrossRef]
22. Stolen, T.; Chamari, K.; Castagna, C.; Wisloff, U. Physiology of soccer. *Sports Med.* **2005**, *3*, 50–60.
23. Krustrup, P.; Mohr, M.; Amstrup, T.; Rysgaard, J.; Johansen, J.; Steensberg, A.; Pedersen, P.K.; Bangsbo, J. The Yo-Yo Intermittent Recovery Test: Physiological Response, Reliability, and Validity. *Med. Sci. Sports Exerc.* **2003**, *35*, 697–705. [CrossRef] [PubMed]
24. Krustrup, P.; Mohr, M.; Nybo, L.; Bangsbo, J. The Yo-Yo IR2 Test: Physiological response, reliability and application to elite soccer. *Med. Sci. Sports Exerc.* **2006**, *38*, 1666–1673. [CrossRef] [PubMed]
25. Buchheit, M.; Bishop, D.; Haydar, B.; Nakamura, F.; Ahmaidi, S. Physiological responses to shuttle repeated sprint running. *Int. J. Sports Med.* **2010**, *31*, 402–409. [CrossRef] [PubMed]
26. Buchheit, M.; Mendez-villanueva, A. Improving Repeated Sprint Ability in Young Elite Soccer Players: Repeated Shuttle Sprints Vs. Explosive Strength Training. *J. Strength Cond. Res.* **2010**, *24*, 2715–2722. [CrossRef] [PubMed]
27. Bishop, D.; Edge, J. Determinants of repeated-sprint ability in females matched for single-sprint performance. *Eur. J. Appl. Physiol.* **2006**, *97*, 373–379. [CrossRef] [PubMed]
28. Bogdanis, G.C.; Nevill, M.E. Contribution of phosphocreatine and aerobic metabolism to energy supply during repeated sprint exercise. *J. Appl. Physiol.* **1996**, *80*, 876–884. [CrossRef]
29. Archiza, B.; Andaku, D.K.; Beltrame, T.; Libardi, C.A.; Borghi-Silva, A. The Relationship between Repeated-Sprint Ability, Aerobic Capacity, and Oxygen Uptake Recovery Kinetics in Female Soccer Athletes. *J. Hum. Kinet.* **2020**, *75*, 115–126. [CrossRef]
30. Datson, N.; Drust, B.; Weston, M.; Gregson, W. Repeated high-speed running in elite female soccer players during international competition. *Sci. Med. Footb.* **2019**, *3*, 150–156. [CrossRef]
31. Doyle, B.; Browne, D.; Horan, D. The relationship of aerobic endurance and linear speed on repeat sprint ability performance in female international footballers. *Int. J. Hum. Mov. Sports Sci.* **2020**, *8*, 147–153. [CrossRef]
32. Pyne, D.B.; Saunders, P.; Montgomery, P.; Hewitt, A.; Sheehan, K. Relationships between repeated sprint testing, speed and endurance. *J. Strength Cond. Res.* **2008**, *22*, 1633–1637. [CrossRef]
33. López-Segovia, M.; Pareja-Blanco, F.; Jiménez-Reyes, P.; González-Badillo, J. Determinant Factors of Repeat Sprint Sequences in Young Soccer Players. *Int. J. Sports Med.* **2014**, *36*, 130–136. [CrossRef]
34. Gunnar, M.; Svein, A.P. The effect of speed training on sprint and agility performance in female youth soccer players. *J. Phys. Educ. Sport* **2015**, *15*, 395–399.
35. Buchheit, M.; Haydar, B.; Ahmaidi, S. Repeated sprints with directional changes: Do angles matter? *J. Sports Sci.* **2012**, *30*, 555–562. [CrossRef]
36. Vescovi, J.D.; Mcguigan, M.R. Relationships between sprinting, agility, and jump ability in female athletes. *J. Sports Sci.* **2008**, *26*, 97–107. [CrossRef] [PubMed]
37. Spencer, M.; Bishop, D.; Dawson, B.; Goodman, C. Physiological and metabolic responses of repeated-sprint activities: Specific to field-based team sports. *Sports Med.* **2005**, *35*, 1025–1044. [CrossRef] [PubMed]
38. Oliveras, R.; Bizzini, M.; Brunner, R.; Maffiuletti, N.A. Field-based evaluation of hip adductor and abductor strength in professional male ice hockey players: Reference values and influencing factors. *Phys. Ther. Sport* **2020**, *43*, 204–209. [CrossRef] [PubMed]
39. Gollin, M.; Scarafiotti, E. The Repeatability of Jump tests measured with the Opto Jump. *Sport Sci. Health* **2012**, *8*, 36.

40. Little, T.; Williams, A.G. Specificity of Acceleration, Maximum Speed, and Agility in Professional Soccer Players. *J. Strength Cond. Res.* **2005**, *19*, 76–78.
41. Bond, C.W.; Willaert, E.M.; Rudningen, K.E.; Noonan, B.C. Reliability of Three Timing Systems Used to Time Short on Ice-Skating Sprints in Ice Hockey Players. *J. Strength Cond. Res.* **2017**, *31*, 3279–3286. [CrossRef]
42. Cipryan, L.; Gajda, V. The influence of aerobic power on repeated anaerobic exercise in junior soccer players. *J. Hum. Kinet.* **2011**, *28*, 63–71. [CrossRef]
43. MacKenzie, B. *101 Performance Evaluation Tests*; Electric Word plc.: London, UK, 2005.
44. Bangsbo, J.; Iaia, F.M.; Krustrup, P. The Yo-Yo Intermittent Recovery Test. *Sports Med.* **2008**, *38*, 37–51. [CrossRef]
45. Granier, P.; Mercier, B.; Mercier, J.; Anselme, F.; Préfaut, C. Aerobic and anaerobic contribution to Wingate test performance in sprint and middle-distance runners. *Eur. J. Appl. Physiol. Occup. Physiol.* **1995**, *70*, 58–65. [CrossRef]
46. Buchheit, M.; Mendez-Villanueva, A.; Simpson, B.M.; Bourdon, P.C. Match Running Performance and Fitness in Youth Soccer. *Int. J. Sports Med.* **2010**, *31*, 818–825. [CrossRef] [PubMed]
47. Castagna, C.; Manzi, V.; Impellizzeri, F.; Weston, M.; Barbero Alvarez, J.C. Relationship between Endurance Field Tests and Match Performance in Young Soccer Players. *J. Strength Cond. Res.* **2010**, *24*, 3227–3233. [CrossRef]
48. Nobari, H.; Alves, A.R.; Clemente, F.M.; Pérez-Gómez, J.; Clark, C.C.T.; Granacher, U.; Zouhal, H. Associations Between Variations in Accumulated Workload and Physiological Variables in Young Male Soccer Players Over the Course of a Season. *Front. Physiol.* **2021**, *12*, 233. [CrossRef] [PubMed]
49. Lesinski, M.; Prieske, O.; Helm, N.; Granacher, U. Effects of soccer training on anthropometry, body composition, and physical fitness during a soccer season in female elite young athletes: A prospective cohort study. *Front. Physiol.* **2017**, *8*, 1093. [CrossRef] [PubMed]
50. Pino-Ortega, J.; Rojas-Valverde, D.; Gómez-Carmona, C.D.; Rico-González, M. Training Design, Performance Analysis, and Talent Identification—A Systematic Review about the Most Relevant Variables through the Principal Component Analysis in Soccer, Basketball, and Rugby. *Int. J. Environ. Res. Public Health* **2021**, *18*, 2642. [CrossRef] [PubMed]
51. Haugen, T.; Tønnessen, E.; Hisdal, J.; Seiler, S. The role and development of sprinting speed in soccer. *Int. J. Sports Physiol. Perform.* **2014**, *9*, 432–441. [CrossRef] [PubMed]
52. Nuell, S.; Illera-Domínguez, V.R.; Carmona, G.; Alomar, X.; Padullés, J.M.; Lloret, M.; Cadefau, J.A. Hypertrophic muscle changes and sprint performance enhancement during a sprint-based training macrocycle in national-level sprinters. *Eur. J. Sport Sci.* **2020**, *20*, 793–802. [CrossRef]
53. Fredericson, M.; Weir, A. Practical management of iliotibial band friction syndrome in runners. *Clin. J. Sport Med.* **2006**, *16*, 261–268. [CrossRef]
54. Tottori, N.; Suga, T.; Miyake, Y.; Tsuchikane, R.; Otsuka, M.; Nagano, A.; Fujita, S.; Isaka, T. Hip Flexor and Knee Extensor Muscularity Are Associated with Sprint Performance in Sprint-Trained Preadolescent Boys. *Pediatr. Exerc. Sci.* **2018**, *30*, 115–123. [CrossRef] [PubMed]
55. Miyake, Y.; Suga, T.; Otsuka, M.; Tanaka, T.; Misaki, J.; Kudo, S.; Nagano, A.; Isaka, T. The knee extensor moment arm is associated with performance in male sprinters. *Eur. J. Appl. Physiol.* **2017**, *117*, 533–539. [CrossRef]
56. Sugisaki, N.; Kobayashi, K.; Tsuchie, H.; Kanehisa, H. Associations Between Individual Lower-Limb Muscle Volumes and 100-m Sprint Time in Male Sprinters. *Int. J. Sports Physiol. Perform.* **2018**, *13*, 214–219. [CrossRef] [PubMed]
57. Gabrys, T.; Stanula, A.; Szmatlan-Gabrys, U.; Garnys, M.; Charvát, L.; Gupta, S. Metabolic and Cardiorespiratory Responses of Semiprofessional Football Players in Repeated Ajax Shuttle Tests and Curved Sprint Tests, and Their Relationship with Football Match Play. *Int. J. Environ. Res. Public Health* **2020**, *17*, 7745. [CrossRef] [PubMed]
58. Granero-Gil, P.; Bastida-Castillo, A.; Rojas-Valverde, D.; Gómez-Carmona, C.D.; de la Cruz Sánchez, E.; Pino-Ortega, J. Accuracy, inter-unit reliability and comparison between GPS and UWB-based tracking systems for measuring centripetal force during curvilinear locomotion. *Proc. Inst. Mech. Eng. Part P J. Sports Eng. Technol.* **2021**. [CrossRef]
59. Granero-Gil, P.; Gómez-Carmona, C.D.; Bastida-Castillo, A.; Rojas-Valverde, D.; de la Cruz, E.; Pino-Ortega, J. Influence of playing position and laterality in centripetal force and changes of direction in elite soccer players. *PLoS ONE* **2020**, *15*, e0232123. [CrossRef] [PubMed]
60. Granero-Gil, P.; Bastida-Castillo, A.; Rojas-Valverde, D.; Gómez-Carmona, C.D.; de la Cruz Sánchez, E.; Pino-Ortega, J. Influence of Contextual Variables in the Changes of Direction and Centripetal Force Generated during an Elite-Level Soccer Team Season. *Int. J. Environ. Res. Public Health* **2020**, *17*, 967. [CrossRef]

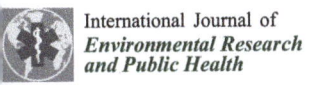

Article

Training Habits of Eumenorrheic Active Women during the Different Phases of Their Menstrual Cycle: A Descriptive Study

Felipe García-Pinillos [1,2], Pascual Bujalance-Moreno [3], Daniel Jérez-Mayorga [4], Álvaro Velarde-Sotres [5,6], Vanessa Anaya-Moix [6,7], Silvia Pueyo-Villa [6,7] and Carlos Lago-Fuentes [5,*]

1. Department of Physical Education, Sports and Recreation, Universidad de La Frontera, Temuco 4811230, Chile; fgpinillos@ugr.es
2. Faculty of Sports Sciences, University of Granada, 18010 Granada, Spain
3. Department of Corporal Expression, University of Jaen, 23071 Jaen, Spain; pascualbujalancemoreno@gmail.com
4. Facultad de Ciencias de la Rehabilitación, Universidad Andrés Bello, Santiago 7591538, Chile; daniel.jerez@unab.cl
5. Faculty of Health Sciences, Universidad Europea del Atlántico, 39011 Santander, Spain; alvaro.velarde@uneatlantico.es
6. Department of Education, Universidad Internacional Iberoamericana, Campeche 24560, Mexico; vanessa.anaya@uneatlantico.es (V.A.-M.); silvia.pueyo@uneatlantico.es (S.P.-V.)
7. Department of Languages and Education, Universidad Europea del Atlántico, 39011 Santander, Spain
* Correspondence: carlos.lago@uneatlantico.es

Abstract: The purpose of this study was to examine the training habits of eumenorrheic active women during their menstrual cycle (MC), and its perceived influence on physical performance regarding their athletic level. A group of 1250 sportswomen filled in a questionnaire referring to demographic information, athletic performance and MC-related training habits. Of the participants, 81% reported having a stable duration of MC, with most of them (57%) lasting 26–30 days. Concerning MC-related training habits, 79% indicated that their MC affects athletic performance, although 71% did not consider their MC in their training program, with no differences or modifications in training volume or in training intensity for low-level athletes (LLA) and high-level athletes (HLA) with hormonal contraceptive (HC) use. However, LLA with a normal MC adapted their training habits more, compared with HLA, also stopping their training (47.1% vs. 16.1%, respectively). Thus, different training strategies should be designed for HLA and LLA with a normal MC, but this is not so necessary for HLA and LLA who use HC. To sum up, training adaptations should be individually designed according to the training level and use or non-use of HC, always taking into account the pain suffered during the menstrual phase in most of the athletes.

Keywords: gender; training load; health surveys; sport participation

1. Introduction

The presence and popularity of physical activity and sport for women has considerably increased in the last few decades, and therefore, the need to improve knowledge about their physiology and adaptations to exercise has become crucial. Traditionally, the physiological responses to exercise were assumed to be equal between the sexes [1], and so the recommendations about sport practice and prescription for women have been generalized for decades without even testing whether these guidelines were correct. A potential rationale for this underrepresentation is the complexities and methodological difficulties related to the menstrual cycle (MC) [1]. Based on that argument, sports sciences have been focused on men, or have included women without considering the MC's influence [2].

A typical MC lasts around 28 days and consists of a follicular phase (i.e., characterized by 12–14 days' duration, high levels of estrogen and low progesterone), ovulation phase (i.e., 1–3 days' duration and preceded by a second increase in estrogen), and a luteal phase (i.e., 12–14 days' duration, with high levels of progesterone and medium levels of estrogen) [3]. Plentiful information has been made available about the role of estrogen and progesterone in the female physiology during the last few decades. Regarding estrogen, it has been demonstrated that it increases the muscle glycogen storage capacity as well as increasing free fatty acid availability, and it is used as a fuel source through the use of oxidative pathways [4]. From a physiological standpoint, this is very important because it leads to decreased carbohydrate use, or glycogen sparing [5], and it therefore decreases the dependence on anaerobic pathways for Adenosine triphosphate (ATP) production. In practical terms, high estrogen levels are associated with lower blood lactate levels and longer times to exhaustion [5]. Progesterone is known to have a sympathetic effect (e.g., it increases resting heart rate [6], basal body temperature and ventilation) [7]. This effect plays a key role during exercise because it seems to increase the perceived exertion and decrease athletic performance, especially in hot and/or humid environments [8]. Beyond these physiological effects, what is crucial to understand about progesterone is its ability to antagonize estrogenic effects [1,9]. In this regard, a previous study showed that high progesterone levels can inhibit the enhancement of the carbohydrate metabolism promoted by estradiol, which is a primary estrogen [10].

Taking into consideration the above information, it seems clear that both hormones have different target organs and create diverse biochemical and physiological environments, which have been suggested to be determinant in exercise capacity and thus adaptations to training [8,11,12]. Nevertheless, there is no consensus about the influence of hormone variations induced by the MC's phases on physical performance, with other works reporting no effect [13,14].

Once the physiological findings are revealed, the next question is to learn the influence of these changes in athletes. For this, the use of questionnaires to analyze vast populations is a common strategy in sports science. In this regard, some previous studies have used self-reported questionnaires to examine topics related to the MC [15,16]. Martin et al. [16] aimed to determine the prevalence of hormonal contraceptive (HC) use and the side effects experienced by users and non-users in elite female athletes, whereas Bruinvels et al. [15] focused on heavy menstrual bleeding (HMB) and its perceived effects on training and performance. However, to the best of the authors' knowledge, no previous studies have examined the influence of their MC and their phases on training habits in eumenorrheic active women.

Since female athletes keep training and competing whilst having to manage hormone alterations and their effects, a description of what female athletes are doing and how they manage the potential effects of the MC might be of interest for coaches, athletes and sports scientists. Although research based on a questionnaire can show some limitations, this is the best option to make a survey with a large sample size, with information directly collected by sportswomen regarding their own MC and its influence on their training habits. For these reasons, the purpose of this study is to examine the training habits of eumenorrheic active women during their MC and its perceived influence on physical performance. The current study also aims to investigate the differences in MC-related training habits regarding the athletic level and the use or non-use of hormonal contraceptives (HC).

2. Materials and Methods

2.1. Subjects

One thousand, two hundred and fifty eumenorrheic active women voluntarily participated in this study (age range: 18-45 years; age mean: 27.8 ± 6.6 years). All participants met the inclusion criteria: (1) older than 18 and younger than 45 years old, and (2) with three or more training sessions per week [17]. This study meets the ethical standards of the World Medical Association's Declaration of Helsinki (2013), and it was approved by the Institutional Review Board (Universidad de La Frontera, Temucho, Chile, 005_19).

2.2. Procedure

A cross-sectional study with a descriptive purpose was performed. An ad-hoc questionnaire was designed for a massive mailshot to physically active women through an online Google Form (https://drive.google.com/open?id=1Pw5AecF3Wqhn-1dn13IhqZxZW2QjiyxTtkmsz55Bs28) (accessed on 15 September 2019). This research project was conducted according to the European General Data Protection Regulation (2018).

After receiving ethical approval from the Institutional Review Board, pilot tests were conducted with a small sample of participants ($n = 40$) to evaluate the clarity and content of the online Google Forms. All participants involved in the pilot test indicated that the questionnaire was appropriate and suitable. Subsequently, sports centers, sports clubs, federations and sports institutes in Spain were contacted through their administrators and asked to publicize the study to their athletes and clients as long as those sports organizations were in line with the current data protection regulations, implying that athletes were informed about the potential use of their personal data for research purposes when they provided such information. Then, athletes who were willing to participate in the study were given a link to the online questionnaire.

According to online informed consent procedures, participants were told of the purpose and details of the study through a participant information sheet. Participants were informed that all responses would be kept strictly confidential and would only be used for the purposes of the study. Having consented to participation in the study, participants filled in seventeen items split into four sections: (i) demographic information (i.e., age), (ii) information about athletic performance in the last 6 months (i.e., to have a coach, to be federated, sport modality and athletic level), (iii) information about their training habits in the last 6 months (i.e., hours and sessions per week), and (iv) information about their MC and MC-related training habits (i.e., age at menarche, duration and regularity of their MC, use of HC, the perceived influence of their MC on physical performance, MC-related modifications in training plans, and pain influence).

2.3. Statistical Analysis

Descriptive data are presented as means and standard deviation for interval variables, and as frequency and percentage for nominal variables. Six level groups were determined according to self-reported athletic level (non-competitive level or level 0, local or level 1, autonomic or level 2, national or level 3, international or level 4, and elite or level 5). To compare differences in the adaptation of the parameters of training during the MC, the six groups were dichotomized into two according to their athletic level: lower-level athletes (LLA) (groups 0, 1 and 2), and higher-level athletes (HLA) (groups 3, 4 and 5). The chi-squared test was conducted to determine differences between level groups with and without HC. All statistical analyses were performed using the software package SPSS (IBM SPSS version 22.0, Chicago, IL, USA). The effect size was calculated following previous studies [18].

3. Results

As general information about this group of 1250 women, the results obtained indicate that participants trained 6.7 ± 3.4 h per week, distributed over 4.3 ± 2.1 sessions per week (Table 1). Among these women, 64.7% had a coach and 33.6% were federated. The most practiced sport modalities were team sports (25.9%), athletics (24.6%) and fitness-related activities (19.7%), whereas other modalities such as CrossFit (9.8%), cycling and dancing (5.8%) also showed moderate levels of practice among active women. The self-reported age at menarche was 12.7 ± 1.7 years.

Table 1. Descriptive data of active women related to sport modality.

	N	Age	Sessions/Week	Hours/Week	Age of Menarche
Athletic	308	29.8 ± 0.4	4.7 ± 0.1	6.7 ± 0.2	13.1 ± 0.1
CrossFit	123	28.4 ± 0.7	4.6 ± 0.3	6.1 ± 0.3	12.6 ± 0.2
Cycling	72	32.4 ± 0.8	4.2 ± 0.2	7.6 ± 0.4	12.4 ± 0.2
Dancing	72	29.5 ± 0.7	5.0 ± 0.5	6.0 ± 0.4	12.2 ± 0.2
Equestrian	6	25.0 ± 1.8	4.5 ± 0.7	8.5 ± 1.6	12.5 ± 0.2
Fight sports	15	26.2 ± 0.7	3.0 ± 0.2	6.0 ± 0.7	12.0 ± 0.3
Fitness	246	27.9 ± 0.4	3.7 ± 0.7	5.6 ± 0.2	12.6 ± 0.1
Gymnastics	18	26.2 ± 0.9	3.0 ± 0.3	5.0 ± 0.9	12.7 ± 0.3
Racquet sports	36	25.2 ± 0.8	3.6 ± 0.2	4.8 ± 0.3	13.0 ± 0.3
Swimming	15	27.4 ± 0.8	4.6 ± 0.2	7.8 ± 0.8	12.6 ± 0.4
Team sports	324	24.5 ± 0.3	4.2 ± 0.9	8.2 ± 0.2	12.7 ± 0.1
Winter sports	9	28.7 ± 1.2	3.0 ± 0.2	5.3 ± 0.3	13.0 ± 0.8

Concerning the athletic level, regardless of sport modality, most of the surveyed women (60.7%) indicated a non-competitive level (level 0), whereas the rest of the participants reported a competitive level (at local level or level 1–9.8%; autonomic or level 2–7.7%; national or level 3–18.7%; international or level 4–2.4%; and elite or level 5–0.6%).

Regarding the profile of the MC in relation to the different athletic levels (Table 2), 81% reported having a stable duration of MC with most of them (57%) lasting 26–30 days. No statistical differences were found in the length of the MC when comparing different athletic levels, except with the elite level ($n = 8$, $p < 0.001$, effect size (ES) = 0.42). Regarding the regularity of the MC, international athletes reported a lower percentage (60% regularity) compared with the rest of the groups. In general, 28% reported using an HC method, showing that 43.8% of the level 2 group used HC.

Table 2. Profile of the menstrual cycle (MC) related to different athletic levels.

Variables		LG0 ($n = 759$)	LG1 ($n = 123$)	LG2 ($n = 96$)	LG3 ($n = 234$)	LG4 ($n = 30$)	LG5 ($n = 8$)	p-Value	ES
Length of MC	21–25 days	153 (20.2)	30 (24.4)	24 (25.0)	51 (21.8)	6 (20.0)	0 (0.0)	<0.001	0.42
	26–30 days	453 (59.7)	54 (43.9)	54 (56.2)	129 (55.1)	9 (30.0)	8 (100.0)		
	31–35 days	81 (10.7)	27 (22.0)	6 (6.2)	18 (7.7)	6 (20.0)	0 (0.0)		
	It varies a lot	72 (9.5)	12 (9.8)	12 (12.5)	36 (15.4)	9 (30.0)	0 (0.0)		
Regularity of MC	Yes	633 (83.4)	99 (80.5)	72 (75.0)	189 (80.8)	18 (60.0)	8 (100.0)	0.008	0.10
	No	126 (16.6)	24 (19.5)	24 (25.0)	45 (19.2)	12 (40.0)	0 (0.0)		
HC	Yes	204 (26.9)	33 (26.8)	42 (43.8)	60 (25.6)	6 (20.0)	0 (0.0)	<0.001	0.26
	No	553 (72.9)	90 (73.2)	54 (56.2)	174 (74.4)	22 (73.3)	8 (100.0)		

Note: percentages are calculated according to the number of sportswomen per level group. ES: effect size, MC: menstrual cycle; HC: hormonal contraceptives; LG0: non-competitive level; LG1: local level; LG2: autonomic level; LG3: national level; LG4: international level; LG5: elite level.

Table 3 includes a comparison between different athletic levels (HLA vs. LLA) with a normal cycle (no HC use). Of the LLA, 80.3% indicated that their MC affects athletic performance, with statistical differences compared to HLA. However, almost 70% did not consider the MC in their training program for both groups. Regarding training volume and intensity, LLA affected both variables more during their menstrual phase (MP) compared with HLA ($p < 0.005$ and $p < 0.001$, respectively). Almost 50% of the LLA stopped their training during their MP, while <20% of HLA did so ($p < 0.001$; ES = 0.84). Lastly, among the sportswomen, 55% to 63% reported that they suffered pain during their MP, without differences between both groups.

Table 3. Influence of the menstrual cycle (MC) on training habits, related to different athletic levels without contraceptive hormones ($n = 905$).

Variables		LLA ($n = 697$)	HLA ($n = 208$)	p-Value	ES
Effect on performance	No	138 (19.8)	48 (23.1)		
	Yes—moderately	397 (57.0)	128 (61.5)	<0.05	0.17
	Yes—strongly	162 (23.2)	32 (15.4)		
Considering MC in training	Yes	210 (30.1)	64 (30.8)	0.86	0.01
	No	487 (69.7)	144 (69.2)		
Adapting volume during MP	Yes	264 (37.9)	55 (26.4)	<0.005	0.29
	No	433 (62.1)	153 (73.6)		
Adapting intensity during MP	Yes	339 (48.6)	64 (30.8)	<0.001	0.42
	No	358 (51.4)	144 (69.2)		
Stopping training during MP	Yes	330 (47.3)	34 (16.3)	<0.001	0.84
	No	367 (52.7)	174 (83.7)		
Pain during MP	Yes	459 (65.9)	128 (61.5)	0.256	0.10
	No	238 (34.1)	80 (38.5)		

Note: percentages are calculated related to the number of sportswomen per level group. ES: effect size; MP: menstrual phase; MC: menstrual cycle; HLA: higher-level athletes, LLA: lower-level athletes.

Table 4 describes the influence of the MC on training habits, comparing HLA and LLA athletes. Both LLA and HLA athletes consuming HC reported their performance being affected. However, only 9.1% of HLA reported no effect, against 28% of LLA ($p < 0.005$; ES = 0.47). Regarding the rest of the variables, no statistical differences were reported when comparing both groups, considering the effect of the MC in their training ($p = 0.669$), neither adapting their volume or training, nor stopping training during their MP ($p = 0.656$, $p = 0.09$ and $p = 0.143$, respectively). Finally, both groups suffered pain during their MP, with between 55 and 63% of athletes reporting it, with no differences between groups.

Table 4. Influence of the menstrual cycle (MC) on training habits, related to different athletic levels with contraceptive hormones ($n = 345$).

Variables		LLA ($n = 279$)	HLA ($n = 66$)	p-Value	ES
Effect on performance	No	78 (28.0)	6 (9.1)		
	Yes—moderately	147 (52.7)	39 (59.1)	<0.005	0.47
	Yes—strongly	54 (19.3)	21 (31.8)		
Considering MC in training	Yes	69 (24.7)	18 (27.3)	0.669	0.06
	No	210 (75.3)	48 (72.7)		
Adapting volume during MP	Yes	81 (29.0)	21 (31.8)	0.656	0.06
	No	198 (71.0)	45 (68.2)		
Adapting intensity during MP	Yes	120 (43.0)	21 (31.8)	0.09	0.22
	No	159 (57.0)	45 (68.2)		
Stopping training during MP	Yes	75 (26.9)	12 (18.2)	0.143	0.20
	No	204 (73.1)	54 (81.8)		
Pain during MP	Yes	156 (55.9)	42 (63.6)	0.254	0.16
	No	123 (44.1)	24 (36.4)		

Note: percentages are calculated related to the number of sportswomen per level group. ES: effect size; MP: menstrual phase; MC: menstrual cycle; HLA: higher-level athletes, LLA: lower-level athletes.

4. Discussion

This study aimed to examine the training habits of eumenorrheic active women during their MC and its perceived influence on their physical performance. The results obtained indicate that, despite a high percentage of the surveyed women confirming that the MC affects physical performance and reporting feeling pain during the MP, most of them reported making no changes to their training programs during the MC, with no modifications in training volume or intensity during the MP. This information is of interest as it reinforces the importance of the MC in the training plans of eumenorrheic active women.

Until now, there has been no clear evidence about the relationship between MC and sports performance in different physical outcomes [13,16,19–21]. Regarding this, almost 80% of athletes indicated that the MC affects their performance, with more influence on LLA with a normal MC and HLA with HC consumption. Athletes also suffered pain during the MP, with no differences between groups, independent of the use or non-use of HC. These results match previous studies that indicated most athletes suffered negative side effects during the early days of the MP, affecting their sports performance throughout the cycle [15,16] because of HMB, stomach cramps, back pain and headaches, among other symptoms. Conversely, exercise has been shown to improve the symptoms of premenstrual syndrome, inter alia [22], so female athletes should consider managing training variables (e.g., volume and intensity) during the MC, especially during the MP, but not stop training.

Given the lack of consensus about the influence of the hormone variations associated with the MC, the results provided by the current work might be of interest for coaches and athletes. For instance, whereas it has been suggested that age at menarche might be influenced by the level of sports practice and specialization in the sport [23], the data provided by this current study indicate that age at menarche was similar for all the sports in the study. About this, a previous study suggested that, in gymnastics, menarcheal age was delayed compared with other athletes [23]. However, the authors could not justify this finding regarding training levels, so according to our results, menarcheal age could not be influenced by training levels [23]. Further longitudinal studies should be performed with young female athletes to analyze possible changes to the menarcheal age and the influence of training levels. In this context, another interesting finding is the lack of differences in the length of the MC between level groups. Martin et al. [16] showed that the length of the MC can vary regarding athletic level, with some negative side effects such as primary dysmenorrhea. However, this does not match our results, with more than 50% of HLA reporting a duration of 26 to 30 days. Furthermore, most groups reported a high regularity of the MC, which is key to female performance and the first step for designing training programs according to their different phases [19]. Lastly, only 27.5% used HCs, which is a low prevalence compared with previous studies, and almost 60% of the British elite athletes [16]. HC can influence the regularity of the MC as well as reducing dysmenorrhea, but it also affects sport performance [16].

Additionally, this study also aimed to investigate the differences in MC-related training habits concerning athletic level, comparing results with and without the use of HC. Regarding this, it has been suggested that athletic level can influence the MC [16]. Firstly, regarding athletes with a natural MC (no HC use), the HLA adapted their training much less according to their MC than did the LLA (i.e., the LLA skipped more training sessions than HLA). Intensity, one of the main factors to control during the MC [20], was modified in 48.6% of the LLA compared with only 30.8% in the HLA group during the MP. That is, the HLA did not modify their workouts, regardless of the negative side effects (such as pain) associated with the MP during their preparation. Okano et al. [24] showed that the athletic level influenced the prevalence of eating disorders in Japanese and Chinese athletes, revealing that HLA are more prone to suffering them. So, training at a high level without considering hormone fluctuations during the MC (and especially the negative side effects before and during the MP) could be dangerous for female health and also increase injury risk [25]. In fact, a recent study stated that periodizing the strength training according to the different phases of the MC improves the gaining of lean body mass compared with traditional training [26]. Secondly, comparing both athletic levels via HC use reported different findings. In general, both groups felt pain during the MP, without statistical differences. No differences were also reported regarding the adaptation of training habits in either variable (intensity and volume) during the MP. Curiously, 90% of HLA with HC reported an effect on their performance, compared with only 72% of LLA. In this sense, a recent systematic review suggested that performance did not differ between the different phases of the MC in HC athletes, but their performance can be slightly inferior compared with a non-HC user [27]. Taking into account that HLA athletes using HC felt more effect on their performance compared with HLA with a natural MC, and the same percentage of pain was reported, HC might not be the best option for top athletes, due to the negative side effects of its use [27].

In summary, the results indicate that, despite a high percentage of the surveyed women confirming that the MC affects physical performance and feeling pain during their MP, most of them reported making no changes to their training programs during the MC, with no modifications in training volume nor intensity during the MP. Comparing HC use to non-use, LLA with a natural MC adapted their training variables more during the MP compared to HLA. On the other hand, athletes using HC did not differ in their training adaptations regarding their athletic level. Apart from these key points, it is relevant to take into account that more than 50% of athletes (in both groups) suffered pain during the MP. This information is essential for coaches and practitioners to understand and adapt training loads when pain is present during the MC. Further strategies should analyze different adaptations of training plans throughout the MC, and particularly during the MP, to as far as possible reduce the pain and optimize their sport performance. For these reasons, monitoring and programming training loads according to athletic level, their type of MC (use or non-use of HC), and the different phases of the MC might be relevant during the training process according to these results. Future studies should apply different intensities and frequencies during the MP to compare the effects on sport performance, especially in a natural MC.

5. Conclusions

The novel aspect of this research regards the level of influence of the menstrual cycle on the performance and training habits of eumenorrheic active women. Defining and knowing the side effects during each phase of the menstrual cycle at different performance levels and sports modalities should be relevant to adapting training programs properly and reducing non-practice times during the menstruation phase, both in HC and non-HC users. For this reason, staff and physical education coaches should be aware of the importance of managing and registering the menstrual phases of women to optimize their training and adapt training loads, especially during the bleeding or menstrual phase. Moreover, these results could also be useful to compare different performances regarding sports modalities.

To sum up, this study provides descriptive information about the MC of eumenorrheic active women, and the modifications performed in their training programs in relation to the different phases of the MC. Given the reported hormonal changes during the different phases of the MC, both sports scientists and coaches must pay special attention to the role of this factor, and also to their negative side effects in some phases, suggesting the need for an educational process and a constant dialog with their athletes about their feelings, negative side effects (if they exist) and pain during the MP, independently of the use or non-use of HC.

Author Contributions: Conceptualization, F.G.-P., P.B.-M. and C.L.-F.; methodology, F.G.-P., D.J.-M. and C.L.-F.; software, C.L.-F. and F.G.-P.; validation, S.P.-V. and V.A.-M.; formal analysis: F.G.-P., P.B.-M. and C.L.-F.; investigation, F.G.-P. and P.B.-M.; resources, F.G.-P.; data curation, F.G.-P. and P.B.-M.; writing—original draft preparation, F.G.-P., Á.V.-S. and D.J.-M.; writing—review and editing, F.G.-P., S.P.-V. and C.L.-F.; visualization, F.G.-P. and P.B.-M.; supervision, F.G.-P. and C.L.-F.; project administration, F.G.-P. and P.B.-M. All authors have read and agreed to the published version of the manuscript.

Funding: This research received no external funding.

Institutional Review Board Statement: This study meets the ethical standards of the World Medical Association's Declaration of Helsinki (2013), and it was approved by the Institutional Review Board (Universidad de La Frontera, Temucho, Chile, 005_19).

Informed Consent Statement: Informed consent was obtained from all subjects involved in the study.

Data Availability Statement: Not applicable.

Acknowledgments: This research was supported by the Pre-competitive Projects for Early Stage Researchers Program from the University of Granada (ref: PPJIA2020.03). The authors would like to thank all the participants.

Conflicts of Interest: The authors declare no conflict of interest.

References

1. Sims, S.T.; Heather, A.K. Myths and Methodologies: Reducing scientific design ambiguity in studies comparing sexes and/or menstrual cycle phases. *Exp. Physiol.* **2018**, *103*, 1309–1317. [CrossRef]
2. Johnson, J.L.; Greaves, L.; Repta, R. Better science with sex and gender: Facilitating the use of a sex and gender-based analysis in health research. *Int. J. Equity Health* **2009**, *8*, 14. [CrossRef]
3. Stricker, R.; Eberhart, R.; Chevailler, M.C.; Quinn, F.A.; Bischof, P.; Stricker, R. Establishment of detailed reference values for luteinizing hormone, follicle stimulating hormone, estradiol, and progesterone during different phases of the menstrual cycle on the Abbott ARCHITECT® analyzer. *Clin. Chem. Lab. Med.* **2006**, *44*, 883–887. [CrossRef]
4. Nicklas, B.J.; Hackney, A.C.; Sharp, R.L. The menstrual cycle and exercise: Performance, muscle glycogen, and substrate responses. *Int. J. Sports Med.* **1989**, *10*, 246–469. [CrossRef]
5. Oosthuyse, T.; Bosch, A.N. The Effect of the Menstrual Cycle on Exercise Metabolism Implications for Exercise Performance in Eumenorrhoeic Women. *Sport. Med.* **2010**, *40*, 207–227. [CrossRef]
6. Sedlak, T.; Shufelt, C.; Iribarren, C.; Merz, C.N.B. Sex hormones and the QT interval: A review. *J. Women's Health* **2012**, *21*, 933–941. [CrossRef]
7. Charkoudian, N.; Hart, E.C.J.; Barnes, J.N.; Joyner, M.J. Autonomic control of body temperature and blood pressure: Influences of female sex hormones. *Clin. Auton. Res.* **2017**, *27*, 140–155. [CrossRef] [PubMed]
8. Janse De Jonge, X.A.K.; Thompson, M.W.; Chuter, V.H.; Silk, L.N.; Thom, J.M. Exercise performance over the menstrual cycle in temperate and hot, humid conditions. *Med. Sci. Sports Exerc.* **2012**, *44*, 2190–2198. [CrossRef] [PubMed]
9. Campbell, S.E.; Febbraio, M.A. Effect of the ovarian hormones on GLUT4 expression and contraction-stimulated glucose uptake. *Am. J. Physiol. Endocrinol. Metab.* **2002**, *282*, E1139–E1146. [CrossRef] [PubMed]
10. D'Eon, T.M.; Sharoff, C.; Chipkin, S.R.; Grow, D.; Ruby, B.C.; Braun, B. Regulation of exercise carbohydrate metabolism by estrogen and progesterone in women. *Am. J. Physiol. Endocrinol. Metab.* **2002**, *5*, E1046–E1055. [CrossRef] [PubMed]
11. Pallavi, L.C.; Souza, U.J.D.; Shivaprakash, G. Assessment of musculoskeletal strength and levels of fatigue during different phases of menstrual cycle in young adults. *J. Clin. Diagnostic Res.* **2017**, *11*, CC11. [CrossRef] [PubMed]
12. Julian, R.; Hecksteden, A.; Fullagar, H.H.K.; Meyer, T. The effects of menstrual cycle phase on physical performance in female soccer players. *PLoS ONE* **2017**, *12*, e0173951. [CrossRef]
13. Romero-Moraleda, B.; Del Coso, J.; Gutiérrez-Hellín, J.; Ruiz-Moreno, C.; Grgic, J.; Lara, B. The influence of the menstrual cycle on muscle strength and power performance. *J. Hum. Kinet.* **2019**, *68*, 123–133. [CrossRef] [PubMed]
14. Sakamaki-Sunaga, M.; Min, S.; Kamemoto, K.; Okamoto, T. Effects of Menstrual Phase-Dependent Resistance Training Frequency on Muscular Hypertrophy and Strength. *J. Strength Cond. Res.* **2016**, *30*, 1727–1734. [CrossRef] [PubMed]
15. Bruinvels, G.; Burden, R.; Brown, N.; Richards, T.; Pedlar, C. The prevalence and impact of heavy menstrual bleeding (Menorrhagia) in elite and non-elite athletes. *PLoS ONE* **2016**, *22*, e0149881. [CrossRef]
16. Martin, D.; Sale, C.; Cooper, S.B.; Elliott-Sale, K.J. Period prevalence and perceived side effects of hormonal contraceptive use and the menstrual cycle in elite athletes. *Int. J. Sports Physiol. Perform.* **2018**, *13*, 926–932. [CrossRef]
17. Piercy, K.L.; Troiano, R.P.; Ballard, R.M.; Carlson, S.A.; Fulton, J.E.; Galuska, D.A.; George, S.M.; Olson, R.D. The physical activity guidelines for Americans. *JAMA J. Am. Med. Assoc.* **2018**, *320*, 2020–2028. [CrossRef]
18. Fritz, C.O.; Morris, P.E.; Richler, J.J. Effect size estimates: Current use, calculations, and interpretation. *J. Exp. Psychol. Gen.* **2012**, *141*, 2. [CrossRef]
19. Constantini, N.W.; Dubnov, G.; Lebrun, C.M. The menstrual cycle and sport performance. *Clin. Sports Med.* **2005**, *24*, e51–e82. [CrossRef]
20. Dokumacı, B.; Hazır, T. Effects of the Menstrual Cycle on Running Economy: Oxygen Cost Versus Caloric Cost. *Res. Q. Exerc. Sport* **2019**, *90*, 1–9. [CrossRef]
21. García-Pinillos, F.; Lago-Fuentes, C.; Bujalance-Moreno, P.; Pérez-Castilla, A. Effect of the Menstrual Cycle When Estimating 1 Repetition Maximum From the Load-Velocity Relationship During the Bench Press Exercise. *J. Strength Cond. Res.* **2020**. [CrossRef]
22. Williams, N.I.; Etter, C.V.; Lieberman, J.L. The Science of Healthy Menstruation in Exercising Women. *Kinesiol. Rev.* **2017**, *6*, 78–90. [CrossRef]

23. Malina, R.M.; Rogol, A.D.; Cumming, S.P.; Coelho E Silva, M.J.; Figueiredo, A.J. Biological maturation of youth athletes: Assessment and implications. *Br. J. Sports Med.* **2015**, *49*, 852–859. [CrossRef] [PubMed]
24. Okano, G.; Holmes, R.A.; Mu, Z.; Yang, P.; Lin, Z.; Nakai, Y. Disordered eating in Japanese and Chinese female runners, rhythmic gymnasts and gymnasts. *Int. J. Sports Med.* **2005**, *26*, 486–491. [CrossRef] [PubMed]
25. McNulty, K.L.; Elliott-Sale, K.J.; Dolan, E.; Swinton, P.A.; Ansdell, P.; Goodall, S.; Thomas, K.; Hicks, K.M. The Effects of Menstrual Cycle Phase on Exercise Performance in Eumenorrheic Women: A Systematic Review and Meta-Analysis. *Sport. Med.* **2020**, 1–15. [CrossRef] [PubMed]
26. Wikstrom-Frisén, L.; Boraxbekk, C.J.; Henriksson-Larsén, K. Increasing training load without risking the female athlete triad: Menstrual cycle based periodized training may be an answer? *J. Sports Med. Phys. Fitness* **2017**, *57*, 1519–1525. [PubMed]
27. Elliott-Sale, K.J.; McNulty, K.L.; Ansdell, P.; Goodall, S.; Hicks, K.M.; Thomas, K.; Swinton, P.A.; Dolan, E. The Effects of Oral Contraceptives on Exercise Performance in Women: A Systematic Review and Meta-analysis. *Sport. Med.* **2020**, *50*, 1785–1812. [CrossRef]

MDPI
St. Alban-Anlage 66
4052 Basel
Switzerland
Tel. +41 61 683 77 34
Fax +41 61 302 89 18
www.mdpi.com

International Journal of Environmental Research and Public Health Editorial Office
E-mail: ijerph@mdpi.com
www.mdpi.com/journal/ijerph

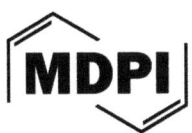

www.ingramcontent.com/pod-product-compliance
Lightning Source LLC
LaVergne TN
LVHW070625100526
838202LV00012B/727